First Aid, CPR, and AED Essentials

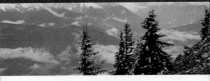

In Loving Memory of
James A. Wilkerson III
Adventurer and Gentleman

Alton L. Thygerson, EdD, FAWM
Medical Writer

Steven M. Thygerson, PhD, MSPH, CIH
Medical Writer

Benjamin Gulli, MD, FAAOS
Medical Editor

Gina Piazza, DO, FACEP
Medical Editor

American College of
Emergency Physicians®
ADVANCING EMERGENCY CARE

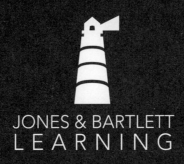

JONES & BARTLETT
LEARNING

World Headquarters
Jones & Bartlett Learning
5 Wall Street
Burlington, MA 01803
978-443-5000
info@jblearning.com
www.jblearning.com

Jones & Bartlett Learning books and products are available through most bookstores and online booksellers. To contact Jones & Bartlett Learning directly, call 800-832-0034, fax 978-443-8000, or visit our website, www.jblearning.com.

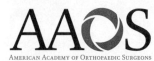

AMERICAN ACADEMY OF ORTHOPAEDIC SURGEONS

Chief Education Officer: Mark W. Wieting
Director, Department of Publications: Marilyn L. Fox, PhD
Managing Editor: Barbara A. Scotese
Associate Senior Editor: Gayle Murray

Production Credits
Chairman, Board of Directors: Clayton Jones
Chief Executive Officer: Ty Field
President: James Homer
SVP, Editor-in-Chief: Michael Johnson
SVP, Chief Operating Officer: Don Jones, Jr.
SVP, Chief Technology Officer: Dean Fossella
SVP, Chief Marketing Officer: Alison M. Pendergast
Executive Publisher: Kimberly Brophy
Executive Vice President—JB Learning: Lawrence D. Newell
VP of Sales, Public Safety Group: Matthew Maniscalco
Executive Acquisitions Editor—EMS: Christine Emerton
Director of Sales, Public Safety Group: Patty Einstein

Associate Editor: Olivia MacDonald
Production Manager: Jenny L. Corriveau
Associate Production Editor: Nora Menzi
Senior Marketing Manager: Brian Rooney
VP, Manufacturing and Inventory Control: Therese Connell
Text Design: Anne Spencer
Composition: Shepherd, Inc.
Cover Design: Kristin E. Parker
Rights and Permissions Manager: Katherine Crighton
Photo Research Supervisor: Anna Genoese
Cover Image: © Jones & Bartlett Learning. Photographed by Sarah Cebulski
Printing and Binding: Courier Corporation
Cover Printing: Courier Corporation

Additional photographic and illustrations credits appear on page 270, which constitutes a continuation of the copyright page.

The first aid, CPR, and AED procedures and protocols in this book are based on the most current recommendations of responsible medical sources. The American Academy of Orthopaedic Surgeons and the publisher, however, make no guarantee as to, and assume no responsibility for, the correctness, sufficiency, or completeness of such information or recommendations. Other or additional safety measures may be required under particular circumstances.

Reviewed by the American College of Emergency Physicians. The American College of Emergency Physicians (ACEP) makes every effort to ensure that its reviewers are knowledgeable content experts. Readers are nevertheless advised that the statements and opinions expressed in this publication are provided as recommendations at the time of publication and should not be construed as official College policy. ACEP is not responsible for, and expressly disclaims all liability for, damages of any kind arising out of use, reference to, reliance on, or performance of such information. The materials contained herein are not intended to establish policy, procedure, or a standard of care. To contact ACEP, write to: PO Box 619911, Dallas, TX 75261-9911; call toll-free 800-798-1822, or 972-550-0911.

Some images in this book feature models. These models do not necessarily endorse, represent, or participate in the activities represented in the images.

Library of Congress Cataloging-in-Publication Data
First aid, CPR, and AED essentials / Steven M. Thygerson ; American Academy of Orthopaedic Surgeons [and] American College of Emergency Physicians—6th ed.
     p. ; cm.
Rev. ed. of: First aid and CPR essentials / Alton Thygerson. 5th ed. c2007.
Related ed. of: Advanced first aid, CPR, and AED. 6th ed.
Includes index.
ISBN 978-1-4496-2662-4
I. Thygerson, Alton L. First aid and CPR essentials. II. American Academy of Orthopaedic Surgeons. III. American College of Emergency Physicians. IV. Title. V. Title: Advanced first aid, CPR, and AED.
[DNLM: 1. First Aid. 2. Cardiopulmonary Resuscitation. 3. Electric Countershock. 4. Emergencies. WA 292]
LC classification not assigned
616.02'52—dc23
                                 2011033474

6048
Printed in the United States of America
15 14 13 12 11   10 9 8 7 6 5 4 3 2 1

brief contents

contents

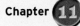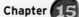

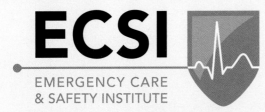

EMERGENCY CARE & SAFETY INSTITUTE

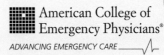

Welcome to the Emergency Care & Safety Institute

Welcome to the Emergency Care & Safety Institute (ECSI), brought to you by the American Academy of Orthopaedic Surgeons (AAOS) and the American College of Emergency Physicians (ACEP).

ECSI is an internationally renowned organization that provides training and certifications that meet job-related requirements as defined by regulatory authorities such as OSHA, The Joint Commission, and state offices of EMS, Education, Transportation, and Health. Our courses are delivered throughout a range of industries and markets worldwide, including colleges and universities, business and industry, government, public safety agencies, hospitals, private training companies, and secondary school systems.

ECSI programs are offered in association with the AAOS and ACEP. AAOS, the world's largest medical organization of musculoskeletal specialists, is known as the original name in EMS publishing with the first EMS textbook ever in 1971, and ACEP is widely recognized as the leading name in all of emergency medicine.

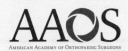

About the AAOS

The AAOS provides education and practice management services for orthopaedic surgeons and allied health professionals. The AAOS also serves as an advocate for improved patient care and informs the public about the science of orthopaedics. Founded in 1933, the not-for-profit AAOS has grown from a small organization serving less than 500 members to the world's largest medical organization of musculoskeletal specialists. The AAOS now serves about 36,000 members internationally.

American College of Emergency Physicians®
ADVANCING EMERGENCY CARE

About ACEP

ACEP was founded in 1968 and is the world's oldest and largest emergency medicine specialty organization. Today it represents more than 28,000 members and is the emergency medicine specialty society recognized as the acknowledged leader in emergency medicine.

ECSI Course Catalog

Individuals seeking training from ECSI can choose from among various traditional classroom-based courses or alternative online courses such as:
- Advanced Cardiac Life Support
- Automated External Defibrillation (AED)
- Bloodborne and Airborne Pathogens
- Babysitter Safety
- Driver Safety
- CPR (Layperson and Health Care Provider Levels)
- Emergency Medical Responder
- First Aid (Multiple Courses Available)
- Oxygen Administration, and more!

ECSI offers a wide range of textbooks, instructor and student support materials, and interactive technology, including online courses. ECSI student manuals are the center of an integrated teaching and learning system that offers resources to better support instructors and train students. The instructor supplements provide practical hands-on, time-saving tools like PowerPoint presentations, DVDs, and web-based distance learning resources. Technology resources provide interactive exercises and simulations to help students become prepared for any emergency.

Documents attesting to ECSI's recognitions of satisfactory course completion will be issued to those who successfully meet the course requirements. Written acknowledgement of a participant's successful course completion is provided in the form of a Course Completion Card, issued by the Emergency Care & Safety Institute.

Visit www.ECSInstitute.org today!

resource preview

This concise student manual is designed to give laypersons the education and confidence they need to effectively provide emergency care. Features that reinforce and expand on essential information include:

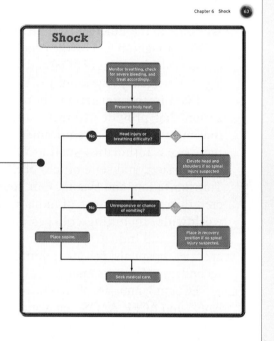

Flowcharts
Pose a central question and organize treatment options by injury or illness type.

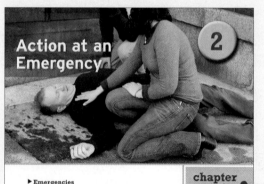

Chapter at a Glance
Guides students through the topics covered in the chapter.

Skill Drills Provide step-by-step explanations and visual summaries of important skills for first aiders.

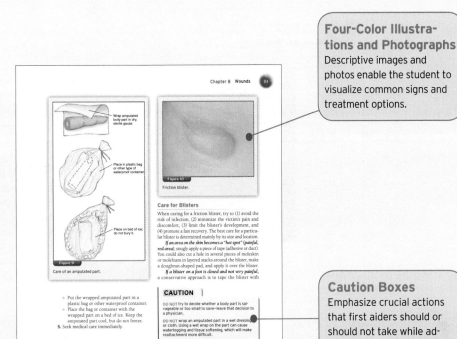

Four-Color Illustrations and Photographs
Descriptive images and photos enable the student to visualize common signs and treatment options.

Caution Boxes
Emphasize crucial actions that first aiders should or should not take while administering treatment.

FYI Boxes Include valuable information related to the injuries or illnesses discussed in that section, including prevention tips and risk factors.

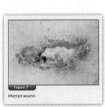

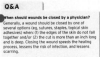

Q&A Boxes
Answer questions common to first aiders.

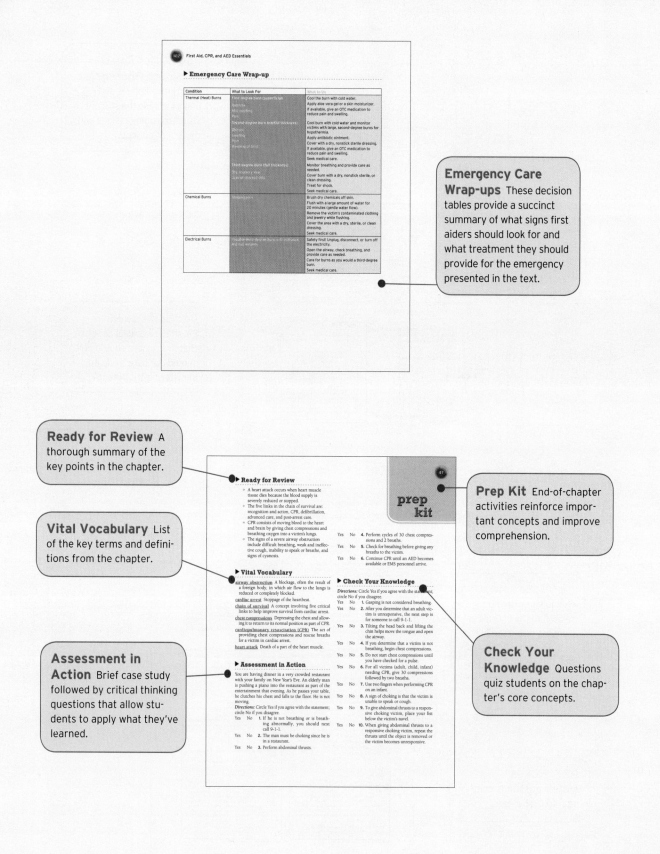

Emergency Care Wrap-ups These decision tables provide a succinct summary of what signs first aiders should look for and what treatment they should provide for the emergency presented in the text.

Ready for Review A thorough summary of the key points in the chapter.

Vital Vocabulary List of the key terms and definitions from the chapter.

Assessment in Action Brief case study followed by critical thinking questions that allow students to apply what they've learned.

Prep Kit End-of-chapter activities reinforce important concepts and improve comprehension.

Check Your Knowledge Questions quiz students on the chapter's core concepts.

Background Information

▶ Why Is First Aid Important?

It is better to know first aid and not need it than to need it and not know it. Everyone should be able to perform first aid, because most people will eventually find themselves in a situation requiring it for another person or for themselves. First aiders do not diagnose (this is what medical doctors do), but they can suspect what the problem is and then give first aid.

▶ Who Needs First Aid?

Although heart disease and cancer continue to be critical health problems in the United States, injuries—both unintentional and intentional—constitute a major threat to public health. This threat has been called the neglected epidemic.

Death statistics do not always reflect the extent or severity of the injury problem. Most people who are injured do not die of their injuries. The scope of injuries can best be appreciated if thought of as a pyramid. Deaths from injuries and hospital discharges, traditionally where the most available data have been, are only the tip of the problem. There are a far greater number of injuries seen in emergency departments, clinics, and physician offices. An even greater number of injuries are treated by first aiders. This supports the need for first aid training (Table 1).

Each year, one in four people experience a nonfatal injury serious enough to need medical care or to restrict activity for at least 1 day.

More sports-related nonfatal injuries are treated in hospital emergency departments than any other type of unintentional injury.

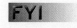

OSHA Regulations

(Standards–29CFR 1910.151) Medical Services and First Aid–General Industry:

"In the absence of infirmary, clinic, or hospital in near proximity to workplace which is used for the treatment of all injured employees, a person or persons shall be adequately trained to render first aid. Adequate first aid supplies shall be readily available."

A delay of as little as 4 minutes when a person's heart stops can mean death. Therefore, what a bystander does can mean the difference between life and death. Fortunately, most injuries do not require lifesaving efforts. During their entire lifetimes, most people will see only one or two situations involving life-threatening conditions. Most injuries do not require lifesaving efforts **Figure 1**. Knowing what to do for less severe injuries demands greater attention during first aid instruction.

Each year, the injuries of millions of Americans go unreported. For many of them, the injury causes temporary pain and inconvenience; for others, however, the injury leads to disability, chronic pain, and a profound change in lifestyle. Given the size of the injury and sudden illness problem, everyone should be prepared to deal with an emergency.

Table 1 10 Leading Causes of Death by Age Group, United States – 2007

Rank	<1	1-4	5-9	10-14	15-24	25-34	35-44	45-54	55-64	65+	Total
1	Congenital Anomalies 5,785	Unintentional Injury 1,588	Unintentional Injury 965	Unintentional Injury 1,229	Unintentional Injury 15,897	Unintentional Injury 14,977	Unintentional Injury 16,931	Malignant Neoplasms 50,167	Malignant Neoplasms 103,171	Heart Disease 496,095	Heart Disease 616,067
2	Short Gestation 4,857	Congenital Anomalies 546	Malignant Neoplasms 480	Malignant Neoplasms 479	Homicide 5,551	Suicide 5,278	Malignant Neoplasms 13,288	Heart Disease 37,434	Heart Disease 65,527	Malignant Neoplasms 389,730	Malignant Neoplasms 562,875
3	Sudden Infant Death Syndrome 2,453	Homicide 398	Congenital Anomalies 196	Homicide 213	Suicide 4,140	Homicide 4,758	Heart Disease 11,839	Unintentional Injury 20,315	Chronic Low Respiratory Disease 12,777	Cerebro-vascular 115,961	Cerebro-vascular 135,952
4	Maternal Pregnancy Complications 1,769	Malignant Neoplasms 364	Homicide 133	Suicide 180	Malignant Neoplasms 1,653	Malignant Neoplasms 3,463	Suicide 6,722	Liver Disease 8,212	Unintentional Injury 12,193	Chronic Low Respiratory Disease 109,562	Chronic Low Respiratory Disease 127,924
5	Unintentional Injury 1,285	Heart Disease 173	Heart Disease 110	Congenital Anomalies 178	Heart Disease 1,084	Heart Disease 3,223	Human Immunodeficiency Virus 3,572	Suicide 7,778	Diabetes Mellitus 11,304	Alzheimer's Disease 73,797	Unintentional Injury 123,706
6	Placenta Cord Membranes 1,135	Influenza & Pneumonia 109	Chronic Low Respiratory Disease 54	Heart Disease 131	Congenital Anomalies 402	HIV 1,091	Homicide 3,052	Cerebro-vascular 6,385	Cerebro-vascular 10,500	Diabetes Mellitus 51,528	Alzheimer's Disease 74,632
7	Bacterial Sepsis 820	Septicemia 78	Influenza & Pneumonia 48	Chronic Low Respiratory Disease 64	Cerebro-vascular 195	Diabetes Mellitus 610	Liver Disease 2,570	Diabetes Mellitus 5,753	Liver Disease 8,004	Influenza & Pneumonia 45,941	Diabetes Mellitus 71,382
8	Respiratory Distress 789	Perinatal Period 70	Benign Neoplasms 41	Influenza & Pneumonia 55	Diabetes Mellitus 168	Cerebro-vascular 505	Cerebro-vascular 2,133	HIV 4,156	Suicide 5,069	Nephritis 38,484	Influenza & Pneumonia 52,717
9	Circulatory System Disease 624	Benign Neoplasms 59	Cerebro-vascular 38	Cerebro-vascular 45	Influenza & Pneumonia 163	Congenital Anomalies 417	Diabetes Mellitus 1,984	Chronic Low Respiratory Disease 4,153	Nephritis 4,440	Unintentional Injury 38,292	Nephritis 46,448
10	Neonatal Hemorrhage 597	Chronic Low Respiratory Disease 57	Septicemia 36	Benign Neoplasms 43	Three Tied* 160	Liver Disease 384	Septicemia 910	Viral Hepatitis 2,815	Septicemia 4,231	Septicemia 26,362	Septicemia 34,828

*The three causes are: Complicated Pregnancy, HIV, Septicema
Source: National Vital Statistics System, National Center for Health Statistics, CDC.
Produced by: Office of Statistics and Programming, National Center for Injury Prevention and Control, CDC.

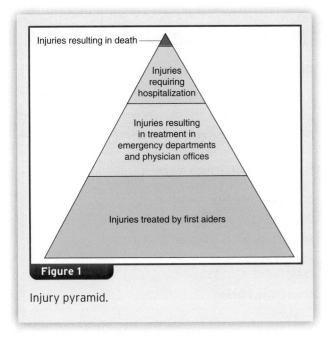

Injuries resulting in death

Injuries requiring hospitalization

Injuries resulting in treatment in emergency departments and physician offices

Injuries treated by first aiders

Figure 1

Injury pyramid.

Q&A

What level of care is a first aider expected to give?

The level of care is also known by the term "standard of care." A first aider cannot provide the same level of care as a physician or an emergency medical technician. To meet the standard of care for a victim, a first aider must: (1) do what is expected of someone with first aid training and experience working under similar conditions, and (2) treat the victim to the best of his or her ability. If the first aid you provide is not up to the expected standard, you may be held liable for your actions.

▶ What Is First Aid?

<u>First aid</u> is the immediate care given to an injured or suddenly ill person. First aid does not take the place of proper medical care. It consists only of giving temporary help until proper medical care, if needed, is obtained or until the chance for recovery without medical care is ensured. Most injuries and illnesses do not require medical care.

Properly applied, first aid might mean the difference between life and death, between rapid recovery and a long hospitalization, or between a temporary and a permanent disability. First aid involves more than doing things for others; it also includes treatments that people can give themselves.

Recognizing a serious medical emergency and knowing how to get help could be crucial in saving a life. Recognition of an emergency can be delayed because neither the victim nor bystanders know basic symptoms (for example, a heart attack victim might wait hours after the onset of symptoms before seeking help). Moreover, too many people do not know first aid; even if they do, they might panic in an emergency.

▶ First Aid Supplies

The supplies in a first aid kit should be customized to include those items likely to be used on a regular basis. A kit for the home is often different than one for the

workplace. A home kit may contain personal medications and a smaller number of items. A workplace kit will need more items (such as bandages) and will not include personal medications. **Table 2** lists the basic items that should be stocked in a workplace first aid kit.

Although a first aid kit may have some medications, such as antihistamines and topical ointments, there might be local requirements that restrict the use of these items by first aiders without prior written approval. For example, teachers, activity leaders, and bus drivers in certain areas might not be able to administer these items to children without specific written permission signed by a child's parent or guardian.

▶ First Aid and the Law

Legal and ethical issues concern all first aiders. For example, is a first aider required to stop and give care at an automobile crash? Can a child with a broken arm be treated even when the parents cannot be contacted for their consent? These and many other legal and ethical questions confront first aiders.

A first aider can be sued. Do not become overly concerned about being sued—it rarely happens. Ways to minimize the risk of a suit include:

- Obtaining the victim's consent before touching him or her.
- Following this book's guidelines and not exceeding your training level.
- Explaining any first aid you are about to give.
- Once starting to care for a victim, stay with that person. You are legally bound to remain with the victim until care is turned over to an equally or better trained person.

Table 2 Sample First Aid Kit

Items	Minimum Quantity	Items	Minimum Quantity
Adhesive strip bandages (1″ × 3″)*	20	Antibiotic ointment, individual packets*	6 packets
Triangular bandages* (muslin, 36″-40″ × 36″-40″ × 52″-56″)	4	Disposable (medical exam) gloves (various sizes)*	2 pairs per size
Sterile eye pads (2″ × 2″)	2	Mouth-to-barrier device (either a face mask with a one-way valve or a disposable face shield)	1
Sterile gauze pads (4″ × 4″)	6		
Sterile gauze pads (3″ × 3″)*	6		
Sterile gauze pads (2″ × 2″)*	6	Disposable instant cold packs	2
Sterile nonstick pads (3″ × 4″)*	6	Sealable plastic bags (quart size)	2
Sterile trauma pads (5″ × 9″)*	2	Padded malleable splint (SAM Splint, 4″ × 36″)	1
Sterile trauma pads (8″ × 10″)	1		
Sterile conforming roller gauze (2″ width)	3 rolls	Emergency blanket	1
		Scissors	1
Sterile conforming roller gauze (4.5″ width)	3 rolls	Tweezers	1
Waterproof tape (1″ × 5 yards)	1 roll	Hand sanitizer (61% ethyl alcohol)	1 bottle
Porous adhesive tape (2″ × 5 yd)*	1 roll	Biohazard waste bag (3.5 gallon capacity)	2
Elastic roller bandages (4″ and 6″)	1 of each		
Antiseptic skin wipes, individually wrapped*	10 packets	Mini flashlight and batteries	1
		List of local emergency telephone numbers	1
		First aid guide*	1

*Item meets the ANSI/ISEA Z308.1-2009 minimum standard for the workplace first aid kit. Optional items and sizes may be added based on the potential hazards.

Consent

A first aider must have the victim's **consent** (permission) before giving first aid. Touching another person without his or her consent is unlawful (known as **battery**) and could be grounds for a lawsuit. Likewise, giving first aid without the victim's consent is unlawful.

Expressed Consent

Consent must be obtained from every alert, mentally competent (able to make a rational decision) person of legal age. Tell the victim that you have first aid training and explain what you will be doing. The victim may give permission verbally or with a nod of the head, which would indicate **expressed consent**.

Implied Consent

Implied consent involves an unresponsive victim with a life-threatening condition. It is assumed or implied that an unresponsive victim would consent to lifesaving interventions. An alert victim who does not resist the administrations of a first aider is also assumed to have given **implied consent**.

Children and Mentally Incompetent Adults

Consent must be obtained from the parent or guardian of a child victim, as legally defined by the state. The same is true for an adult who is mentally incompetent. When life-threatening situations exist and a parent or legal guardian is not available for consent, first aid should be given based on implied consent. Do not withhold first aid from a minor just to obtain consent from a parent or guardian.

Psychiatric emergencies present difficult problems of consent. Under most conditions, a police officer is the only person with the authority to restrain and transport a person against that person's will. A first aider should not intervene unless directed to do so by a police officer or unless it is obvious that the victim is about to do life-threatening harm to himself or herself or to others.

Refusing Help

Although it seldom happens, a person might refuse assistance for countless reasons, such as religious grounds, avoidance of possible pain, or the desire to be examined by a physician rather than by a first aider. Whatever the reason for refusing medical care, or even if no reason is given, the alert and mentally competent adult can reject help.

Generally, the wisest approach is for you to inform the victim of his or her medical condition, what you propose to do, and why the help is necessary. If the victim understands the consequences and still refuses treatment, there is little else you can do. Call 9-1-1 and, while awaiting arrival:

- Try again to persuade the victim to accept care and encourage others at the scene to persuade the victim. A victim could change his or her mind after a short time.
- Make certain you have witnesses. A victim could refuse consent and then deny having done so.
- Consider calling for law enforcement assistance. In most locations, the police can place a person in protective custody and require him or her to go to a hospital.

Abandonment

Abandonment means leaving a victim after starting to give help without first ensuring that the victim will receive continued care at the same level or higher. Once you have responded to an emergency, you must not leave a victim who needs continuing first aid until another competent and trained person takes responsibility for the victim. This might seem obvious, but there have been cases in which critically ill or injured victims were left unattended and then died. Thus, a first aider must stay with the victim until another equally or better trained person takes over.

Q&A

How can I avoid a lawsuit resulting from giving first aid?
Before giving first aid, get the victim's consent or permission. Then provide good care, keep within your training level, be nice to the victim, have witnesses, and afterward, write down what you did, names of witnesses, and who took over the victim's care from you.

Negligence

Negligence means not following the accepted standards of care, resulting in further injury to the victim. Negligence involves:

1. Having a duty to act (required to give first aid)
2. Breaching that duty (either by giving no care or by giving substandard care)
3. Causing injury and damages
4. Exceeding your level of training

Duty to Act

No one is required to give first aid unless a legal **duty to act** exists. For example, you do not have to help a stranger unless you have a legal obligation to that person, or you were involved in the events that led to the victim's injuries, regardless of who was at fault. The decision to help in an emergency is usually an ethical (moral) one. Duty to act could apply in the following situations:

- When employment requires it. If your employer designates you as the person responsible for providing first aid to meet Occupational Safety and Health Administration (also known as OSHA) requirements and you are called to an injury scene, you have a duty to act. Examples of occupations that involve a legal obligation to give first aid include law enforcement officers, park rangers, athletic trainers, lifeguards, flight attendants, and fire fighters.
- When on duty (and sometimes when off duty). Some states require certain people who are licensed by the state to give emergency care regardless of their on- or off-duty status. In other words, these people are considered to be always on duty. Other states require them to act when on duty but not generally

when they are off duty, unless they are in uniform or have other visible insignia and appear to be on duty—in which case these people must respond.

- When a preexisting responsibility exists. You might have a preexisting relationship with other persons that makes you responsible for them, which means that you must give first aid should they need it. For example, a parent has a preexisting responsibility for a child, and a driver for a passenger.

Breach of Duty

A **breach of duty** happens when a first aider fails to provide the type of care that would be given by a person having the same or similar training. There are two ways to breach one's duty: acts of omission and acts of commission. An **act of omission** is the failure to do what a reasonably prudent person with the same or similar training would do in the same or similar circumstances. An **act of commission** is doing something that a reasonably prudent person would not do under the same or similar circumstances. Forgetting to put on a dressing is an act of omission; cutting a snake-bite site is an act of commission.

Injury and Damages Inflicted

In addition to physical damage, injury and damage can include physical pain and suffering, mental anguish, medical expenses, and sometimes loss of earnings and earning capacity.

Confidentiality

First aiders might learn confidential information. It is important that you be extremely cautious about revealing information you learn while caring for someone.

The law recognizes that people have the right to privacy. Do not discuss what you know with anyone other than those who have a medical need to know. The exception to this is when state laws require the reporting of certain incidents, such as rape, abuse, and gunshot wounds.

Good Samaritan Laws

Good Samaritan laws encourage people to assist others in distress by granting them immunity against lawsuits. Although the laws vary from state to state, Good Samaritan immunity generally applies only when the rescuer is (1) acting during an emergency; (2) acting in good faith, which means he or she has good intentions; (3) acting without compensation; and (4) not guilty of malicious misconduct or gross negligence toward the victim (deviating from rational first aid guidelines).

Although Good Samaritan laws primarily cover health care providers, many states have expanded them to include laypersons serving as first aiders. In fact, some states have several Good Samaritan laws that cover different types of people in various situations. Many legal experts believe Good Samaritan laws have given first aiders a false sense of security. These laws will not protect first aiders who have caused further injury to a victim. Good Samaritan laws are not a protection for poorly given first aid or for exceeding the scope of your training. Fear of lawsuits has made some people hesitant of becoming involved in emergency situations. First aiders, however, are rarely sued.

▶ Ready for Review

- Everyone should be able to perform first aid because most people will eventually find themselves in a situation requiring it for another person or for themselves.
- First aid is the immediate care given to an injured or suddenly ill person. First aid does not take the place of proper medical care.
- The supplies in a first aid kit should be customized to include those items likely to be used on a regular basis.
- Legal and ethical issues concern all first aiders.
- A first aider must have the victim's consent (permission) before giving first aid.
- First aiders might learn confidential information. It is important that you be extremely cautious about revealing information you learn while caring for someone.
- Varying from state to state, Good Samaritan laws encourage people to assist others in distress by granting them immunity against lawsuits.

▶ Vital Vocabulary

abandonment Failure to continue first aid until relieved by someone with the same or a higher level of training.

act of commission Doing something that a reasonably prudent person would not do under the same or similar circumstances.

act of omission Failure to do what a reasonably prudent person with the same or similar training would do in the same or similar circumstances.

battery Touching a person or providing first aid without consent.

breach of duty When a first aider fails to provide the type of care that would be given by a person having the same or similar training.

consent An agreement by a patient or victim to accept treatment offered as explained by medical personnel or first aiders.

duty to act A person's responsibility to provide victim care.

expressed consent Permission for care that a victim gives verbally or with a head nod.

first aid Immediate care given to an injured or suddenly ill person.

Good Samaritan laws Laws that encourage people to voluntarily help an injured or suddenly ill person by minimizing the liability for errors made while rendering emergency care in good faith.

implied consent An assumed consent given by an unconscious adult when emergency lifesaving treatment is required.

negligence Deviation from the accepted standard of care that results in further injury to the victim.

prep kit

▶ Assessment in Action

Toward the end of the ski season you hear that a ski resort in a neighboring state is almost vacant of skiers, and the resort is offering reduced fees during weekdays. You decide to take advantage of reduced ski fees and take a few days off to go skiing. As you ski down the mountain on a run with trees bordering on both sides, you come across a man lying motionless in the snow near a tree he may have crashed into. No other skiers are in sight and you are alone. As you approach the victim, you see no obvious injuries. You have no first aid supplies. Your first aid certification is still current.

Directions: Circle Yes if you agree with the statement; circle No if you disagree.

Yes　No　**1.** You have to stop to help the man.

Yes　No　**2.** You have implied consent to help this man.

Yes　No　**3.** After tapping on the man's shoulder to see if he is OK, he remains unresponsive but breathing. You can leave and assume that the ski patrol will be coming shortly.

Yes　No　**4.** You decide to help. Before assessing the victim, you roll him over, causing him to slide down the hill and hit a tree. Good Samaritan laws protect you even if you cause further harm to the victim.

▶ Check Your Knowledge

Directions: Circle Yes if you agree with the statement; circle No if you disagree.

Yes　No　**1.** Because an ambulance can arrive within minutes in most locations, most people do not need to learn first aid.

Yes　No　**2.** Correct first aid can mean the difference between life and death.

Yes　No　**3.** During your lifetime, you are likely to encounter many life-threatening emergencies.

Yes　No　**4.** All injured victims need medical care.

Yes　No　**5.** Before giving first aid to an alert, competent adult, you must get consent (permission) from the victim.

Yes　No　**6.** If you ask an injured adult if you can help, and she says "No," you can ignore her and proceed to provide care.

Yes　No　**7.** People who are designated as first aiders by their employers must give first aid to injured employees while on the job.

Yes　No　**8.** First aiders who help injured victims are rarely sued.

Yes　No　**9.** Good Samaritan laws provide a degree of protection for first aiders who act in good faith and without compensation.

Yes　No　**10.** You are required to provide first aid to any injured or suddenly ill person you encounter.

2

Action at an Emergency

▶ Emergencies

Emergencies have distinctive characteristics. They are:

- Dangerous—people's lives, well-being, or property are threatened.
- Unusual and rare events—the average person will probably encounter fewer than a half a dozen serious emergencies in a lifetime.
- Different from one another—each presents a different set of problems.
- Unforeseen—they happen suddenly and without warning.
- Urgent—if the emergency is not dealt with immediately, the situation will escalate.

▶ What Should Be Done?

Victims would benefit if bystanders could quickly and reliably do the following:

1. Recognize the emergency.
2. Decide to help.
3. Call 9-1-1 if emergency medical service is needed.
4. Check the victim.
5. Give first aid.

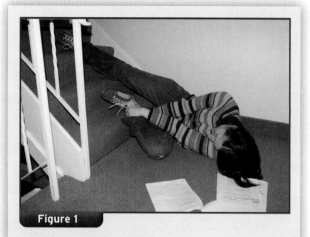

Figure 1

It is not always clear at first glance whether an emergency exists.

Recognize the Emergency

To help in an emergency, the bystander first has to notice that something is wrong. Noticing that something is wrong is related to four factors (**Figure 1**):

- *Severity.* Severe, catastrophic emergencies such as a motor vehicle crash involving an overturned car or several vehicles attract attention.
- *Physical distance.* The closer a bystander is to an emergency situation, the more likely he or she will notice it.
- *Relationship.* Knowing the victim increases the likelihood of noticing an emergency. For example, you would notice your child's injuries before you might notice the same injuries on a stranger.
- *Time exposed.* Evidence indicates that the longer a bystander is aware of the situation, the more likely he or she will notice it as an emergency.

Decide to Help

At some time, everyone will have to decide whether to help another person. Unless the decision to act in an emergency is considered well in advance of an actual emergency, the many obstacles that make it difficult or unpleasant for a bystander to help a stranger are almost certain to impede action. One important strategy that people use to avoid action is to refuse (consciously or unconsciously) to acknowledge the emergency. Many emergencies do not look like the ones portrayed on television, and the uncertainty of the real event can make it easier for the bystander to avoid acknowledging the emergency.

Making a quick decision to get involved at the time of an emergency is more likely to occur if the bystander has previously considered the possibility of helping others. Thus, the most important time to make the decision to help is before you ever encounter an emergency. Deciding to help is an attitude about emergencies and about one's ability to deal with emergencies. It is an attitude that takes time to develop and is affected by a number of factors.

Call 9-1-1 if EMS Is Needed

Wrong decisions about calling 9-1-1 can be made. Examples include a delay in calling 9-1-1 until callers are absolutely sure that an emergency exists, or deciding to bypass EMS and to transport the victim to medical care in a private vehicle. Such actions can endanger a victim. Fortunately, most injuries and sudden illnesses do not require medical care—only first aid.

Check the Victim

You must decide whether life-threatening conditions exist and what kind of help a victim needs. See the chapter entitled Finding Out What's Wrong for details.

Give First Aid

Often the most critical life support measures are effective only if started immediately by the nearest available person. That person usually will be a layperson—a bystander.

▶ Seeking Medical Care

Knowing when to call 9-1-1 for help from EMS is important. To know when to call, you must be able to tell the difference between a minor injury or illness and a life-threatening one. For example, upper abdominal pain can be indigestion, ulcers, or an early sign of a heart attack. Wheezing could be related to a person's asthma, for which the person can use his or her prescribed inhaler for quick relief, or it can be as serious as a severe allergic reaction from a bee sting.

Not every cut needs stitches, nor does every burn require medical care. It is, however, always best to err on the side of caution. According to the American College of Emergency Physicians (ACEP), if the answer to any of the following questions is "yes," or if you are unsure, call 9-1-1 for help.

- Is the victim's condition life threatening?
- Could the condition get worse and become life threatening on the way to the hospital?
- Does the victim need the skills or equipment of EMS?
- Could the distance or traffic conditions cause a delay in getting the victim to the hospital?
- Is a spinal injury suspected?

ACEP also recommends immediate transport to the hospital emergency department, by EMS or by private vehicle, for the following conditions that are warning signs of more serious conditions:

- Chest pain lasting 2 minutes or more
- Uncontrolled bleeding (see the following list of wounds needing immediate medical care)
- Any sudden or severe pain
- Coughing or vomiting blood
- Difficulty breathing, shortness of breath
- Sudden dizziness, weakness, fainting
- Changes in vision
- Difficulty speaking
- Severe or persistent vomiting or diarrhea
- Change in mental status (for example, confusion, difficulty arousing)
- Suicidal or homicidal feelings
- Wounds needing immediate medical care include (see the chapter entitled Wounds for additional wounds needing medical care) those in which:
  - Bleeding from a cut does not slow during the first 15 minutes of steady direct pressure.
  - Signs of shock occur.
  - Breathing is difficult because of a cut to the neck or chest.
  - A deep cut to the abdomen causes moderate to severe pain.
  - There is a cut to the eyeball.
  - A cut amputates or partially amputates an extremity.

When a serious situation occurs, call 9-1-1 first. Do not call your doctor, the hospital, a friend, relatives, or neighbors for help before you call 9-1-1. Calling anyone else first only wastes time.

If the situation is not an emergency, call your doctor. However, if you have any doubt about whether the situation is an emergency, call 9-1-1.

▶ How to Call EMS

In most communities, to receive emergency assistance of any kind, call 9-1-1 **Figure 2**. Check to see if this is true in your community. Emergency telephone numbers are usually listed on the inside front cover of telephone directories. Keep these numbers near or on every telephone. Dial 0 (the operator) if you do not know the emergency number.

When you call 9-1-1, speak slowly and clearly. Be ready to give the dispatcher the following information:

1. The victim's location. Give the address, names of intersecting roads, and other landmarks, if possible. This information is the most important thing you can give. Also, tell the specific location of the victim. (For example, "in the basement" or "in the backyard.")
2. The phone number you are calling from and your name. This allows dispatchers to detect false reports, thus minimizing their frequency, and it allows a dispatch center without the enhanced 9-1-1 system to call back if disconnected or for additional information if needed.
3. What happened. State the nature of the emergency. (For example, "My husband fell off a ladder and is not moving.")
4. Number of persons needing help and any special conditions. (For example, "There was

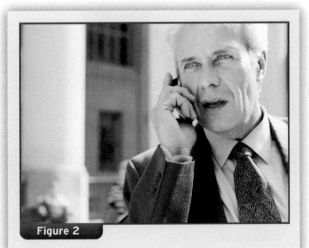

Figure 2

For help, call 9-1-1 or the local emergency number.

a car crash involving two cars. Three people are trapped.")

5. Victim's condition. (For example, "My husband's head is bleeding.") List any first aid you have tried (such as pressing on the site of the bleeding).

Do *not* hang up the phone unless the dispatcher instructs you to do so. Enhanced 9-1-1 systems can track a call, but some communities lack this technology. Also, the EMS dispatcher could tell you how best to care for the victim. If you send someone else to call, have the person report back to you so you can be sure the call was made.

▶ Scene Size-up

If you are at the scene of an emergency situation, do a 10-second <u>scene size-up</u> ⬤ Figure 3, looking for three things: (1) hazards that could be dangerous to you, the victim(s), or bystanders; (2) the cause of the injury or illness; and (3) the number of victims. As you approach an emergency scene, scan the area for immediate dangers to yourself or to the victim ⬤ Figure 4.

If the scene is dangerous, stay away and call 9-1-1. You are not being cowardly, merely realistic. Never attempt a rescue that you have not been specifically trained to do. You cannot help another person if you also become a victim.

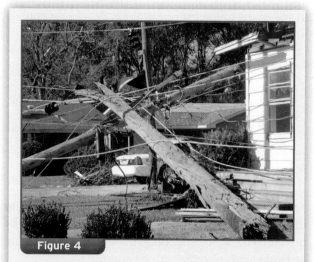

Figure 4

The scene size-up includes evaluating the scene for hazardous conditions.

The second step is to try to determine the cause of the injury. For example, if the emergency department physician knows that a victim was thrown against a steering wheel, he or she will check for liver, spleen, and cardiac injuries. Be sure to tell EMS personnel about your findings so they can identify the extent of any injuries. Finally, determine how many people are involved. There could be more than one victim, so look around and ask about others involved.

▶ Disease Precautions

First aiders must understand the risks from infectious diseases, which can range in severity from mild to life threatening. First aiders should know how to reduce the risk of contamination to themselves and to others.

An <u>infectious disease</u> is a medical condition caused by the growth and spread of small, harmful organisms within the body. A <u>communicable disease</u> is a disease that can spread from one person to another. Immunizations, protective techniques, and handwashing can minimize the risk of infection. Because there are so many different infectious diseases to be concerned about, the Centers for Disease Control and Prevention (CDC) developed a set of <u>standard precautions</u>, which advise you to assume that all victims are infected and can spread an organism that poses a risk for transmission of infectious diseases. These protective measures are designed to prevent first aiders from coming into direct contact with infectious agents.

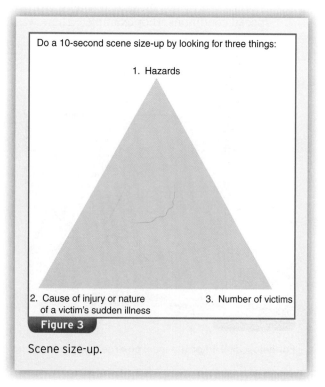

Do a 10-second scene size-up by looking for three things:

1. Hazards

2. Cause of injury or nature of a victim's sudden illness

3. Number of victims

Figure 3

Scene size-up.

Handwashing

Handwashing is one of the simplest yet most effective ways to control disease transmission. Even if you are wearing gloves, you should wash your hands before, if possible, and definitely after every victim contact. The longer the germs remain with you, the greater their chance of infecting you.

The proper procedure for washing your hands is as follows:

1. Use soap and warm water, if possible. All types of soap are acceptable when washing with water.
2. Rub your hands together for 15 to 20 seconds to work up a lather. Wash all surfaces well, including wrists, palms, backs of hands, and fingers. Clean the dirt from under your fingernails.
3. Rinse the soap from your hands.
4. Dry your hands completely with a clean towel if possible (this helps remove the germs). If towels are not available, however, it is okay to allow your hands to air dry.

If soap and water are not available, use an alcohol-based hand sanitizer to clean your hands **Figure 5**. Apply the gel to one hand and rub hands together, covering all surfaces of hands and fingers, until the hands are dry. If your mucous membranes (for example, your eyes, nose, or mouth) are splashed by a bloody fluid, immediately flush the area with clean water.

Personal Protective Equipment

<u>Personal protective equipment (PPE)</u> includes exam gloves, mouth-to-barrier devices, eye protection, and gowns. PPE provides a barrier between the first aider and infectious diseases.

Exam Gloves

Exam gloves are the most common type of PPE and should always be worn when there is any possibility of exposure to blood or body fluids. All first aid kits should contain several pairs of gloves. Because some rescuers have allergic reactions to latex, latex-free gloves should also be available. You might consider putting on a second pair of gloves over the first if there is major, significant external bleeding or body fluid. If the gloves are cut or torn, replace them.

Mouth-to-Barrier Devices

Mouth-to-barrier devices are recommended **Figure 6**. Although there are no documented cases of disease transmission to rescuers as a result of performing unprotected mouth-to-mouth resuscitation on a victim with an infection, you should use a barrier device such as a pocket mask when providing CPR.

Other Personal Protective Equipment

Other PPE includes eye protection and gowns and aprons. OSHA requires these to be available in some workplaces, especially for health care workers. These are not required for first aiders and usually will not be available.

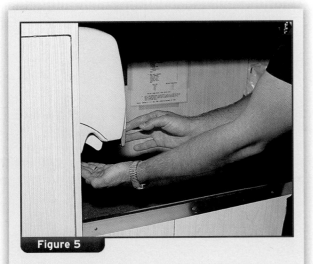

Figure 5
Use a waterless handwashing solution if there is no running water available.

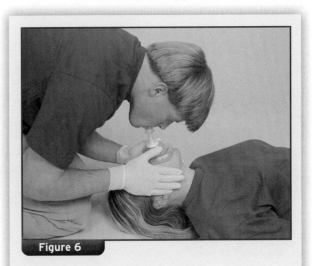

Figure 6
Pocket face mask, one-way valve.

Cleaning Up After an Emergency

When cleaning up blood or other body fluids, protect yourself and others against disease transmission by following these steps:

1. Wear heavier gloves than lightweight latex or vinyl.
2. If you have been trained in the correct procedures, use absorbent barriers to soak up blood or other infectious materials.
   Clean the spill area using soap and water. After cleaning, disinfect with a bleach and water solution at a 1:10 dilution. Isopropyl alcohol also can be used to disinfect. These solutions can corrode or discolor certain fabrics, leathers, vinyl, or other synthetic materials.
3. Discard contaminated materials in an appropriate waste disposal container.

If you have been exposed to blood or body fluids:

1. Use soap and water to wash the parts of your body that have been contaminated.
2. If the exposure happened at work, report the incident to your supervisor. Otherwise, contact your personal physician. If the exposure was significant, seek medical care. Early action can prevent the development of certain infections.

The best protection against disease is using the safeguards described here. By following these guidelines, first aiders can decrease their chances of contracting bloodborne illnesses.

▶ Ready for Review

- Emergencies are dangerous, unusual, rare, unforeseen, and must be dealt with before the situation becomes worse.
- A bystander is a vital link between EMS and the victim.
- Victims would benefit if bystanders could quickly and reliably do the following:
  – Recognize the emergency.
  – Decide to help.
  – Call 9-1-1 if EMS is needed.
  – Check the victim.
  – Give first aid.
- Knowing when to call 9-1-1 is important. To do so, you must be able to tell the difference between a minor injury or illness and a life-threatening one.
- In most communities, call 9-1-1 to receive emergency assistance.
- The sight of blood and the cries of victims can be upsetting, but it is essential that first aiders remain alert and working at an injury scene.
- If you are at the scene of an emergency situation, do a 10-second scene size-up looking for hazards, the cause of the injury or illness, and the number of victims.
- First aiders should take precautions to protect against infectious diseases.
- There are few incidents that involve emotional stress like the life-and-death situations that you might face.

▶ Vital Vocabulary

communicable disease A disease that can spread from person to person, or from animal to person.

infectious disease A medical condition caused by the growth of small, harmful organisms within the body.

personal protective equipment (PPE) Equipment, such as exam gloves, used to block the entry of an organism into the body.

scene size-up Steps taken when approaching an emergency scene. Steps include checking for hazards, noting the cause of the injury or illness, and determining the number of victims.

standard precautions Protective measures that have traditionally been developed by the Centers for Disease Control and Prevention (CDC) for use in dealing with objects, blood, body fluids, or other potential exposure risks of communicable disease.

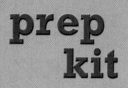

prep kit

▶ Assessment in Action

You are walking from house to house in an unfamiliar neighborhood collecting donated clothing for a local charitable organization. You find no one home at a particular house but hear a loud explosion in the garage. You decide to see what happened. Upon entering the garage you find a teenage boy lying on the ground.

There is a strong gasoline odor. You have a cellular telephone with you.

Directions: Circle Yes if you agree with the statement; circle No if you disagree.

Yes   No   **1.** This scene could be dangerous.

Yes   No   **2.** You should not be concerned about other possible victims.

Yes   No   **3.** In most communities, 9-1-1 can be used to contact EMS.

Yes   No   **4.** If you do not know the exact address of the emergency, be prepared to give a description of the location as best as you can.

▶ Check Your Knowledge

Directions: Circle Yes if you agree with the statement; circle No if you disagree.

Yes   No   **1.** A scene survey should be done before giving first aid to an injured victim.

Yes   No   **2.** For a severely injured victim, call the victim's doctor before calling for an ambulance.

Yes   No   **3.** Dial 0 (for the telephone operator) if you do not know the emergency telephone number.

Yes   No   **4.** First aiders should assume that blood and all body fluids are infectious.

Yes   No   **5.** If you are exposed to blood while on the job, report it to your supervisor, and if off the job, to your personal physician.

Yes   No   **6.** First aid kits should contain exam gloves.

Yes   No   **7.** Wash your hands with soap and water after giving first aid.

Yes   No   **8.** Exam gloves can be made of almost any material as long as they fit the hand well.

Finding Out What's Wrong

3

▶ Victim Assessment Overview

During emergency situations when panic exists, knowing what to do and what not to do is crucial. A victim assessment is a sequence of actions that helps determine what is wrong and thus helps provide safe and appropriate first aid. Becoming familiar with the process of victim assessment will enable you to act quickly and decisively in hectic emergency situations. Victim assessment is an important first aid skill. It requires an understanding of each assessment step as well as decision-making skills.

Finding out what is wrong with a person will be influenced by whether the victim is suffering from an illness or an injury, whether the victim is responsive or unresponsive, and whether life-threatening conditions exist. A key point is to conduct a **primary check** first and to care for any problems you uncover before going on with the assessment.

Different problems and conditions require different approaches for determining what is wrong. Not all parts of an assessment apply to every victim, and the sequencing can vary depending on the victim's problem. Most victims do not require a complete assessment. For example, a victim who cut a finger while whittling a stick will not require a complete assessment, but a victim who slipped and fell 20 feet down a mountainside and cut a finger will, because other injuries might be present. **Table 1** and the flowchart give a preview of the sequence for the different types of victim you may encounter.

Table 1 Sequence of Victim Assessment

Injured Victim			Suddenly Ill Victim	
	Responsive			
Unresponsive	With Significant COI	Without Significant COI	Unresponsive	Responsive
• Primary check	• Primary check	• Primary check	• Primary check	• Primary check
• Secondary check using the DOS parts of DOTS	• Secondary check using DOTS	• Examine chief complaint using DOTS	• Secondary check using the DOS parts of DOTS	• SAMPLE history
• SAMPLE history from others	• SAMPLE history	• SAMPLE history	• SAMPLE history from others	• Examine chief complaint

COI = cause of injury; also known as mechanism of injury. DOTS = deformity, open wounds, tenderness, swelling. SAMPLE = symptoms, allergies, medications, pertinent history, last oral intake, and events leading up to the illness or injury

A victim assessment can provide important information about a problem and help you determine how to treat it and whether medical care is needed. If the victim requires medical care, pass what you found during the assessment to the emergency medical service (EMS) personnel or health care providers. Call 9-1-1 for any victim with a significant **cause of injury (COI)** or **nature of illness**, and for any unresponsive victim.

You should check the victim systematically. You can do this by performing these five steps:

1. Perform a scene size-up (see the chapter entitled Action at an Emergency).
2. Perform a primary check.
3. Perform a secondary check, also known as a physical exam or head-to-toe exam.
4. Obtain the victim's SAMPLE history.
5. Perform a reassessment.

The scene size-up helps determine the safety of the scene and the general condition of the victim. It is followed by the primary check, in which the first aider identifies and treats immediate life-threatening conditions involving problems with the victim's breathing and severe bleeding. Victims with immediate life-threatening conditions can die within minutes unless their problems are quickly recognized and treated.

A **secondary check**, consisting of a physical examination, follows the primary check. These procedures can reveal information that will help identify the injury or illness, its severity, and what first aid is needed. Detailed information is gained about the victim's injury (eg, a painful ankle or bleeding nose) or chief complaint (eg, chest pain or itchy skin).

Performing the secondary check right after the primary check and before doing the **SAMPLE history** allows an injury to be found and cared for sooner than if the SAMPLE history comes before the secondary check. In some cases, especially when caring for a stranger, performing the SAMPLE history before the secondary check involves a conversation with the stranger, which may ease the victim's anxiety about having a first aider conduct a secondary check. Also, in cases of illness, performing the SAMPLE history before the secondary check can indicate which part of the secondary check should be performed first.

▶ Primary Check

The second part of a victim assessment sequence is always the primary check. The purpose of the primary check is to identify life-threatening conditions so you can immediately take action to treat the conditions. The primary check includes checking the victim's responsiveness, checking circulation, checking for breathing, and checking for severe bleeding.

First Impression of the Victim

While approaching the victim, form an immediate **first impression** of the victim. This also has been

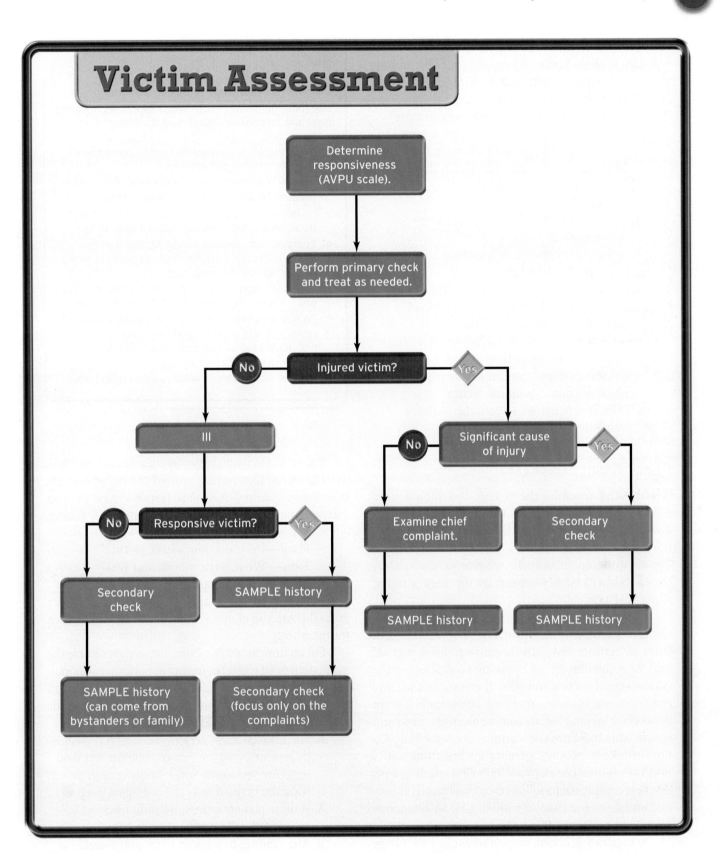

Victim Assessment

Determine responsiveness (AVPU scale).

Perform primary check and treat as needed.

Injured victim?

No → Ill

Yes → Significant cause of injury

Ill branch:
Responsive victim?
- No → Secondary check → SAMPLE history (can come from bystanders or family)
- Yes → SAMPLE history → Secondary check (focus only on the complaints)

Injured branch — Significant cause of injury:
- No → Examine chief complaint. → SAMPLE history
- Yes → Secondary check → SAMPLE history

referred to as a general impression, look test, or gut reaction. Both the scene size-up and your first impression of the victim should help determine:

1. Does the victim appear to have an injury or an illness? If you are unable to determine whether the victim is ill or injured, treat the situation as though he or she were injured. Impressions can come from such things as the victim's position and the victim's breathing sounds.
2. Is the victim obviously responsive or unresponsive?
3. Is the victim obviously breathing adequately or normally? Talking?
4. Are there signs of obvious bleeding—blood spurting, blood-soaked clothing, blood pooled on the ground or floor?
5. Is there a chance of exposure to the victim's blood or other body fluids? If so, be sure to use standard precautions before making physical contact with the victim.
6. Is there any danger to you, the victim, or bystanders at the scene?

Check Responsiveness

Shortly after reaching the victim, you should have a good idea of whether the victim is responsive or unresponsive. If the victim is motionless, gently tap the victim's shoulder and ask loudly, "Are you okay?" Beyond this point, how and in what order you conduct the checks will largely depend on the answer to the above question.

If the victim answers, moans, or moves, the victim is responsive. If the victim does not respond, call 9-1-1 to activate EMS. In the unresponsive victim, look for regular breathing by taking a quick look at the chest to see if it rises and falls. If you cannot see any chest movement and cannot hear any sounds (except occasional gasping) of air coming from the nose and mouth, this indicates the victim is not breathing. Do not mistake occasional gasping for breathing—it is not! Take immediate steps to begin CPR, starting with 30 chest compressions followed by two breaths (1 second each). See the chapter entitled CPR for directions on how to perform CPR.

A victim's level of responsiveness can range from fully responsive (conscious) to unresponsive (unconscious). Not all responsive victims are fully alert, and they may respond to different levels of stimulation.

For an alert victim, begin by introducing yourself. Tell the victim that you are trained in first aid and ask permission to help. For an alert, responsive victim, you can evaluate the victim's ability to remember by asking:

- Person—What is your name?
- Place—Do you know where you are?
- Time—What is the month and year?
- Event—What happened?

For a motionless victim, tap his or her shoulder and ask, "Are you okay?" If there is no response, check for breathing.

For an unresponsive victim, the steps resemble the same steps used when beginning to perform cardiopulmonary resuscitation (CPR)—RAP-CAB—although most unresponsive victims do not need CPR (see the chapter entitled CPR) **Skill Drill 1**:

R For any motionless person, check responsiveness by gently tapping the victim's shoulder and shouting, "Are you okay?" Speak loudly enough to wake the victim if he or she is sleeping (**Step ❶**).

A If there is no response, activate EMS by calling 9-1-1 (**Step ❷**).

P After calling to activate EMS, you should position the victim onto his or her back on a flat, firm surface. If the victim is breathing, place him or her in the recovery position and check for severe bleeding (**Step ❸**).

CAB Immediately begin CPR for adult victims who are unresponsive and not breathing or not breathing normally (only gasping) (**Step ❹**). If you are alone and the victim is a child or an infant, perform CPR for five cycles before calling 9-1-1. If a bystander is present for any victim, have him or her call 9-1-1 while you begin CPR. (See the chapter entitled CPR for directions.)

An unresponsive, breathing victim can receive other first aid, especially to control severe bleeding. Providing care would be covered by implied consent. (Refer to the chapter entitled Background Information.)

The steps for an alert, responsive victim are RAP-ABC. A first aider is more likely to see this type of victim. Responsive victims rarely need the type of primary check used in unresponsive victims. However, a responsive victim may be developing an airway obstruction, may have severe bleeding, may be having a heart attack, or may be in the early stages of shock or some other serious condition. Each of these conditions is considered a medical emergency, and immediate care must be provided if you suspect any of them. Follow these steps to care for an alert, responsive victim:

R While approaching a responsive victim, make eye contact, introduce yourself as a trained first aider, and give your name. Next, ask if you can help—this is asking for the victim's consent to help. With permission from the victim, perform a victim assessment.

A If the victim appears to be severely injured or ill, activate EMS.

P Position the victim in a comfortable position (eg, lying down, tripod position, leaning against stable object).

A Make sure that the airway stays open.

B Check breathing—are there abnormal breathing sounds (eg, wheezing, gurgling) or is the victim breathing fast?

C Check circulation—is there severe bleeding?

Check Breathing

Check for adequate breathing by looking for chest rise and fall, listening for normal or abnormal breath sounds, and feeling for adequate air movement. Distinguish between effective and ineffective breathing efforts. Cyanosis and ashen (grey) skin are signs of inadequate oxygenation. See **Table 2** for breathing sounds that indicate a breathing problem.

Table 2 Breathing Sounds

Breathing Sound	Possible Cause
Snoring	Airway partially blocked (usually by tongue)
Gurgling (breaths passing through liquid)	Fluids in throat
Crowing (noisy creak or squeak)	Spasm of the larynx; foreign body
Wheezing	Spasm or partial obstruction in bronchi (asthma, emphysema)
Occasional gasping breaths (known as agonal respirations)	Breathing after the heart has stopped

Check for Severe Bleeding

Check for severe bleeding by quickly looking over the victim's entire body for blood (eg, blood-soaked clothing or blood pooling on the floor or the ground). This is not a head-to-toe examination, but a search for large amounts of blood around the victim or in the victim's clothing. In most cases, placing a sterile dressing over the wound and applying direct pressure with a hand or a pressure bandage controls the bleeding. Life-threatening external bleeding is rare, but when found, it must be controlled immediately or the victim can bleed to death. Avoid contact with the victim's blood whenever possible by using exam gloves or extra layers of dressings or cloth.

Position the Victim

Most victims should not be moved, especially if a spinal injury is suspected. The exceptions to this "rule of thumb" include:

- When the victim and first aider(s) are in an unsafe location.
- When an unresponsive victim is face down (prone position) and needs CPR, the victim should be turned to face up (supine position) on a firm, flat surface to be in a position to receive CPR.
- When the victim has difficulty breathing because of vomiting or secretions, or if the

skill drill

1   Primary Check: RAP-CAB for Unresponsive Victim

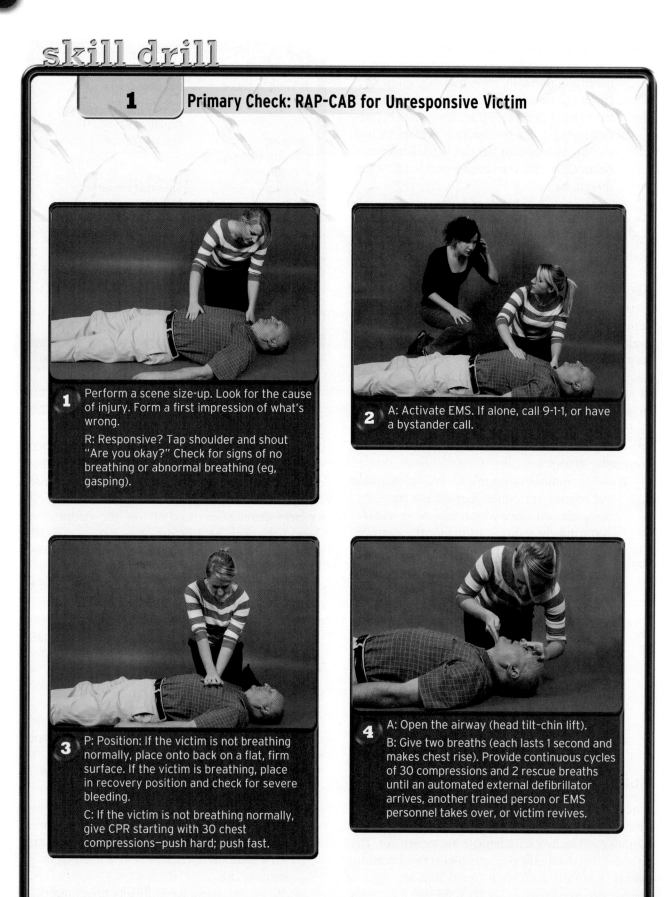

1 Perform a scene size-up. Look for the cause of injury. Form a first impression of what's wrong.
R: Responsive? Tap shoulder and shout "Are you okay?" Check for signs of no breathing or abnormal breathing (eg, gasping).

2 A: Activate EMS. If alone, call 9-1-1, or have a bystander call.

3 P: Position: If the victim is not breathing normally, place onto back on a flat, firm surface. If the victim is breathing, place in recovery position and check for severe bleeding.
C: If the victim is not breathing normally, give CPR starting with 30 chest compressions—push hard; push fast.

4 A: Open the airway (head tilt–chin lift).
B: Give two breaths (each lasts 1 second and makes chest rise). Provide continuous cycles of 30 compressions and 2 rescue breaths until an automated external defibrillator arrives, another trained person or EMS personnel takes over, or victim revives.

first aider is alone and must leave to get help. The victim can be placed in a modified High Arm IN Endangered Spine (HAINES) recovery position. It is best for the victim to rest on his or her left side. While rolling the victim into the side position, keep the victim's nose and navel pointing in the same direction to avoid twisting the spine. Roll the victim onto the left side using the following steps:

1. Keeping the victim's left arm straight, extend it above the head with the upper part of the arm next to the head.
2. Bring the right arm across the chest and place the back of the victim's right hand against the left cheek; hold it there.
3. Hold the victim's hand against the cheek to support the head. Bend the victim's far leg at the knee and pull the bent leg to roll the victim toward you.
4. The victim's head remains on top of the left arm while rolling and the right hand stabilizes the head. The right bent knee prevents rolling.

- When signs of shock develop, place the victim on his or her back (supine position). Do not move the victim if suspected leg fractures or head or spine injuries exist.

Most victims with no suspected spine injuries may be placed in a position in which they are most comfortable. Victims with chest pain, nausea, or difficulty breathing fare better if in a half-sitting (semi-sitting) position at about a 45° angle. During an asthma attack, a victim may prefer the tripod position, which is sitting up, leaning forward with hands on knees and elbows out.

Q&A

When should a first aider interrupt a primary check?

When a life-threatening condition is identified during the primary check, first aid should begin immediately. For example, if a victim has an obstructed airway, this should be treated before going through the other assessment steps. Once the life-threatening condition (eg, choking) has been cared for and/or corrected, the primary check of the victim should continue until completed.

Q&A

Do I have to perform a complete victim assessment for every injured or suddenly ill victim?

No. Perform a primary check for every victim and acquire as much of each victim's SAMPLE history as you can. Performing a complete secondary check, which includes a head-to-toe physical exam, is crucial for the unresponsive, ill, or significantly injured victim. However, for the responsive ill person and the nonsignificantly injured victim, the secondary check focuses primarily on the victim's chief complaint.

▶ Secondary Check

A first aider should complete a secondary check following the primary check. Immediately treat any life-threatening problems found during a secondary check.

The goal of doing a hands-on secondary check is to identify any potentially life-threatening illness or injury needing first aid. A good secondary check is essential in discovering what is wrong. The adage of "find it; fix it" stresses the fact that you cannot provide first aid unless you know what is wrong. And you will not know what is wrong until you do a victim assessment.

Most of the victims a first aider will encounter require a secondary check of only the chief complaint, and a full secondary check (described below) is not needed. Nevertheless, first aiders should know how to perform one. In addition to the questions, "What's wrong?" or "What happened to you?" another important question to ask of the victim who has been injured is, "Do you hurt anywhere?" Many victims view a physical examination with apprehension and anxiety—they feel vulnerable and exposed. Maintain dignity throughout the assessment. Show compassion toward the victim and family members. If possible, the victim should be sitting or lying down.

Start by reconsidering the cause or mechanism of injury that you identified during the scene size-up. Ask the victim to describe what happened in detail, so that you can use the mechanism or cause of injury to predict possible injured areas—especially head, neck, spine, and internal injuries (see the chapter entitled Action at an Emergency). This helps to determine which first aid procedures to use.

Determine whether the cause or mechanism of injury was significant Table 3 . In addition to the significant causes of injury, assume that a victim with a head injury also has a spinal injury until proven otherwise. About 15% to 20% of head injury victims also have a spinal injury.

For a responsive victim, check for a spinal injury by asking the victim the following questions (refer to Skill Drill 1 in the chapter entitled Head and Spinal Injuries):

- Can you feel me squeezing your fingers and toes? (Before doing this, have the victim look away or close his or her eyes.) While you are squeezing, ask the victim which finger or toe you are squeezing.
- Can you wiggle your fingers and toes?
- Can you squeeze my hand, and can you push your foot against my hand?

For an unresponsive victim, check the spinal cord by stroking the bottom of the foot firmly toward the big toe with a key or similar blunt object. This is known as the Babinski reflex test. The normal response is an involuntary reflex that makes the big toe go down (except in infants, in whom it goes in the opposite direction). If the spinal cord or brain is injured, the toe will flex upward for both adults and children.

If you suspect a spinal injury, do not move the victim's head or neck. Stabilize the victim against any movement, and tell him or her not to move.

A secondary check assesses the victim's entire body from head to toe; you will note the victim's signs and symptoms:

- **Signs**—victim's conditions you can see, feel, hear, or smell.
- **Symptoms**—things the victim feels and is able to describe; known as the chief complaint.

To check a part of the body, look and feel (mnemonic is LAF) for the following signs and symptoms of injury: deformities, open wounds, tenderness, and swelling. The mnemonic **DOTS** is helpful for

Q&A

When might an assessment be unreliable?
Use caution when assessing any victim who has an altered mental status, a distracting painful injury (eg, femur fracture), or who has ingested alcohol or drugs.

Table 3 Significant Causes of Injury

- Falls of more than 15' for adults, more than 10' for children, or more than three times the victim's height
- Falls head-first from the victim's height or greater distance
- Vehicle collisions involving ejection, a rollover, high speed, a pedestrian, a motorcycle, or a bicycle
- Head trauma with altered mental status (V, P, or U on AVPU scale)
- Penetrations of the head, chest, or abdomen (for example, stab or gunshot wounds)
- Major burn injury
- Death of an occupant in the same vehicle
- Pedestrian hit by a vehicle

remembering the signs and symptoms of an injury Figure 1 :

- D = Deformity—abnormal shape of the body part (compare with the opposite uninjured part). Deformities occur when bones are broken or joints are dislocated.
- O = Open wounds—the skin is broken and there is bleeding.
- T = Tenderness—sensitivity, discomfort, or pain when touched.
- S = Swelling—area looks larger than usual. Caused by excess fluid in the tissue. When possible, compare one side of the body with the other side (eg, if an ankle appears swollen, look at the other one).

Victim With a Significant Cause of Injury

This is a hands-on, full-body, head-to-toe assessment and should take no more than 2 minutes to complete. The victim may be responsive or unresponsive. Assume that an unresponsive victim has a spinal injury and stabilize the head and neck against movement. When a male examines a female, it is wise, if possible, to have another female present. Follow the steps in Skill Drill 2 to perform a secondary check:

1. **Check the head**. Use both hands to check the scalp for DOTS. A deformity may be a bump or a depression. Do not move the victim's head during this procedure. Check

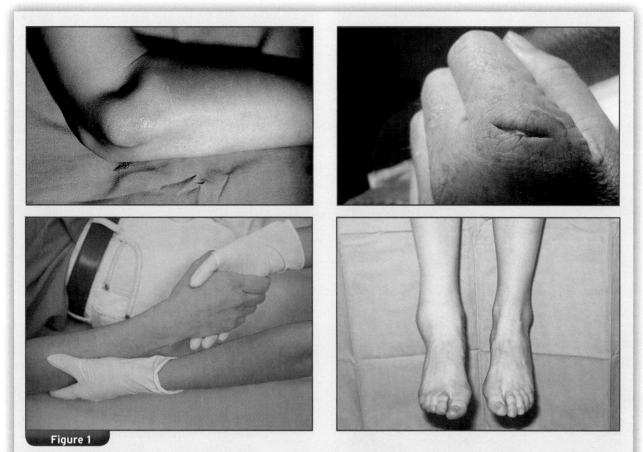

Figure 1

Examine an area by looking and feeling for: D = deformity; O = open wounds; T = tenderness; S = swelling.

the skin condition for temperature, color, and moisture.

2. **Check the eyes.** Compare the pupils, the dark part at the center of the eye. They should be the same size and react to light. The mnemonic PERRL helps you to remember what to look for **Figure 2** :
   - P = pupils
   - E = equal
   - R = round
   - R = react
   - L = light

   Use a flashlight to determine whether the pupils are reactive. If there is no flashlight, cover an eye with your hand and notice the pupil reaction when the eye is uncovered. Normally, the pupil constricts (gets smaller) within 1 second. No pupil reaction to light could mean death, coma, cataracts (in older persons), or an artificial eye. Pupil dilation happens within 30 to 60 seconds of cardiac arrest.

   Look for unequal pupils. A difference in the size of the two pupils is almost always a sign of a medical emergency, such as a stroke or a brain injury. However, the unequal condition occurs normally in 2% to 4% of the population. Also, an artificial eye may give the appearance of unequal pupils. Look at the inner eyelid surface—pink is normal in all healthy people regardless of skin pigmentation. A pale color may indicate poor blood circulation.

3. **Check the ears and nose** for clear or blood-tinged fluid. Check the nose for DOTS.

4. **Check the mouth** for swelling or objects (eg, broken teeth, dentures, chewing gum, vomit, food, and foreign objects), which could block the airway (**Step ❶**).

5. **Check the neck for DOTS.** Look for a medical identification necklace chain and tag (**Step ❷**).

6. **Check the chest for DOTS.** Warn the victim that you are going to apply pressure to the

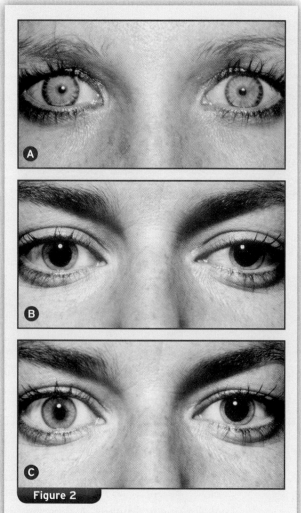

Figure 2

A. Constricted pupils. B. Dilated pupils. C. Unequal pupils.

abnormal lumps and hardened areas. Do not push too deeply. The victim may "guard" an area if it is tender by tightening abdominal muscles or protecting that area with his or her hands. Anything protruding from the abdomen will be obvious, but be sure to check for penetrating objects (**Step ❹**).

8. **Check the pelvis for DOTS**. If the victim does not report pain, gently press inward on the tops of the hip bones and then, if there was no pain, press downward on the same bones. Warn the victim before pressing about possible tenderness (**Step ❺**).

9. **Check all four extremities for DOTS**. Use both hands to encircle an extremity and gently but firmly squeeze each part of the extremity for any sign of tenderness. Compare the two sides of the body with each other. Look for a medical identification bracelet on a wrist (**Step ❻**).

   Check all four extremities for circulation, sensation, and movement (CSM):
   - C = Circulation—for arms, feel for radial (on the wrist's thumb side) pulse, and for legs, feel the posterior tibial pulse behind the ankle bone (malleolus) on the inner (medial) side of the ankle.
   - S = Sensation—pinch the end of fingers and toes (have victim close his or her eyes and tell you which finger or toe is being squeezed).
   - M = Movement—have the victim wiggle fingers and toes.

10. **Check the back**. If no spinal injury is suspected, turn the victim onto his or her side and check for DOTS. You may have to turn the victim toward one side to check half of the back and then turn the victim the other direction to check the other half of the back (**Step ❼**).

If you suspect a neck or spinal injury and the victim's position is stable, tell the victim not to move while you are performing the check. If the victim is uncooperative or in an unstable position, you may have to stop at that point and stabilize the victim's head and neck manually until more help arrives.

Victim With No Significant Cause of Injury

When a victim has no significant cause (mechanism) of injury, a full body physical exam from head to toe is

sides of the chest. Gently squeeze the chest inward and ask if doing so is painful. Pain from squeezing or compressing the sides may indicate a rib fracture (**Step ❸**).

7. **Check the abdomen for DOTS**. Feel the abdomen for tenderness by pushing gently downward in all four of the abdominal quadrants (divide the abdomen into four parts by two imaginary lines intersecting at right angles at the navel). If a chief complaint is abdominal pain, ask the victim to point to where it hurts. Do not push on the area that hurts. Begin on the opposite side from the spot, and press gently on each abdominal quadrant to see if it hurts. As you press on an area, ask the victim if it hurts. Feel for

skill drill

2 **Perform a Secondary Check**

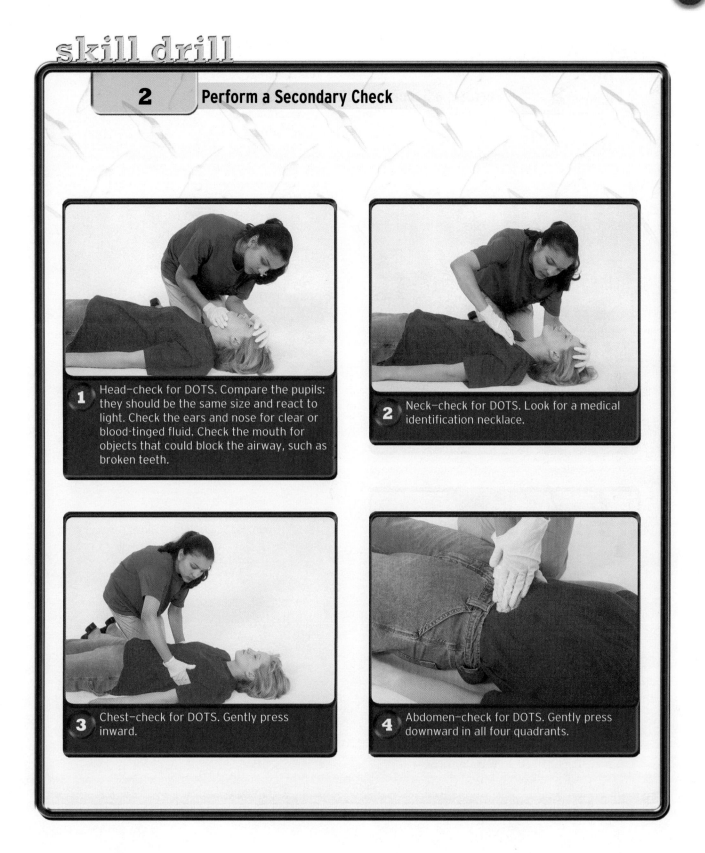

1 Head–check for DOTS. Compare the pupils: they should be the same size and react to light. Check the ears and nose for clear or blood-tinged fluid. Check the mouth for objects that could block the airway, such as broken teeth.

2 Neck–check for DOTS. Look for a medical identification necklace.

3 Chest–check for DOTS. Gently press inward.

4 Abdomen–check for DOTS. Gently press downward in all four quadrants.

skill drill

2 | **Perform a Secondary Check (*continued*)**

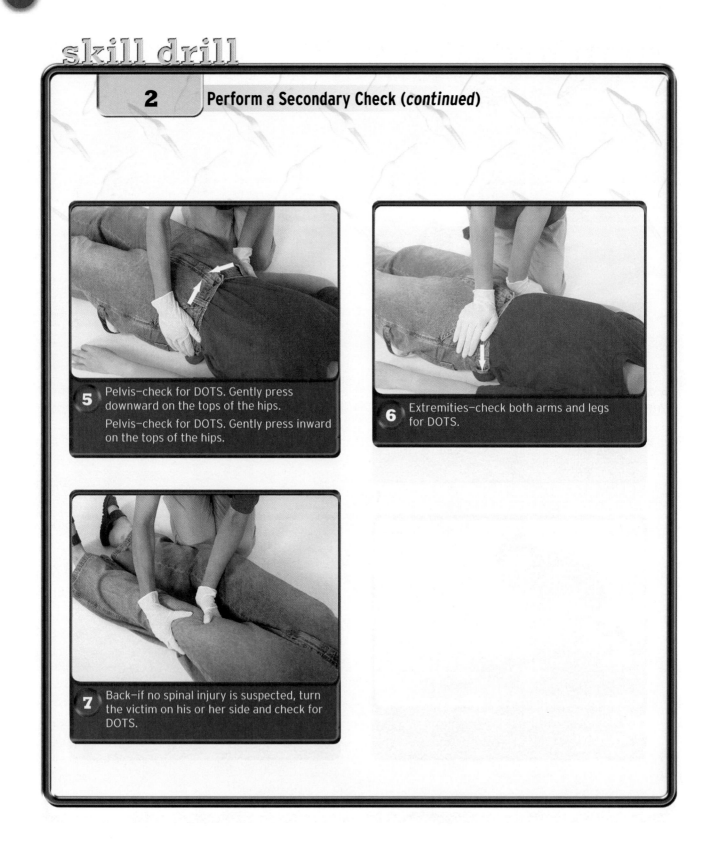

5 Pelvis—check for DOTS. Gently press downward on the tops of the hips.
Pelvis—check for DOTS. Gently press inward on the tops of the hips.

6 Extremities—check both arms and legs for DOTS.

7 Back—if no spinal injury is suspected, turn the victim on his or her side and check for DOTS.

Table 4 Skin Color

Skin Color	Possible Cause
Pink	Normal color in nonpigmented areas regardless of skin complexion–lining of the eyelids, inside mouth, fingernail beds
Red (flushed)	Dilated blood vessels; excess circulation to that part of the body
White (pale)	Constricted blood vessels from blood loss, shock, hypothermia, emotional distress
Blue (cyanosis)	Lack of oxygen in the blood from breathing or heart problems
Yellow (jaundice)	Liver disease or failure

Table 5 Skin Temperature

Skin Temperature/ Moisture	Possible Cause
Warm and dry	Normal
Hot and dry or moist	Excessive body heat (heat stroke, high fever)
Cool and moist (clammy)	Poor circulation, heat exhaustion, shock, acute stress reaction
Cold and moist	Body is losing heat
Cold and dry	Exposed to cold and has lost considerable heat (hypothermia)

not needed. Instead, focus the assessment on the chief complaints (the areas that the victim complains about). For most first aiders, this will be the more frequently performed type of assessment.

Special Considerations

Skin Condition

A quick check of the victim's skin can also provide information about the victim's condition. When assessing the head, check skin temperature, color, and moisture. Skin color, especially in light-skinned people, reflects the circulation under the skin as well as oxygen status **Table 4**. For those with dark complexions, changes might not be readily apparent but can be assessed by the appearance of the nail beds, the inside of the mouth, and the inner eyelids.

You can get a rough idea of skin temperature by putting the back of your hand or wrist on the victim's forehead to determine whether the temperature is elevated or decreased. Dry skin is normal. Skin that is wet, moist, or excessively dry and hot suggests a problem **Table 5**.

Expose the Injury

Clothing might have to be removed to check for an injury and to give proper first aid. If you need to remove clothing, explain what you intend to do

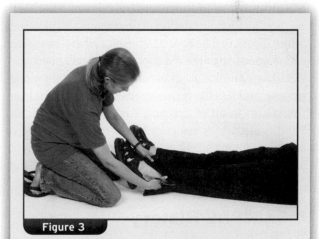

Figure 3

Expose the injury. Remove as much clothing as necessary while trying to maintain privacy.

(and why) to the victim and any family members or bystanders. Remove as much clothing as necessary, try to maintain privacy, and prevent exposure to cold. Damage clothing only if necessary—cut along the seams **Figure 3**.

Check for Medical Identification Tags

Look for a medical identification tag or for a medical information card in the victim's wallet or purse (this might be illegal in some states). It can be beneficial in identifying allergies, medications, or medical history **Figure 4**. A medical identification tag, worn as a

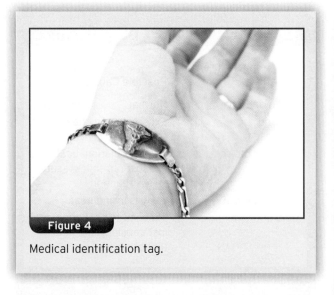

Figure 4

Medical identification tag.

Table 6 SAMPLE History

Description	Questions
S = Symptoms	What's wrong? Where do you hurt? (known as the chief complaint)
A = Allergies	Are you allergic to anything?
M = Medications	Are you taking any prescription or nonprescription medications? What are they for?
P = Past medical history	Have you had this problem before? Have you had recent medical problems?
L = Last oral intake	When did you last eat or drink anything? What was it? How much?
E = Events leading up to the illness or injury	Injury: How did you get hurt? Illness: What led to this problem?

necklace or as a bracelet, contains the wearer's medical problem(s) and a 24-hour telephone number that offers, in case of an emergency, access to the victim's medical history plus names of physicians and close relatives. These can be especially useful when the wearer is unresponsive or not old enough to answer questions. Necklaces and bracelets are durable, instantly recognizable, and less likely than cards to be separated from the victim in an emergency. Always look for victim identification in a wallet or purse in the presence of another person at the scene to protect you against later accusations should money or credit cards be missing.

▶ SAMPLE History

The information in a SAMPLE history could help you identify what is wrong with the victim and can indicate the needed first aid. It is called a SAMPLE history because the letters in SAMPLE stand for the elements of the history .

In the best of circumstances, the victim will be able to answer all questions about his or her chief complaint and medical history. In other cases, this information may be obtained from family, friends, bystanders, medical identification jewelry, or other medical information sources.

FYI

Check for Clues

In addition to a medical identification tag, there may be other clues to what might be wrong with a victim. A medicine bottle label gives the medication's name, but most first aiders will not know why the medication was prescribed. For example, suspect a diabetic emergency if you find glucose tablets or gel or insulin with a victim. An inhaler indicates that a victim has asthma. An auto-injector could point to a person's susceptibility for anaphylaxis caused by one of several things.

The cause (mechanism) of injury (such as a sharp object, broken glass, or bent steering wheel) can alert a first aider about an injury. Additionally, objects at the scene that are not the cause of an injury can offer a clue as to what may be wrong with a victim. Examples include a fallen ladder or an open medicine bottle.

▶ What to Do Until Medical Help Is Available

The primary and secondary checks and SAMPLE history are done quickly so that injuries and illnesses can be identified and given first aid. After the most serious problems have been cared for, regularly recheck an alert victim who has a serious injury or illness every 15 minutes, and at least every 5 minutes for an unresponsive victim or one having breathing difficulties, major blood loss, or who has experienced a significant cause of injury. When in doubt, keep checking the victim every 5 minutes or as frequently as possible.

▶ Triage: What to Do With Multiple Victims

You might encounter emergency situations in which there are two or more victims. This is often the case in multiple-car collisions or disasters. After making a quick scene size-up, decide who must be cared for and transported first. This process of prioritizing victims is called triage.

Various systems have been used to establish priorities. To find those needing immediate care for life-threatening conditions, tell all victims who can get up and walk to move to a specific area. Victims who can get up and walk rarely have life-threatening injuries. These victims are known as "the walking wounded." Do not force a victim to move if he or she complains of pain.

Find the life-threatened victims by performing only the primary check on all remaining victims. Go to motionless victims first. You must move rapidly (spend less than 60 seconds with each victim) from one victim to the next until all have been checked. Classify victims according to the following care and transportation priorities:

1. Immediate care. Victims who have life-threatening injuries but can be saved.
   a. Breathing difficulties (abnormal breath sounds or not breathing)
   b. Severe bleeding
   c. Severe burns
   d. Signs of shock
   e. Open chest or abdominal injuries
2. Delayed care. Victims who do not fit into the immediate or "walking wounded" categories. Care and transportation can be delayed up to 1 hour.
3. Walking wounded. Victims with minor injuries. Care and transportation can be delayed up to 3 hours.
4. Dead. Victims who are obviously dead, or unlikely to survive.

Recheck victims regularly for changes in their condition. Only after those with immediate life-threatening conditions receive care should those with less serious conditions be given care. You will usually be relieved from triage responsibility when more highly trained emergency personnel arrive on the scene. You might then be asked to provide first aid, to help move victims, or to help with ambulance or helicopter transportation.

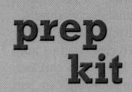

prep kit

▶ Ready for Review

- Victim assessment is a sequence of actions that helps determine what is wrong and thus ensures safe and appropriate first aid.
- Every time you encounter a victim, first check out the scene.
- Victim assessment will be influenced by whether the victim is suffering from an illness or an injury, whether the victim is responsive or unresponsive, and whether life-threatening conditions are present.
- The primary check determines whether there are life-threatening problems requiring quick care.
- The goal of a hands-on secondary check is to identify immediately any potentially life-threatening illness or injury.
- Look for medical identification tags on the victim.
- The information in a SAMPLE history can help you identify what is wrong with the victim and can indicate the needed first aid.
- Triage is the process of prioritizing victims.

▶ Vital Vocabulary

cause of injury (COI) The force that causes an injury.

DOTS A mnemonic for assessment in which each area of the body is evaluated for deformities, open wounds, tenderness, and swelling.

first impression The part of the victim assessment that helps identify any immediately or potentially life-threatening conditions.

nature of illness The general type of illness a victim is experiencing.

primary check A step of the victim assessment process in which a first aider checks for life-threatening injuries and gives care for any that are found.

SAMPLE history A brief history of a victim's condition to determine symptoms, allergies, medications, pertinent past history, last oral intake, and event leading to the illness/injury.

secondary check Part of the victim assessment process in which a detailed, area-by-area exam is performed on victims whose problems cannot be readily identified or when more specific information is needed about a problem.

signs Evidence of an injury or disease that can be seen, heard, or felt.

symptoms What a victim tells a first aider about what he or she feels.

triage A system of placing priorities for first aid and/or transportation in cases when two or more people are injured or suddenly ill.

▶ Assessment in Action

You are in a crowded mall doing some last-minute holiday shopping. You hear someone yelling for help at a nearby store. You are the first to arrive on the scene. Bystanders begin to approach and ask what is going on. The person who called for help witnessed the victim collapse.

Directions: Circle Yes if you agree with the statement; circle No if you disagree.

Yes No **1.** The first thing you should do is conduct a secondary check.

Yes No **2.** Your primary check of the victim includes identifying and treating immediate life-threatening conditions such as problems with the victim's breathing and severe bleeding.

Yes No **3.** When conducting the secondary check, use the AVPU scale to determine physical injuries.

Yes No **4.** The victim is responsive and alert. Ask permission from him before beginning first aid.

Yes No **5.** The victim asks you to stay until medical help arrives. You should continue to do regular checks of the victim every 15 minutes until medical help arrives.

▶ Check Your Knowledge

Directions: Circle Yes if you agree with the statement; circle No if you disagree.

Yes No **1.** The purpose of a primary check is to find life-threatening conditions.

Yes No **2.** A quiet, motionless victim could indicate a breathing problem.

Yes No **3.** Most injured victims require a complete secondary check.

Yes No **4.** For a secondary check, you usually begin at the head and work down the body.

Yes No **5.** If the victim is not breathing, give two breaths before giving chest compressions.

Yes No **6.** The mnemonic DOTS helps in remembering what information to obtain about the victim's history that could be useful.

Yes No **7.** For all injured and suddenly ill persons, look for a medical identification tag during a secondary check.

Yes No **8.** The mnemonic SAMPLE can remind you how to examine an area for signs of an injury.

Yes No **9.** If there is more than one victim, go to the quiet, motionless victim first.

Yes No **10.** A gurgling sound heard while checking for breathing indicates possible fluid in the throat.

CPR

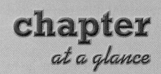

▶ Heart Attack and Cardiac Arrest

A **heart attack** occurs when heart muscle tissue dies because its blood supply is severely reduced or stopped. This often occurs because of a clot in one or more coronary arteries. The signs of a heart attack and the steps for caring for a heart attack are discussed in detail in the *Automated External Defibrillation* chapter.

If damage to the heart muscle is too severe, the victim's heart can stop beating—a condition known as cardiac arrest. Sudden **cardiac arrest** is a leading cause of death in the United States.

▶ Caring for Cardiac Arrest

Few victims experiencing sudden cardiac arrest outside of a hospital survive unless a rapid sequence of events takes place. One way of describing the ideal sequence of care that should take place when a cardiac arrest occurs is to think about the links in a chain. Each link is dependent on the others for strength and success. In this way, the links form a **chain of survival**.

The five events (links) that must occur rapidly and in an integrated manner during cardiac arrest are as follows:

1. *Recognition and Action* Recognizing the early warning signs of cardiac arrest and immediately calling 9-1-1 to activate emergency medical services (EMS)

2. *CPR* The chest compressions delivered during **cardiopulmonary resuscitation (CPR)** circulate blood to the heart and

brain. Effective chest compressions are critical to buying time until a defibrillator and EMS personnel are available.

3. *Defibrillation* Administering a shock to the heart can restore the heartbeat in some victims. Time is a critical factor. The earlier the shock, the better the chance of success.

4. *Advanced Care* Paramedics provide advanced cardiac life support to victims of sudden cardiac arrest. This includes providing IV fluids, medications, advanced airway devices, and rapid transportation to the hospital.

5. *Post-Arrest Care* The hospital can provide lifesaving medications, surgical procedures, and advanced medical care to enable the victim of sudden cardiac arrest to survive and recover.

▶ Performing CPR

When a victim's heart stops beating, he or she needs CPR, defibrillation, and EMS professionals quickly. CPR consists of moving blood to the heart and brain by giving **chest compressions** and providing periodic breaths to place oxygen into the victim's lungs. CPR techniques are similar for infants (birth to 1 year), children (1 year to puberty), and adults (puberty and older), with just slight variations.

Check for Responsiveness and Breathing

In a motionless victim, check for responsiveness by tapping the victim's shoulder and asking if he or she is okay. If the victim does not respond (ie, answers, moves, or moans), he or she is said to be unresponsive.

At the same time you check for responsiveness, you should look at the victim to see whether he or she is breathing. If the victim is not breathing or is only gasping, EMS professionals are needed. Ask a bystander to call 9-1-1. If you are alone with an adult victim and a phone is nearby, call 9-1-1 yourself. If you are alone with a child or infant, give CPR for five cycles of 30 compressions and two breaths (2 minutes); then call 9-1-1.

Give Chest Compressions

Chest compressions are the most important step in CPR and, whenever possible, should be performed on a firm, flat surface. Perform chest compressions with two hands for an adult, one or two hands for a child, and two fingers for an infant. Effective compressions require rescuers to push hard and push fast. The chest of an adult should be compressed at least 20; the chest of a child about 20; and the chest of an infant about 1½. The desired hand position for chest compressions is in the center of the chest (lower half of the sternum [breast bone]) **Figure 1**.

Give compressions at a rate of at least 100 compressions per minute for adults, children, and infants. The 100-compression rate is not the actual number of compressions given in a minute; it is the speed of compressions. Give 30 compressions in about 18 seconds and then give two rescue breaths. Continue CPR until an automated external defibrillator (AED) becomes available, the victim shows signs of life, EMS personnel take over, or you are too tired to continue. Interruptions in compressions should be kept to a minimum. If other rescuers are available, they can rotate performing chest compressions after every five

Q&A

For CPR purposes, what defines an adult, child, and infant victim?

- Infants are those less than 1 year of age.
- A child ranges from 1 year to puberty. (Puberty can be recognized by hair in the armpits of males and breast development in females.)
- Adults include those at puberty and older.

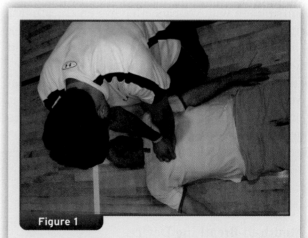

Figure 1

The hand position for chest compressions is in the center of the chest.

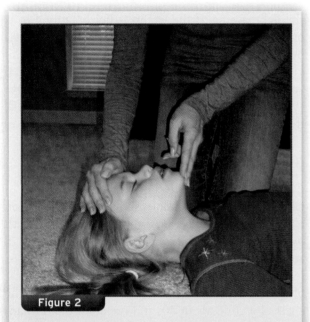

Figure 2

Tilt the victim's head back and lift the chin to open the airway.

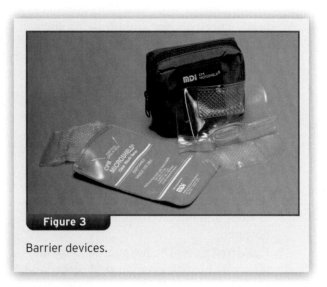

Figure 3

Barrier devices.

cycles of 30 compressions and two breaths (2 minutes) or after an AED delivers a shock.

Give Rescue Breaths

Tilt the victim's head back and lift the chin to open the airway **Figure 2**. This moves the tongue away from the back of the throat. Lay rescuers should use this method for all victims—even for those with a possible spinal injury. With the airway open, pinch the victim's nose and make a tight seal over the victim's mouth with your mouth. Give one breath lasting 1 second, take a normal breath for yourself, and then give the victim another breath lasting 1 second. Each rescue breath should make the victim's chest rise. Rescue breaths can cause stomach distention. Minimize this problem by limiting the force of your breath—you need only to make the victim's chest gently rise.

Other methods of rescue breathing are as follows:
- Mouth-to-breathing device
- Mouth-to-nose method
- Mouth-to-stoma method

Mouth-to-Breathing Device

A breathing device is placed in the victim's mouth or over the victim's mouth and nose as a precaution against disease transmission. There are several different types of barrier devices **Figure 3**.

Mouth-to-Nose Method

If you cannot open the victim's mouth, the victim's mouth is severely injured, or you cannot make a good seal with the victim's mouth (for example, because there are no teeth), use the mouth-to-nose method. With the head tilted back, push up on the victim's chin to close the mouth. Make a seal with your mouth over the victim's nose and provide rescue breaths.

Mouth-to-Stoma Method

Some diseases of the vocal cords may result in surgical removal of the larynx. People who have this surgery breathe through a small permanent opening in the neck called a stoma. To perform mouth-to-stoma breathing, close the victim's mouth and nose and breathe through the opening in the neck.

Adult CPR

To perform adult CPR, follow the steps in **Skill Drill 1**.

Child CPR

To perform CPR on a child, follow the steps in **Skill Drill 2**.

Infant CPR

To perform CPR on an infant, follow the steps in **Skill Drill 3**.

skill drill

1 | **Adult CPR**

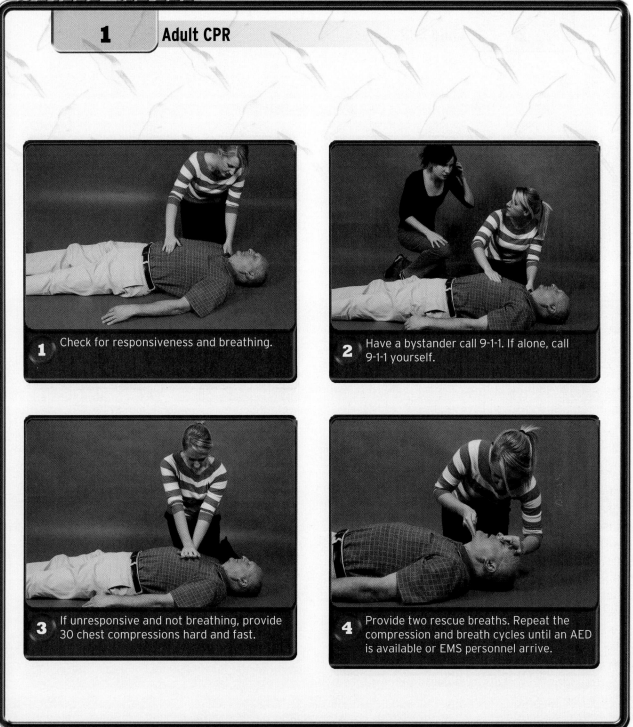

1. Check for responsiveness and breathing.

2. Have a bystander call 9-1-1. If alone, call 9-1-1 yourself.

3. If unresponsive and not breathing, provide 30 chest compressions hard and fast.

4. Provide two rescue breaths. Repeat the compression and breath cycles until an AED is available or EMS personnel arrive.

skill drill

2 Child CPR

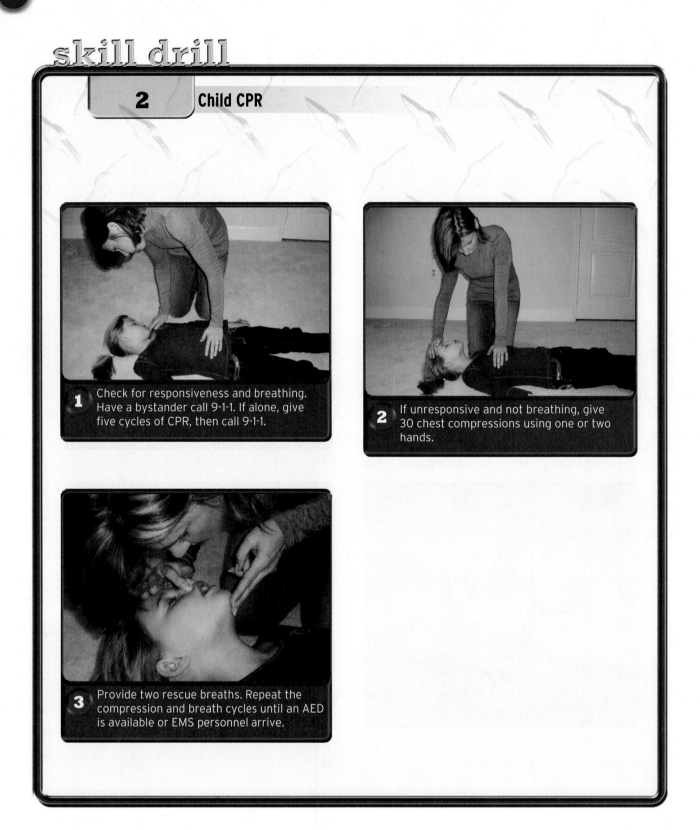

1 Check for responsiveness and breathing. Have a bystander call 9-1-1. If alone, give five cycles of CPR, then call 9-1-1.

2 If unresponsive and not breathing, give 30 chest compressions using one or two hands.

3 Provide two rescue breaths. Repeat the compression and breath cycles until an AED is available or EMS personnel arrive.

skill drill

3 | **Infant CPR**

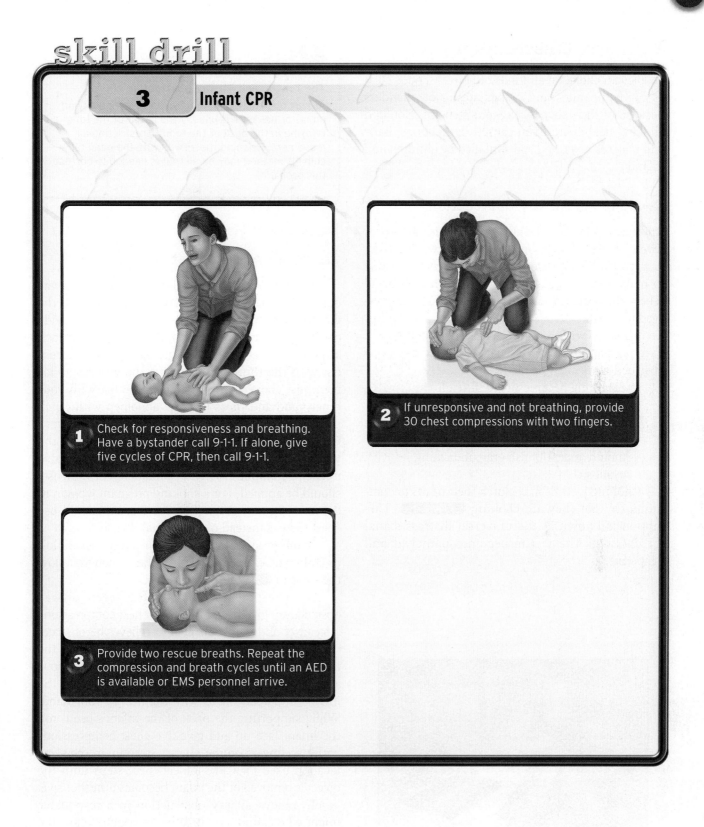

1 Check for responsiveness and breathing. Have a bystander call 9-1-1. If alone, give five cycles of CPR, then call 9-1-1.

2 If unresponsive and not breathing, provide 30 chest compressions with two fingers.

3 Provide two rescue breaths. Repeat the compression and breath cycles until an AED is available or EMS personnel arrive.

▶ Airway Obstruction

People can choke on all kinds of objects. Foods such as candy, peanuts, and grapes are major offenders because of their shapes and consistencies. Nonfood choking deaths are often caused by balloons, balls and marbles, toys, and coins inhaled by children and infants.

Recognizing Airway Obstruction

An object lodged in the airway can cause a mild or severe <u>airway obstruction</u>. In a mild airway obstruction, good air exchange is present. The victim is able to make forceful coughing efforts in an attempt to relieve the obstruction. The victim should be encouraged to cough.

A victim with a severe airway obstruction will have poor air exchange. The signs of a severe airway obstruction include the following:

- Breathing becomes more difficult
- Weak and ineffective cough
- Inability to speak or breathe
- Skin, fingernail beds, and the inside of the mouth appear bluish gray (indicating cyanosis)

Choking victims may clutch their necks to communicate that they are choking Figure 4 . This motion is known as the universal distress signal for choking. The victim becomes panicked and desperate.

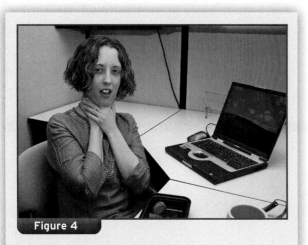

Figure 4

The universal sign of choking.

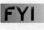

The Tongue and Airway Obstruction
Airway obstruction in an unresponsive victim lying on his or her back is usually the result of the tongue relaxing in the back of the mouth, restricting air movement. Opening the airway with the head tilt–chin lift method may be all that is needed to correct this problem.

Caring for Airway Obstruction

For a responsive adult or child with a severe airway obstruction, ask the victim "Are you choking?" If the victim is unable to respond, but nods yes, provide care for the victim. Move behind the victim and reach around the victim's waist with both arms. Place a fist with the thumb side against the victim's abdomen, just above the navel. Grasp the fist with your other hand and press into the abdomen with quick inward and upward thrusts (Heimlich maneuver). Continue thrusts until the object is removed or the victim becomes unresponsive. If a rescuer is unable to encircle an obese victim's abdomen, chest thrusts should be applied. For a choking pregnant woman in the late stages of pregnancy, the rescuer should use chest thrusts instead of abdominal thrusts.

To relieve airway obstruction in a responsive adult or child who cannot speak, breathe, or cough, follow the steps in Skill Drill 4 .

For a responsive infant with a severe airway obstruction, give back blows and chest compressions instead of abdominal thrusts to relieve the obstruction. Support the infant's head and neck and lay the infant face down on your forearm, then lower your arm to your leg. Give five back blows between the infant's shoulder blades with the heel of your hand. While supporting the back of the infant's head, roll the infant face up and give five chest compressions with two fingers on the infant's sternum in the same location used for CPR. Repeat these steps until the object is removed or the infant becomes unresponsive.

To relieve airway obstruction in a responsive infant who cannot cry, breathe, or cough, follow the steps in Skill Drill 5 .

If a choking victim becomes unresponsive, immediately call 9-1-1 and begin CPR. Each time the airway is opened during CPR, the rescuer should look for an object in the victim's mouth and, if seen, remove it.

skill drill

4   Airway Obstruction in a Responsive Adult or Child

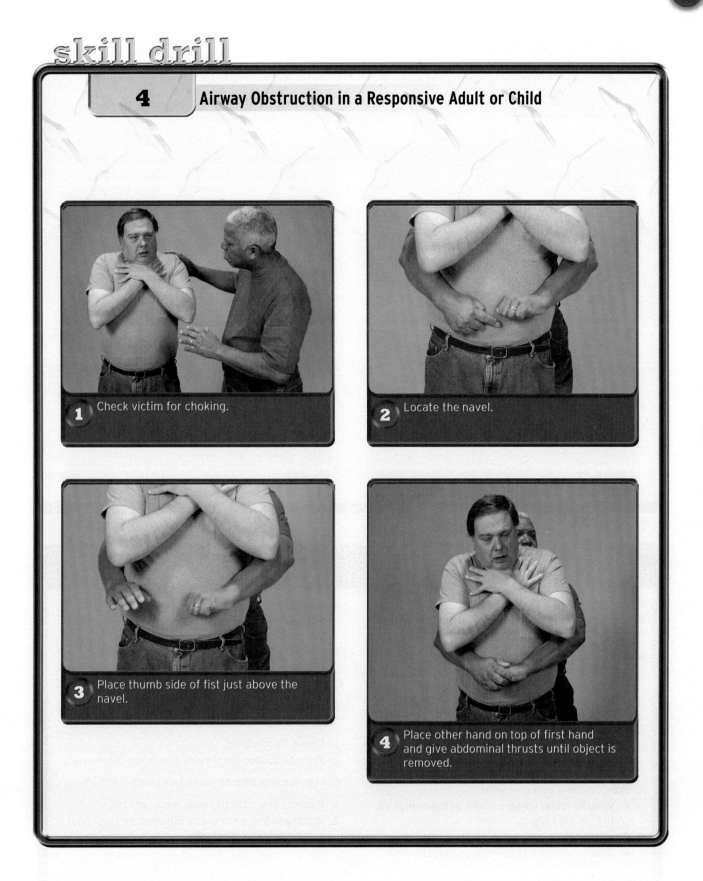

1 Check victim for choking.

2 Locate the navel.

3 Place thumb side of fist just above the navel.

4 Place other hand on top of first hand and give abdominal thrusts until object is removed.

skill drill

5   Airway Obstruction in a Responsive Infant

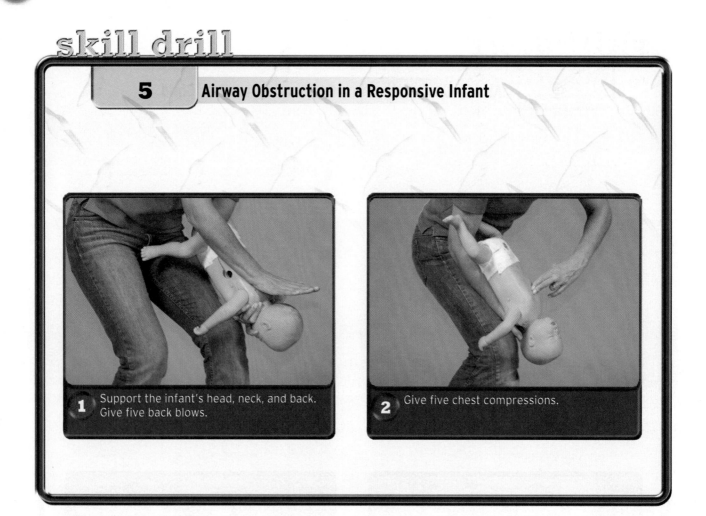

1 Support the infant's head, neck, and back. Give five back blows.

2 Give five chest compressions.

CPR and Airway Obstruction Review

CPR

These steps are the same for all victims regardless of age:

1. Check for responsiveness and look for signs of breathing and gasping.
   - If the victim is unresponsive and has normal breathing, place the victim in the recovery position, and have someone call 9-1-1.
   - If the victim is unresponsive and has abnormal breathing (not breathing or only gasping), have someone call 9-1-1, and retrieve an AED if available. Perform Steps 2 through 5.
2. Provide chest compressions:
   - Give 30 chest compressions in the center of the victim's chest.
3. Open the airway:
   - Tilt the victim's head back and lift the chin.

4. Give 2 breaths:
   - Each breath lasts 1 second to produce visible chest rise.
5. Continue CPR until an AED is available, EMS personnel take over, or the victim starts to move.

Airway Obstruction

For responsive adults and children (anyone older than 1 year):

1. Check for choking.
2. Provide abdominal thrusts (Heimlich maneuver).

For responsive infants (birth to 1 year):

1. Support the infant's head, neck, and back.
2. Alternate five back blows followed by five chest compressions repeatedly.

Q&A

Why change the sequence from A-B-C to C-A-B?

Chest compressions are critical to resuscitating a cardiac arrest victim. The A-B-C sequence involved opening the airway, giving rescue breaths, and per-haps getting and placing a mouth-to-barrier device. This delayed the giving of chest compressions. The C-A-B shortens the time for giving the first chest compressions. Giving chest compressions first may also encourage rescuers to begin CPR, because most victims of out-of-hospital cardiac arrest do not receive any bystander CPR.

Q&A

Why isn't the pulse checked?

Studies show that lay rescuers as well as health care providers take too long to check for a pulse and have difficulty determining whether a pulse is present. Taking too long delays giving chest compressions.

Lay Rescuer Adult CPR

Use the mnemonic RAP-CAB to remember what to do. Start as soon as possible!

R: Responsive? Tap shoulder and shout, "Are you OK?" Check for breathing and gasping.	
If . . .	Then . . .
Unresponsive and gasping or not breathing	Go to next step (A). Gasping is a sign of cardiac arrest.
Unresponsive and breathing normally	Place victim in recovery position (on victim's side with lower arm in front of body). For a suspected spinal injury, extend arm above head and roll body to the side so victim's head rests on extended arm.

A: Activate EMS. Call 9-1-1.	
If . . .	Then . . .
Alone	Immediately call 9-1-1 (EMS) and get AED, if available. Then, return to the victim to attach and use AED.
Second rescuer is available	While one calls 9-1-1 and gets an AED, if available, the other goes to steps (P) and (C).

P: Position victim on back, on a flat, firm surface.
C: Chest compressions. Push hard and fast.

Where to place hands?	How deep?	How fast?	How many?
Place the heel of your hand in center of chest with the other hand on top and fingers interlaced.	Push down on chest at least 2". Allow chest to recoil completely before the next compression.	Push chest at rate of at least 100 pushes per minute (the same beat of the Bee Gee's song, "Stayin' Alive").	Give 30 compressions without interruption unless AED arrives. (AED should be used immediately.)

A: Airway open. Open the victim's airway using the head tilt–chin lift method for all victims.
B: Breaths. Pinch the victim's nose and make an airtight mouth-to-mouth seal. Use a CPR mask if available. Give two breaths (1 second each) that make chest rise.

If . . .	Then . . .
Two breaths make chest rise	Begin CPR: • 30 compressions (push hard and fast). • Two breaths (1 second each). Take a regular breath, not a deep breath, between the two breaths. • Continue 30:2 compression-breath ratio until AED arrives and is ready to use, or until trained person or EMS provider takes over. • Do not stop to check for breathing.
First breath does not make chest rise; the airway may be blocked.	Retilt head, give a second breath: • If second breath does not make chest rise, begin CPR (30 compressions and two breaths). Each time the airway is opened during CPR, look for an object in the victim's mouth and, if found, remove it.

Quick Review of Lay Rescuer Basic Life Support Using the RAP-CAB Steps

Steps/Action	Adults (at or above puberty)	Child (1 year to puberty)	Infant (<1 year)
R = Responsive?			
Technique	Tap shoulder and shout "Are you OK?" If the victim does not answer, move, or moan, he/she is unresponsive.		
Breathing?	If not breathing or only gasping, CPR is needed. If normal breathing is seen, no CPR is needed; place in recovery position and monitor breathing		
A = Activate Emergency Medical Service (EMS) and get AED (if nearby and accessible; use as soon as possible)			
When	If one rescuer: Call immediately If two rescuers: One calls immediately	If one rescuer: Call after five cycles (2 minutes) of CPR If two rescuers: One calls immediately	
Who to call	In a community: Call 9-1-1 In a facility or institution: Call its emergency number		
P = Position on back (on firm, flat surface)			
C = Chest compressions			
Where to place hand	Center of chest		Two fingers, with one touching and below nipple line
Technique: • Push hard and fast • Allow complete recoil	Two hands: Heel of one hand on breastbone; other hand on top	One hand: Heel of one hand only Two hands: Heel of one hand with second on top	Two fingers
Depth	At least 2" (5 cm)	About 2" (5 cm)	At least 1½" (4 cm)
Rate	At least 100 per minute (same beat as the Bee Gee's song, "Stayin' Alive")		
Ratio of chest compressions to breaths	30:2		
A = Airway open			
Technique	Head tilt-chin lift		

	• Pinch nose and make airtight mouth-to-mouth seal
	• Give two breaths:
	  • Each breath lasting 1 second
	  • Blow enough to make chest rise
	• If first breath does not cause chest to rise, retilt head and give second breath. If second breath does not make chest rise, begin CPR (30 compressions and two breaths). Each time the airway is opened, look for an object in mouth and, if seen, remove it.
			• Cover the infant's mouth and nose with your mouth, making an airtight seal. If this does not work, try either mouth-to-mouth or mouth-to-nose
			• Same procedures as for an adult and child.

(continues)

Steps/Action	Adults (at or above puberty)	Child (1 year to puberty)	Infant (<1 year)
Continue CPR until:			
1. Victim begins breathing 2. Other rescuer(s) (ie, trained lay person, EMS personnel) take over 3. AED arrives and is used 4. Rescuer is physically exhausted and unable to continue			
Defibrillation			
• Use AED as soon as possible. • Expose chest, turn on AED, attach appropriate pads. • Follow voice directions			
If no shock advised	Resume CPR immediately (five sets of 30 compressions and two breaths)		
If shock advised	Do not touch victim; give one shock. Or, shock as advised by AED. Resume immediately 30 compressions and two breaths.		

prep kit

▶ Ready for Review

- A heart attack occurs when heart muscle tissue dies because the blood supply is severely reduced or stopped.
- The five links in the chain of survival are: recognition and action, CPR, defibrillation, advanced care, and post-arrest care.
- CPR consists of moving blood to the heart and brain by giving chest compressions and breathing oxygen into a victim's lungs.
- The signs of a severe airway obstruction include difficult breathing, weak and ineffective cough, inability to speak or breathe, and signs of cyanosis.

▶ Vital Vocabulary

airway obstruction A blockage, often the result of a foreign body, in which air flow to the lungs is reduced or completely blocked.

cardiac arrest Stoppage of the heartbeat.

chain of survival A concept involving five critical links to help improve survival from cardiac arrest.

chest compressions Depressing the chest and allowing it to return to its normal position as part of CPR.

cardiopulmonary resuscitation (CPR) The act of providing chest compressions and rescue breaths for a victim in cardiac arrest.

heart attack Death of a part of the heart muscle.

▶ Assessment in Action

You are having dinner in a very crowded restaurant with your family on New Year's Eve. An elderly man is pushing a piano into the restaurant as part of the entertainment that evening. As he passes your table, he clutches his chest and falls to the floor. He is not moving.

Directions: Circle Yes if you agree with the statement; circle No if you disagree.

Yes No **1.** If he is not breathing or is breathing abnormally, you should next call 9-1-1.

Yes No **2.** The man must be choking since he is in a restaurant.

Yes No **3.** Perform abdominal thrusts.

Yes No **4.** Perform cycles of 30 chest compressions and 2 breaths.

Yes No **5.** Check for breathing before giving any breaths to the victim.

Yes No **6.** Continue CPR until an AED becomes available or EMS personnel arrive.

▶ Check Your Knowledge

Directions: Circle Yes if you agree with the statement; circle No if you disagree.

Yes No **1.** Gasping is not considered breathing.

Yes No **2.** After you determine that an adult victim is unresponsive, the next step is for someone to call 9-1-1.

Yes No **3.** Tilting the head back and lifting the chin helps move the tongue and open the airway.

Yes No **4.** If you determine that a victim is not breathing, begin chest compressions.

Yes No **5.** Do not start chest compressions until you have checked for a pulse.

Yes No **6.** For all victims (adult, child, infant) needing CPR, give 30 compressions followed by two breaths.

Yes No **7.** Use two fingers when performing CPR on an infant.

Yes No **8.** A sign of choking is that the victim is unable to speak or cough.

Yes No **9.** To give abdominal thrusts to a responsive choking victim, place your fist below the victim's navel.

Yes No **10.** When giving abdominal thrusts to a responsive choking victim, repeat the thrusts until the object is removed or the victim becomes unresponsive.

Automated External Defibrillation

5

▶ Public Access Defibrillation

A victim's chance of survival dramatically improves through early cardiopulmonary resuscitation (CPR) and early <u>defibrillation</u> with the use of an <u>**automated external defibrillator (AED)**</u>. To be effective, defibrillation must be used in the first few minutes following cardiac arrest. The implementation of state public access defibrillation (PAD) laws and the Food and Drug Administration's (FDA) approval of "home use" AEDs have made this important care step available to many rescuers in many places, including the following **Figure 1** :

- Airports and airplanes
- Stadiums
- Health clubs
- Golf courses
- Schools
- Government buildings
- Offices
- Homes
- Shopping centers/malls

▶ How the Heart Works

The heart is an organ with four hollow chambers. The two chambers on the right side receive blood from the body and send it to the lungs for oxygen. The two chambers on the left side of the heart receive freshly oxygenated blood from the lungs and send it back out to the body 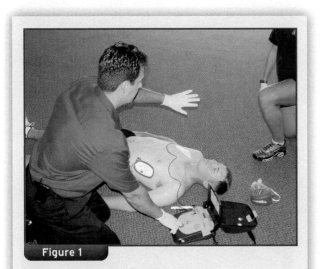 Figure 2 .

The heart has a unique electrical system that controls the rate at which the heart beats and the amount of work the heart performs. In the right upper chamber of the heart, there is a collection of special pacemaker cells. These cells emit electrical impulses about 60 to 100 times a minute that cause the other heart muscle cells to contract in a coordinated manner.

Because the heart contracts approximately every second, it needs an abundant supply of oxygen, which it gets through the coronary arteries. These arteries run along the outside of the heart muscle and branch into smaller vessels. These arteries sometimes become diseased (atherosclerosis), resulting in a lack of oxygen to the pacemaker cells, which can cause abnormal electrical activity in the heart.

When Normal Electrical Activity Is Interrupted

Ventricular fibrillation (also known as V-fib) is the most common abnormal heart rhythm in cases of sudden cardiac arrest in adults Figure 3 .

The organized wave of electrical impulses that cause the heart muscle to contract and relax in a regular fashion is lost when the heart is in ventricular fibrillation. As a result, the lower chambers of the heart quiver and cannot pump blood, so circulation is lost (no pulse).

A second, potentially life-threatening, electrical problem is ventricular tachycardia (V-tach), in which the heart beats too fast to pump blood effectively Figure 4 .

Figure 1

AEDs are available in many places for use by trained rescuers.

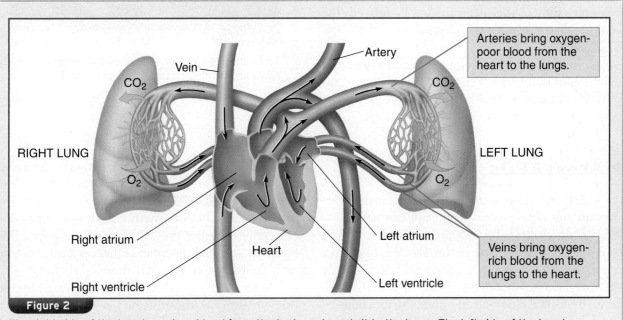

Figure 2

The right side of the heart receives blood from the body and sends it to the lungs. The left side of the heart receives the oxygenated blood and sends it to the body.

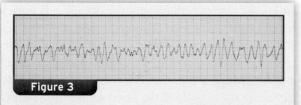

Figure 3

Ventricular fibrillation is disorganized electrical activity.

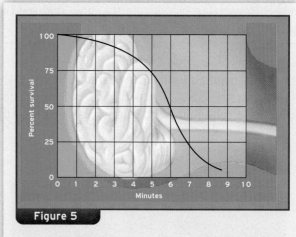

Figure 5

A victim's chance of survival decreases with every minute that passes without proper care.

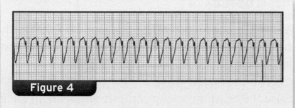

Figure 4

Ventricular tachycardia is very rapid electrical activity.

▶ Care for Cardiac Arrest

When the heart stops beating, the blood stops circulating, cutting off all oxygen and nourishment to the entire body. In this situation, time is a crucial factor. For every minute that defibrillation is delayed, the victim's chance of survival decreases by 7% to 10% **Figure 5**.

CPR is the initial care for cardiac arrest until a defibrillator is available. Perform cycles of chest compressions and breaths until an AED is ready to be connected to the victim.

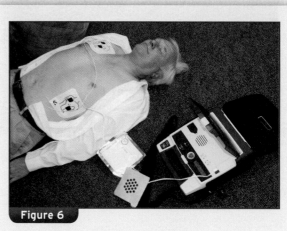

Figure 6

Two adhesive pads are placed on the victim's chest and connected by a cable to the AED.

▶ About AEDs

An AED is an electronic device that analyzes the heart rhythm and if necessary (such as in cardiac arrest) delivers an electric shock, known as defibrillation, to the heart. The purpose of this shock is to correct one of the abnormal electrical disturbances previously discussed and to reestablish a heart rhythm that will result in normal electrical and pumping function.

All AEDs are attached to the victim by a cable connected to two adhesive pads (electrodes) placed on the victim's chest. The pad and cable system sends the electrical signal from the heart into the device for analysis and delivers the electric shock to the victim when needed **Figure 6**.

AEDs have built-in rhythm analysis systems that determine whether the victim needs a shock. This system enables first aiders and other rescuers to deliver early defibrillation with only minimal training.

AEDs also record the victim's heart rhythm (known as an electrocardiogram, or ECG), shock data, and other information about the device's performance (for example, the date, time, and number of shocks supplied) **Figure 7**.

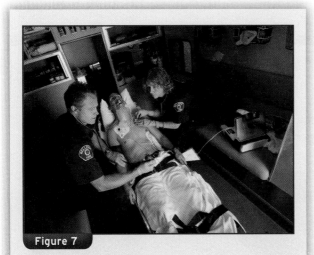

Figure 7

AEDs store data, including heart rhythms and shocks.

Q&A

How does an AED work?

A microprocessor inside the defibrillator interprets (analyzes) the victim's heart rhythm through adhesive electrodes. The computer analyzes the heart rhythm and advises the rescuer whether a shock is needed. AEDs advise a shock to only ventricular fibrillation and fast ventricular tachycardia.

Common Elements of AEDs

Many different AED models exist. The principles for use are the same for each, but the displays, controls, and options vary slightly. You will need to know how to use your specific AED. All AEDs have the following elements in common:

- Power on/off mechanism
- Cable and pads (electrodes)
- Analysis capability
- Defibrillation capability
- Prompts to guide you
- Battery operation for portability

▶ Using an AED

Once you have determined the need for the AED (victim unresponsive and not breathing), the basic

operation of all AED models follows the sequence in **Skill Drill 1**.

1. Some AEDs power on by pressing an on/off button. Others power on when opening the AED case lid. Once the power is on, the AED will quickly go through some internal checks and will then begin to provide voice and screen prompts (**Step ❶**).

2. Expose the victim's chest. The skin must be fairly dry so that the pads will adhere and conduct electricity properly. If necessary, dry the skin with a towel. Because excessive chest hair may also interfere with adhesion and electrical conduction, you may need to shave quickly the area where the pads are to be placed.

3. Remove the backing from the pads and apply them firmly to the victim's bare chest according to the diagram on the pads (**Step ❷**). One pad is placed to the right of the breastbone, just below the collarbone and above the right nipple. The second pad is placed on the left side of the chest, left of the nipple and above the lower rib margin.

4. Make sure the cable is attached to the AED, and stand clear for analysis of the heart's electrical activity (**Step ❸**). No one should be in contact with the victim at this time, or later if a shock is indicated.

5. Verify that no one is in contact with the victim. The AED will advise of the need to shock and, depending on the device, will either advise the rescuer to push a button to administer the shock, or will deliver the shock automatically. Begin CPR immediately following the shock and follow the prompts that include reanalyzing the rhythm (**Step ❹**). If the shock worked, the victim may begin to regain signs of life. Continue providing care until EMS personnel arrive and take over.

▶ Special Considerations

There are several special situations that you should be aware of when using an AED. These include the following:

- Water
- Children
- Medication patches
- Implanted devices

skill drill

1   **Using an AED**

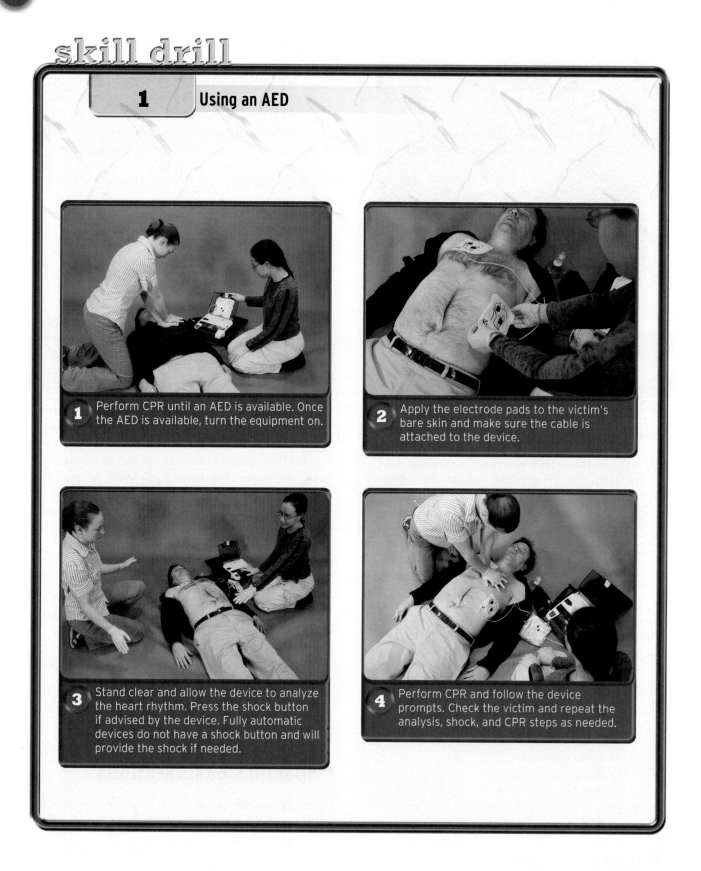

1 Perform CPR until an AED is available. Once the AED is available, turn the equipment on.

2 Apply the electrode pads to the victim's bare skin and make sure the cable is attached to the device.

3 Stand clear and allow the device to analyze the heart rhythm. Press the shock button if advised by the device. Fully automatic devices do not have a shock button and will provide the shock if needed.

4 Perform CPR and follow the device prompts. Check the victim and repeat the analysis, shock, and CPR steps as needed.

Will I get zapped if a victim is shocked in the rain or near water?

It is remotely possible to get shocked or to shock bystanders if there is standing water around and under the victim. Try to move the victim to a dry area and cut off wet clothing. Also be sure that the skin has been dried off so that the electrode pads will stick to the skin. No one should be touching any part of the victim while the device emits an electrical current.

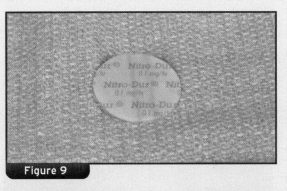
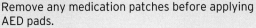

Figure 9

Remove any medication patches before applying AED pads.

Water

Because water conducts electricity, it may provide an energy pathway between the AED and the rescuer or bystanders. Remove the victim from free-standing water. Quickly dry the chest before applying the pads. The risk to the rescuers and bystanders is very low if the chest is dry and the pads are secured to the chest.

Children

Cardiac arrest in children is usually caused by an airway or breathing problem, rather than a primary heart problem as in adults. AEDs can deliver energy levels appropriate for children aged 1 year or older. If your AED has special pediatric pads and cable, use these for the child   Figure 8 . If the pediatric equipment is not available, use the adult equipment.

Medication Patches

Some people wear an adhesive patch containing medication (such as nitroglycerin, nicotine, or pain medication) that is absorbed through the skin. Because these patches may block the delivery of energy from the pads to the heart, they need to be removed and the skin wiped dry before attaching the AED pads   Figure 9 .

Implanted Devices

Implanted pacemakers and defibrillators are small devices placed underneath the skin of people with certain types of heart disease   Figure 10 . These devices often can be seen or felt when the chest is exposed. Avoid placing the pads directly over these devices whenever possible. If an implanted defibrillator is discharging, you may see the victim twitching periodically. Allow the implanted unit to stop before using your AED.

AED Maintenance

Periodic inspection of your AED can ensure that the device has the necessary supplies and is in proper

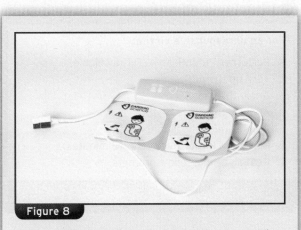

Figure 8

If your AED has pediatric pads, use them according to the manufacturer's instructions.

AED Use on an Infant

For infants (children younger than 1 year), a manual defibrillator can be used. If a manual defibrillator is not available, an AED with a pediatric dose attenuation can be used. If neither is available, an AED without a dose attenuator may be used.

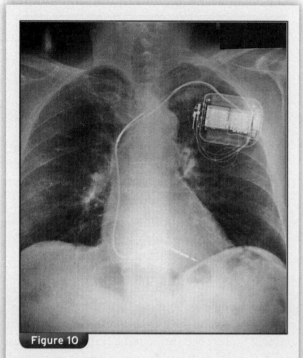

Figure 10

Implanted defibrillator.

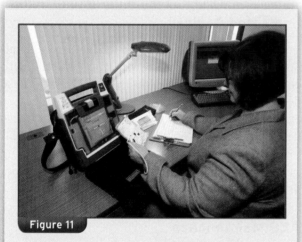

Figure 11

Periodic inspection of your AED supplies can ensure that all items are in working condition.

working condition **Figure 11**. AEDs conduct automatic internal checks and provide visual indications that the unit is ready and functioning properly. You do not need to turn the device on daily to check it as part of any inspection. Doing so will only wear down the battery.

AED supplies should include items such as the following:

- Two sets of electrode pads with expiration dates that are not expired
- An extra battery
- Razor
- Hand towel

Other items that should be considered are a breathing device (for example, a mask or shield) and exam gloves.

▶ AED Manufacturers

AED devices and related supplies are available from different manufacturers **Figure 12**.

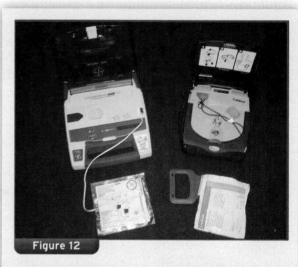

Figure 12

Various AED devices.

AED Review

For an unresponsive victim:

1. Perform CPR until an AED is available.
2. Turn on the AED.
3. Apply the pads.
4. Analyze the heart rhythm.
5. Administer a shock if needed.
6. Perform CPR for five cycles (2 minutes).
7. Reanalyze and follow prompts.

AED Skill Checklist

Student's Name _____ Date _____

Skills	Satisfactory	Unsatisfactory
Check for Scene Safety	○	○

Primary check and care:
If two rescuers are involved, one assesses and performs CPR while the other applies the AED.

	Satisfactory	Unsatisfactory
• Establish unresponsiveness and breathing status (not breathing or is gasping).	○	○
• Begin 30 chest compressions (regardless of the compression number, interrupt compressions to apply an AED when it arrives).	○	○
• Open airway.	○	○
• Give two breaths (1 second each).	○	○
• Continue cycles of 30 compressions and two breaths until an AED becomes available.	○	○

Defibrillation:

	Satisfactory	Unsatisfactory
• Turn AED power on.	○	○
• Ensure skin surface is dry.	○	○
• Apply electrode pads correctly.	○	○
• Ensure electrode cable is plugged in.	○	○
• Stand clear while analyzing.	○	○
• If shock is indicated:	○	○
a. Remain clear.	○	○
b. Deliver shock.	○	○
c. Perform 2 minutes of CPR.	○	○
d. Reanalyze.	○	○
• If shock is indicated, repeat steps a through d.	○	○
• If no shock is indicated:	○	○
a. Check victim for breathing.	○	○
b. If victim is not breathing, perform 5 cycles of CPR and reanalyze.	○	○

Pass _____   Fail _____

prep kit

▶ Ready for Review

- A victim's chances for survival are dramatically improved through early CPR and early defibrillation.
- Because the heart contracts approximately every second, it needs an abundant supply of oxygen.
- CPR is the initial care for cardiac arrest until a defibrillator is available.
- An AED is an electronic device that analyzes the heart rhythm and delivers an electrical shock to the heart of a person in cardiac arrest.
- There are several special situations to be aware of when using an AED, including: water, children, medication patches, and implanted devices.
- Periodic inspection of the AED can ensure that the device has the necessary supplies and is in proper working condition.

▶ Vital Vocabulary

<u>automated external defibrillator (AED)</u> Device capable of analyzing the heart rhythm and providing a shock.

<u>defibrillation</u> The electrical shock administered by an AED to reestablish a normal heart rhythm.

▶ Assessment in Action

Your workplace has recently implemented an AED program. You and several other employees have been trained to locate and use an AED. While at work, a coworker collapses. She is around 50 years old and you know she has a history of heart problems. You tell a coworker to call 9-1-1 and to bring the AED.

Directions: Circle Yes if you agree with the statement; circle No if you disagree.

Yes   No   1. You should establish unresponsiveness before starting anything else.

Yes   No   2. Chest compressions should begin as soon as possible and stop only to apply the AED pads to the chest or to give two breaths.

Yes   No   3. AED pads can be applied over the top of the victim's blouse.

Yes   No   4. The AED will alert you about improper pad placement and connection.

Yes   No   5. You should deliver a shock even if the AED has not alerted you to do so.

▶ Check Your Knowledge

Directions: Circle Yes if you agree with the statement; circle No if you disagree.

Yes   No   1. The earlier defibrillation occurs, the better the victim's chance of survival.

Yes   No   2. An AED is to be applied only to a victim who is unresponsive and not breathing.

Yes   No   3. CPR is not needed if you are sure an AED will be available in 3 to 4 minutes.

Yes   No   4. AEDs require the operator to know how to interpret heart rhythms.

Yes   No   5. Because all AEDs are different, the basic steps of operation are also different.

Yes   No   6. The AED pads (electrodes) need to be attached to a dry chest.

Yes   No   7. Two electrode pads are placed on the left side of the victim's chest.

Yes   No   8. Batteries and pads have expiration dates of which you should be aware.

Yes   No   9. An AED still can be used if an implanted pacemaker is present.

Yes   No   10. You need to turn the AED on daily as part of a routine inspection.

Shock

▶ Shock

Perfusion is when adequate blood and oxygen are provided to all cells in different tissues and organs in the body. Shock occurs when the body's tissues do not receive enough oxygen-rich blood. Do not confuse this with electric shock or being shocked, as in being scared or surprised. <u>Shock</u> (hypoperfusion) describes a state of collapse and failure of the cardiovascular system in which blood circulation decreases and eventually ceases. Shock can be associated with a wide variety of conditions—from a heart attack to a severe allergic reaction.

▶ Causes of Shock

Understanding the basic physiologic causes of shock will better prepare you to treat it. The damage caused by shock depends on which body part is deprived of oxygen and for how long. For example, without oxygen, the brain will be irreparably damaged in 4 to 6 minutes, the abdominal organs in 45 to 90 minutes, and the skin and muscle cells in 3 to 6 hours.

To understand shock, think of the circulatory system as having three components: a working pump (the heart), a network of pipes (the blood vessels), and an adequate amount of fluid (the blood) pumped through the pipes. Damage to any of these components can deprive tissues of blood and produce the condition known as shock. These

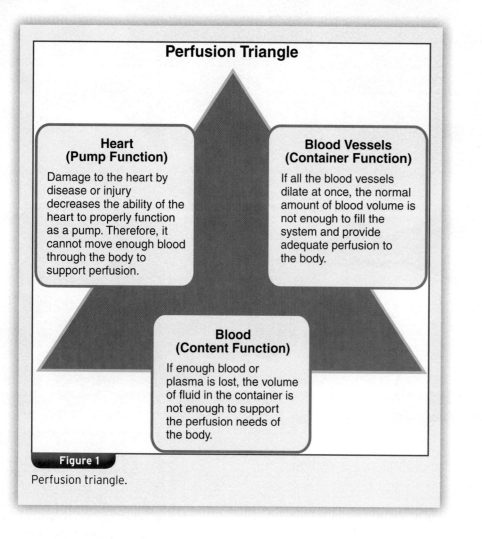

Perfusion Triangle

Heart (Pump Function)

Damage to the heart by disease or injury decreases the ability of the heart to properly function as a pump. Therefore, it cannot move enough blood through the body to support perfusion.

Blood Vessels (Container Function)

If all the blood vessels dilate at once, the normal amount of blood volume is not enough to fill the system and provide adequate perfusion to the body.

Blood (Content Function)

If enough blood or plasma is lost, the volume of fluid in the container is not enough to support the perfusion needs of the body.

Figure 1

Perfusion triangle.

three parts can be referred to as the perfusion triangle **Figure 1**. When a victim is in shock, one or more of the three sides is not working properly.

Causes of shock can be both cardiovascular and noncardiovascular. The noncardiovascular causes of shock are respiratory insufficiency, psychogenic shock, and **anaphylaxis**, an extreme allergic reaction to a foreign substance **Figure 2**.

Cardiovascular Causes of Shock

- *Pump failure.* Cardiogenic shock is caused by inadequate function of the heart, or pump failure. Circulation requires the constant pumping action of a normal heart muscle. Many diseases can cause destruction or inflammation of this muscle. The heart can adapt somewhat to these problems, but if too much muscle damage occurs, as sometimes happens in a heart attack, the heart no longer

functions well. The major effect is the backup of blood into the lungs. The resulting buildup of fluid in the lungs is called pulmonary edema.

- *Content failure.* In injuries, shock is most often the result of fluid or blood loss. This type of shock is called hypovolemic (low-volume) shock or hemorrhagic shock. The loss can be due to internal or external bleeding. Hypovolemic shock also occurs with severe thermal burns. Plasma, the fluid portion of the blood, leaks from the circulatory system into burned tissues adjacent to the injury. Dehydration aggravates shock. In all these circumstances, the common factor is an insufficient volume of blood within the vascular system to provide adequate perfusion to the tissues.

- *Poor vessel function.* Spinal cord damage can injure the part of the nervous system that controls blood vessel size and muscle tone. Neurogenic shock can result. Cut off from their impulses to contract, muscles in the blood vessels dilate (relax) widely, increasing the size and capacity of the vascular system. The blood in the body can no longer fill the enlarged vessels **Figure 3**.

- *Combined vessel and content failure.* Septic shock is seen in victims who have severe bacterial infections that produce toxins (poisons). The toxins damage the vessel walls, causing them to become leaky and making them unable to contract well. Widespread vessel dilation, combined with the loss of plasma through injured vessel walls, results

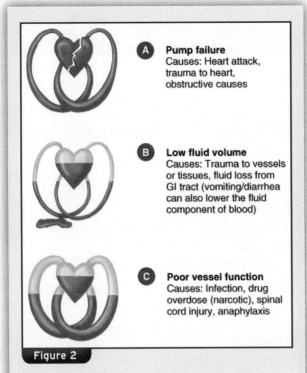

A **Pump failure**
Causes: Heart attack, trauma to heart, obstructive causes

B **Low fluid volume**
Causes: Trauma to vessels or tissues, fluid loss from GI tract (vomiting/diarrhea can also lower the fluid component of blood)

C **Poor vessel function**
Causes: Infection, drug overdose (narcotic), spinal cord injury, anaphylaxis

Figure 2

There are three basic causes of shock and impaired tissue function. **A.** Pump failure occurs when the heart is damaged by disease, injury, or obstructive causes. The heart may not generate enough energy to move the blood through the system. **B.** Low fluid volume, often a result of bleeding, leads to inadequate perfusion. **C.** The blood vessels can dilate excessively so that the blood within them, even though it is of normal volume, is in adequate to fill the system and provide efficient perfusion.

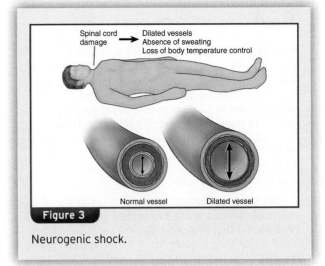

Spinal cord damage → Dilated vessels / Absence of sweating / Loss of body temperature control

Normal vessel   Dilated vessel

Figure 3

Neurogenic shock.

in shock. Septic shock is almost always a complication of a serious illness, injury, or surgery. Septic shock also occurs with anaphylaxis.

Noncardiovascular Cause of Shock

- *Respiratory insufficiency.* A severe chest injury or an airway obstruction can make a victim unable to breathe adequately. Insufficient oxygen in the blood can produce shock as rapidly as vascular causes, even when cardiovascular function is normal. Circulation of nonoxygenated blood will not benefit the victim.
- *Anaphylactic shock.* Anaphylaxis, or anaphylactic shock, occurs when the immune system reacts violently to a substance to which it has already been sensitized. Severe allergic reactions commonly follow exposure by one of these:

- Medications (penicillin and related drugs, aspirin, sulfa drugs)
- Food (shellfish, nuts—especially peanuts, eggs)
- Insect stings (honeybee, wasp, yellow jacket, hornet, fire ant)

Anaphylactic reactions can develop in minutes or even seconds after contact with the substance to which a victim is sensitized. The signs of such allergic reactions are distinct from those of other forms of shock. **Table 1** shows the signs and symptoms of anaphylactic shock.

In anaphylactic shock, although there is no loss of blood, no vascular damage, and only a slight possibility of cardiac muscular injury, the widespread vascular dilation causes poor oxygenation and poor perfusion of tissues, which can easily cause death.

- *Psychogenic shock.* Psychogenic shock is a sudden nervous system reaction that produces a temporary vascular dilation, resulting in fainting, or syncope. Blood pools in the dilated vessels, reducing the blood supply to the brain, and the victim becomes unresponsive. Causes of fainting (psychogenic shock) include fear, bad news, or unpleasant sights (often the sight of blood).

▶ The Progression of Shock

Although shock itself cannot be seen, you can see its signs and symptoms progress. The early stage of hemorrhagic (blood loss) shock, when the body can still compensate for blood loss, is called compensated

Q&A

What is the optimal position for a person in shock? Does elevating the legs improve outcome?

Most victims should not be moved. However, first aiders are often taught to raise the feet of a suspected victim of shock in theory to return blood volume to the victim's central circulation, thus raising cardiac output and blood pressure. While the evidence is mixed on the effects of leg elevation, no studies in the medical literature demonstrate improved victim outcome.

The elevation of the legs for a victim suffering potential pelvic or lower extremities injuries may not be apparent to a first aider and the elevation of the legs may cause a greater harm. Therefore, the legs should not be raised if a leg is injured or if moving an injured leg causes pain.

Table 1 Signs and Symptoms of Anaphylactic Shock

Skin

- Flushing, itching, or burning, especially over the face and upper chest
- Hives, which can spread over large areas of the body
- Swelling, especially of the face, tongue, and lips
- Bluish lips (cyanosis)

Circulatory system

- Weak pulse (you might be barely able to feel it)
- Dizziness
- Fainting and unresponsiveness

Respiratory system

- Sneezing or itching in the nostrils
- Tightness in the chest, with a persistent, dry cough
- Breathing difficulty
- Secretions of fluid and mucus into the throat and lungs
- Wheezing (forced expirations during breathing)
- Breathing stops

shock. The late stage, when blood pressure is falling, is decompensated shock. The final stage, when shock is terminal, is called irreversible shock. Even transfusion will not save the victim's life at this point.

▶ Care for Shock

Because every injury affects the circulatory system to some degree, first aiders should automatically treat injured victims for shock. Shock is one of the most common causes of death in an injured victim. Even if an injured victim does not have signs or symptoms of shock, first aiders should care for shock. You can prevent shock from getting worse; first aiders cannot reverse it.

General Care for Shock

1. Monitor breathing and, if absent, begin CPR.
2. Control all obvious external bleeding.
3. Place the victim on his or her back (supine position). Those having a heart attack or those with lung disease breathe easier in a half-sitting position **Figure 4**.
4. Do not move the victim if there are suspected fractures or head, spine, or torso injuries. Loosen tight clothing at the neck, chest, and waist.
5. Splint any bone or joint injuries to minimize pain and bleeding. This also prevents further damage to tissues.

CAUTION

DO NOT place victims with breathing difficulties, chest injuries, penetrating eye injuries, or heart attacks on their backs. Place them in a half-sitting position to help breathing.

DO NOT give the victim anything to eat or drink. It could cause nausea and vomiting. It could also cause complications if surgery is needed.

DO NOT lift the foot of a bed or stretcher—breathing will be affected, and the blood flow from the brain could be impeded and lead to brain swelling.

DO NOT raise the legs of a victim with head injuries, stroke, chest injuries, breathing difficulty, or those of a victim in whom a heart attack is suspected.

DO NOT use external heat sources (such as hot water bottles or heating pads).

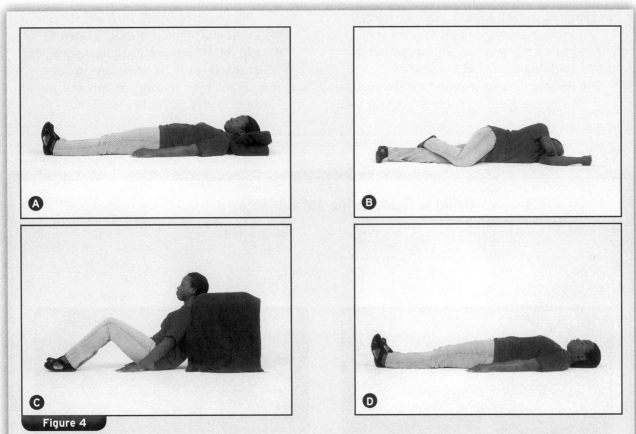

Figure 4

Shock positions. **A.** For a victim with head injury, elevate the head (if spinal injury is not suspected). **B.** Position an unresponsive or stroke victim in the recovery position. **C.** Use a half-sitting position for victims with breathing difficulties, chest injuries, or a heart attack. **D.** Keep the victim flat if a spinal injury or leg fracture is suspected.

6. Keep the victim warm. Place blankets under and over the victim. Do not use external heat sources (for example, hot water bottles or heating pads).
7. Handle the victim gently.
8. Seek immediate medical care. Depending on the problem, it might require calling 9-1-1 or transporting a victim using a private vehicle if EMS is not available.

Care for Anaphylaxis

1. Call 9-1-1 immediately.
2. Monitor breathing and, if absent, begin CPR.
3. If the victim has his or her own physician-prescribed epinephrine, help him or her use it. Some people have an **epinephrine auto-injector**, which allows them to

administer an emergency dose of epinephrine. If you are assisting with or using an auto-injector, follow these steps **Skill Drill 1**:

a. Obtain the victim's physician-prescribed epinephrine. Determine that the prescription is the victim's and has not expired.
b. Remove the safety cap from the auto-injector (**Step ❶**).
c. Support the victim's thigh against movement.
d. Prepare to thrust the tip of the auto-injector against the victim's outer thigh, midway between the hip and the knee. It is designed to work through light clothing.

e. Using a quick motion, push the injector firmly against the thigh and hold it in place for 10 seconds. This will inject the medication (**Step ❷**).

f. Remove the auto-injector from the thigh. Using one hand, carefully reinsert the used auto-injector, needle first, into the carrying tube and properly dispose it (**Step ❸**).

4. Help the victim take an antihistamine (eg, Benadryl)—it is not life saving because it takes too long to work (20 minutes), but it can help prevent further reactions.

skill drill

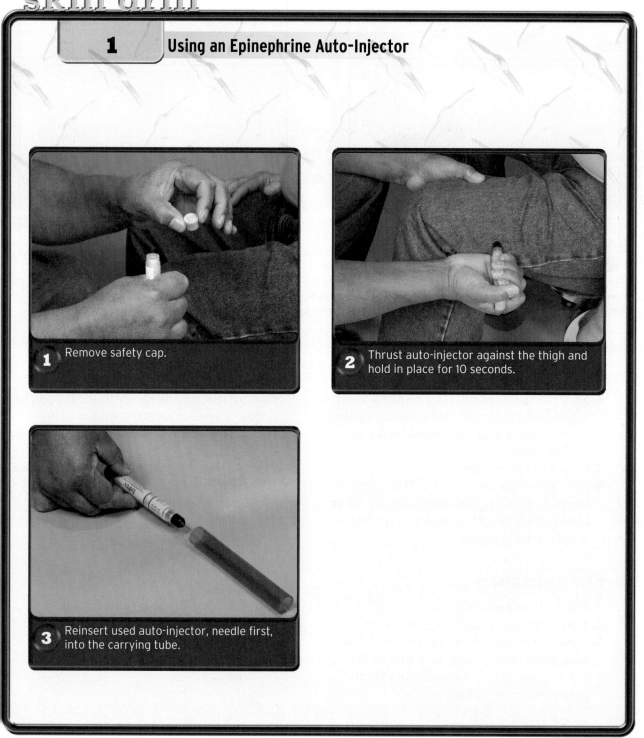

| 1 | **Using an Epinephrine Auto-Injector** |

1 Remove safety cap.

2 Thrust auto-injector against the thigh and hold in place for 10 seconds.

3 Reinsert used auto-injector, needle first, into the carrying tube.

Shock

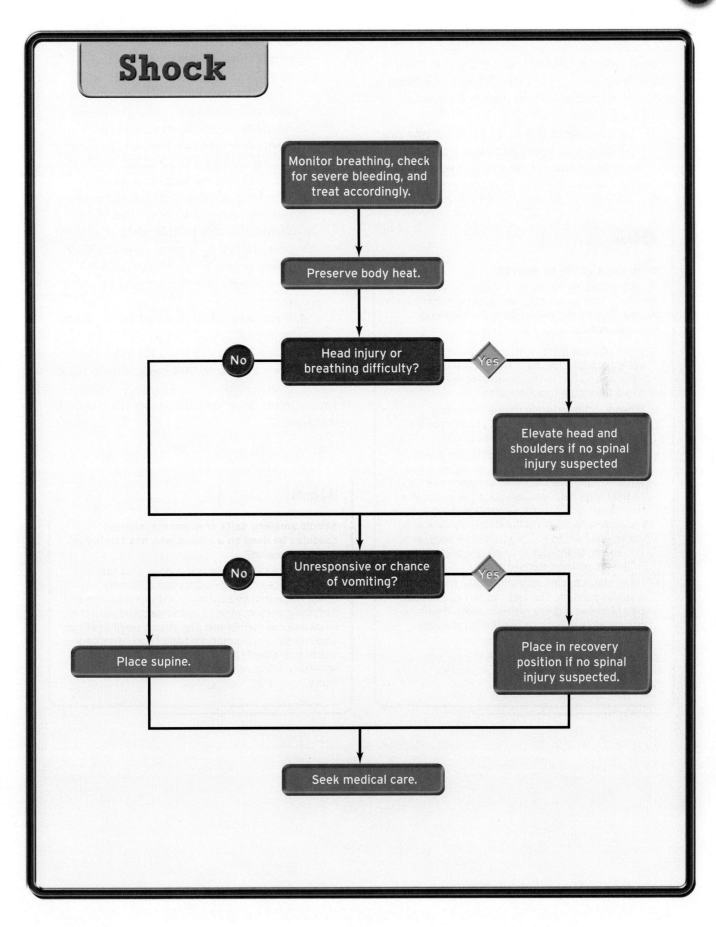

Care for Fainting (Psychogenic Shock)

In most cases of fainting, once the victim collapses and is lying down, blood circulation to the brain is restored and responsiveness usually returns.

If you feel faint:

- Lie down or sit down. Do not place your head between your knees because if you faint you may fall. Some believe that this position also kinks the body and inhibits blood flow returning from the legs to the heart.

If someone else faints:

1. Check for breathing and, if absent, begin CPR and call 9-1-1.
2. Keep the victim flat in a comfortable position or on his or her back. Consider raising the legs 6 to 12 inches unless there are head or spine injuries suspected.
3. Check for possible head and spine injuries, especially in older victims. If the victim is unable to walk without weakness, dizziness, or pain, suspect a head injury or another problem. Call 9-1-1 immediately and treat for possible spine injury.
4. If the person fell, check for and treat any injuries.
5. Allow fresh air to reach the victim (eg, open a window). Ask bystanders to stand clear.

For more information on fainting, see the *Sudden Illness* chapter.

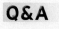

When can a victim be moved?

When possible, do not move a victim. This is especially true for a victim whose spine might be injured. Victims can be moved in the following circumstances:

- When hazards exist (eg, burning building, potential explosion, hazardous materials, vehicular traffic, landslide, avalanche), you can move the victim to a safer area.

- When a victim is facing downward (prone position) and is unresponsive, you can roll the victim to face upward (supine position).

- When a victim has breathing difficulty due to vomit or other body fluids (eg, blood) or if you are alone and must leave an unresponsive victim to get help, you can place the victim in a modified HAINES recovery position (High Arm IN Endangered Spine). Do this by placing one arm above and next to the head. Roll the body, as a single unit, to the victim's side. Support the head, which lies on the extended arm.

- When shock begins appearing, keep the victim in a supine position. The feet can be raised about 6 to 12 inches if there are no injuries. If pain occurs while moving or positioning the victim, do not raise the feet.

Source: Markenson D, et al. 2010. Part 13: First Aid: 2010 Consensus on First Aid Science. *Circulation.* 122(suppl):S532-S605.

Q&A

Should smelling salts or ammonia inhalant capsules be used on a person who has fainted or is unresponsive?

No. You shouldn't splash water on or slap the person's face either. Inhalants can adversely affect the victim by causing an asthma attack in an asthmatic person. Inhaled ammonia could burn the nasal mucous membrane. The strong smell of either smelling salts or ammonia inhalants could cause a victim to suddenly jerk his or her head, which could adversely affect any pre-existing cervical spine injury.

▶ Emergency Care Wrap-up

Condition	What to Look For	What to Do
Shock (cardiogenic, hemorrhagic, septic, neurogenic)	Agitation Anxiety Restlessness Feeling of impending doom Altered mental status Weak, rapid, or absent pulse Clammy (pale, cool, moist) skin* Paleness, with cyanosis about the lips Shallow, rapid breathing Shortness of breath Nausea or vomiting	Monitor breathing and provide care if needed. Control all obvious bleeding. Place the victim on his or her back. (Those having a heart attack or those with lung disease breathe easier in a half-sitting position). Do not move the victim if there are suspected fractures or head, spine, or torso injuries. Splint any bone or joint injuries. Place blankets under and over the victim. Handle the victim gently. Seek medical care by calling 9-1-1 if signs of shock are present.
Anaphylaxis	**Skin** Flushing, itching, or burning, especially over the face and upper chest Hives, which can spread over large areas of the body Swelling, especially of the face, tongue, and lips Bluish lips (cyanosis) **Circulatory system** Weak pulse (you might be barely able to feel it) Dizziness Fainting and unresponsiveness **Respiratory system** Sneezing or itching in the nostrils Tightness in the chest, with a persistent dry cough Breathing difficulty Secretions of fluid and mucus into the throat and lungs Wheezing (forced expirations during breathing) Breathing stops	Call 9-1-1 immediately. Monitor breathing, and if necessary, give CPR. If the victim has his or her own prescribed epinephrine, help the victim use it. If you are assisting with or using an auto-injector, follow the container's instructions. Give an antihistamine (such as Benadryl)—it is not life saving because it takes too long to work (20 minutes), but can prevent further reactions.

*Victims of neurogenic shock have warm, pink skin.

prep kit

▶ Ready for Review

- Shock is a state of collapse and failure of the cardiovascular system in which blood circulation decreases and eventually ceases.
- The damage caused by shock depends on which body part is deprived of oxygen and for how long.
- Causes of shock can be both cardiovascular and noncardiovascular.
- Anaphylaxis occurs when the immune system reacts violently to a substance to which it has already been sensitized.
- Although shock itself cannot be seen, you can see its signs and symptoms progress.
- First aiders should automatically treat victims for shock.

▶ Vital Vocabulary

anaphylaxis A life-threatening allergic reaction.

epinephrine auto-injector Prescribed device used to administer an emergency dose of epinephrine to a victim experiencing anaphylaxis.

shock Inadequate tissue oxygenation resulting from serious injury or illness.

▶ Assessment in Action

You are walking up a popular canyon trail on a cool fall afternoon. You hear someone call for help further up the trail, near a cliff. You jog up the trail and find a hiker bent over another person at the base of a cliff.

The hiker says the person lying motionless fell about 20 feet while climbing the cliff with no ropes or harness. There are no obvious signs of injury. The victim appears to be breathing and no serious bleeding is seen. *Directions:* Circle Yes if you agree with the statement; circle No if you disagree.

Yes No 1. You should suspect spinal injury.

Yes No 2. You should preserve the victim's body heat, but do not use external heat sources.

Yes No 3. You should offer the victim something to eat and drink.

Yes No 4. There is no need to seek medical care for this situation.

▶ Check Your Knowledge

Directions: Circle Yes if you agree with the statement; circle No if you disagree.

Yes No 1. Place all severely injured victims in the recovery position.

Yes No 2. Prevent body heat loss by putting blankets under and over the victim.

Yes No 3. A shock victim with possible spinal injuries should be placed in a seated position.

Yes No 4. A shock victim with breathing difficulty or chest injury should be placed on his or her back.

Yes No 5. Anxiety and restlessness are signs of shock.

Yes No 6. An epinephrine auto-injector requires a doctor's prescription.

Yes No 7. All severely injured or ill victims should be treated for shock.

Yes No 8. Treat severely injured victims for shock even if there are no signs of it.

Yes No 9. Anaphylaxis is a life-threatening breathing emergency.

Yes No 10. Victims in shock have hot skin.

Bleeding

▶ Bleeding

The average-size adult has 5 to 6 quarts (10–12 pints) of blood and can safely donate a pint. However, rapid blood loss of 1 quart or more can lead to shock and death. A child who loses 1 pint of blood is in extreme danger.

▶ External Bleeding

External bleeding refers to blood coming from an open wound. The term <u>hemorrhage</u> refers to a large amount of bleeding in a short time. External bleeding can be classified into three types according to the type of blood vessel that is damaged: an artery, vein, or capillary Figure 1 . In arterial bleeding, blood spurts (up to several feet) from the wound. <u>Arterial bleeding</u> is the most serious type of bleeding because a large amount of blood can be lost in a very short period of time. Arterial bleeding also is less likely to clot because blood can clot only when it is flowing slowly or not at all. Arterial bleeding is dangerous and must be controlled. Unless a very large artery has been cut, however, it is unlikely that a person will bleed to death before the flow can be controlled.

In <u>venous bleeding</u>, blood from a vein flows steadily or gushes. Venous bleeding is easier to control than arterial bleeding. Most veins collapse when cut. Bleeding from deep veins, however, can be as massive and as hard to control as arterial bleeding. In <u>capillary bleeding</u>,

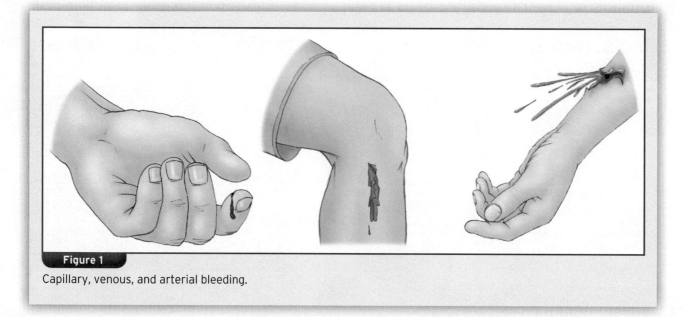

Figure 1

Capillary, venous, and arterial bleeding.

the most common type of bleeding, blood oozes from capillaries. It usually is not serious and can be controlled easily. Quite often, this type of bleeding will clot and stop by itself. Each type of blood vessel—artery, vein, or capillary—contains blood of a different shade of red. An inexperienced person may have difficulty detecting the color difference but would still be able to identify the type of bleeding by its flow.

Care for External Bleeding

Regardless of the type of bleeding or the type of wound, the first aid is the same. First, and most important, you must control the bleeding **Skill Drill 1** :

1. Protect yourself against disease by wearing exam gloves. If they are not available, use several layers of gauze pads, clean cloths, plastic wrap, a plastic bag, or waterproof material. If those are unavailable, you can have the victim apply pressure on the wound with his or her hand.
2. Expose the wound by removing or cutting the victim's clothing to find the source of the bleeding (Step **1**).
3. Place a sterile gauze pad or a clean cloth such as a handkerchief, washcloth, or towel over the entire wound and apply direct pressure with your fingers for small wounds and with the palm of your hand for large wounds (**Step 2**). Hold steady, firm, and

CAUTION

DO NOT come in contact with blood with your bare hands. Protect yourself with exam gloves, extra gauze pads, or clean cloths, or have the victim apply the direct pressure. If you must use your bare hands, do so only as a last resort. After the bleeding has stopped and the wound has been cared for, vigorously wash your hands with soap and water.

DO NOT use direct pressure on an eye injury, a wound with an embedded object, or a skull fracture.

DO NOT remove a blood-soaked dressing. Doing so can pull off clots that have already formed. Apply another dressing on top and continue putting pressure over the wound.

uninterrupted pressure on the wound for at least 5 minutes. The gauze or cloth allows you to apply even pressure. Direct pressure stops most bleeding. Applying direct pressure to the wound compresses the sides of the torn vessel and helps the body's natural clotting mechanisms work. Be sure the pressure remains constant, is not too light, and is applied to the bleeding source. Do not remove blood-soaked dressings; simply add new dressings over the old ones.

4. To free you to attend to other injuries or victims, use a pressure bandage to hold the

skill drill

1   Care for External Bleeding

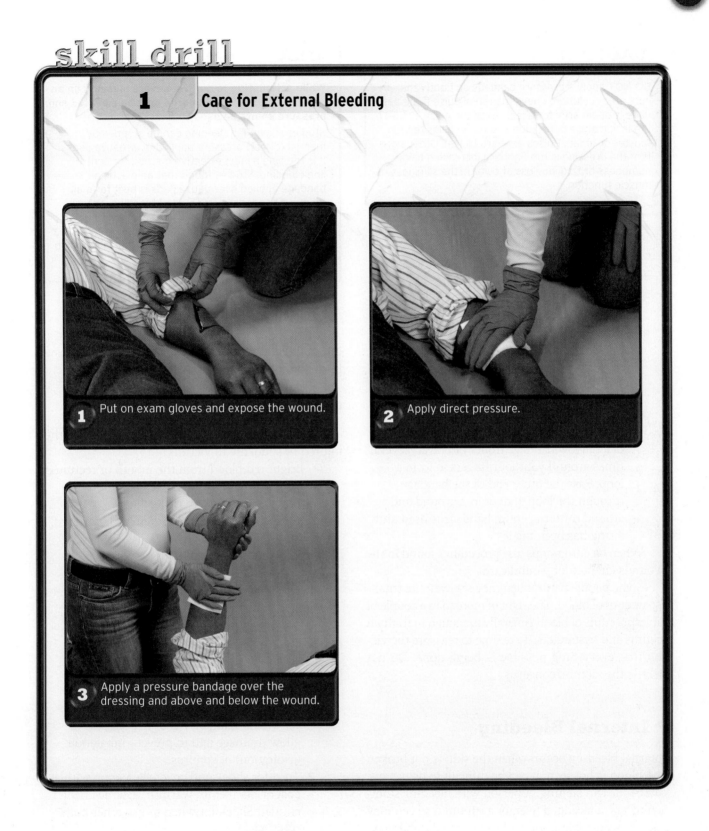

1. Put on exam gloves and expose the wound.

2. Apply direct pressure.

3. Apply a pressure bandage over the dressing and above and below the wound.

CAUTION

DO NOT apply a pressure bandage so tightly that it cuts off circulation. Check the radial pulse if the bandage is on an arm; for a leg, check the pulse between the inside ankle bone knob and the Achilles tendon (posterior tibial). Pulses are hard to feel. Other signs that the dressing is too tight are increasing pain, numbness or tingling, loss of color in the skin, loss of muscle function.

Q&A

While attempting to control severe bleeding on an arm or leg, should the injured part be elevated and pressure points be used?
Studies show that bleeding can be stopped by manual (direct) pressure applied over gauze pads. It is the single most effective method for controlling bleeding. Studies found that an elastic adhesive bandage applied over gauze pads is best for maintaining a hands-free stopping of bleeding. No evidence exists that pressure points eliminated distal pulses—blood flow continued. No evidence exists that elevation of a bleeding part has any role in stopping bleeding.

dressing on the wound. Wrap a roller gauze bandage tightly over the dressing and above and below the wound site (Step **3**). Do not wrap it so tightly that it cuts off circulation.

5. When direct pressure cannot be applied, such as in the case of a protruding bone, skull fracture, or embedded object, use a doughnut-shaped (ring) pad to control bleeding. To make a ring pad, wrap one end of a narrow bandage (roller or cravat) several times around your four fingers to form a loop. Pass the other end of the bandage through the loop and wrap it around and around until the entire bandage is used and a ring has been made.

When bleeding stops, use procedures found in the Wounds chapter for wound care.

Some people panic when they see even the smallest amount of blood. The sight of more than a couple of tablespoonfuls of blood generally is enough to frighten victims and bystanders. Take time to reassure the victim that everything possible is being done. Do not belittle the victim's concerns.

▶ Internal Bleeding

Internal bleeding occurs when the skin is not broken and blood is not seen. It can be difficult to detect and can be life threatening. A person with bleeding stomach ulcers, a lacerated liver, or a ruptured spleen may lose a considerable amount of blood into the abdomen with no outward sign of bleeding other than the presence of shock. Broken bones can also cause serious

internal blood loss. A broken femur can easily result in a loss of 1 or more quarts of blood.

Recognizing Internal Bleeding

The signs of internal bleeding may be seen in either injured or suddenly ill victims:

- Bright red blood from the mouth or rectum or blood in the urine
- Nonmenstrual vaginal bleeding
- Vomited blood; may be bright red, dark red, or look like coffee grounds
- Black, foul-smelling, tarry stools
- Pain, tenderness, bruising, or swelling
- Broken ribs, bruises over the lower chest, or a rigid abdomen

Care for Internal Bleeding

For severe internal bleeding, follow these steps:

1. Monitor breathing.
2. Expect vomiting. If vomiting occurs, keep the victim lying on his or her left side to allow drainage and to prevent inhalation (aspiration) of vomitus.
3. Treat for shock and cover the victim with a coat or blanket for warmth. See the chapter entitled Shock for when to use other body positions.
4. Treat suspected internal bleeding in an extremity by applying a splint.
5. Seek immediate medical care.

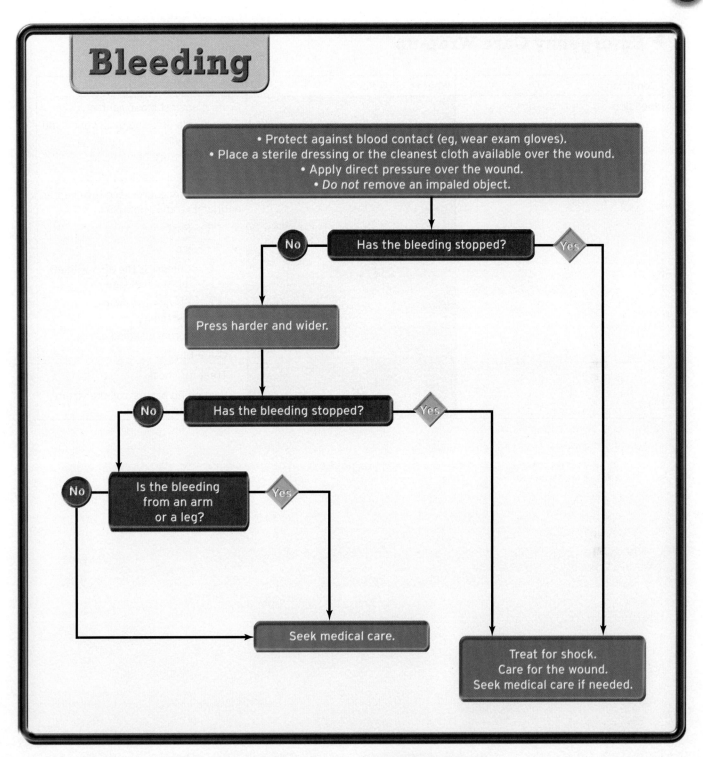

Bleeding

• Protect against blood contact (eg, wear exam gloves).
• Place a sterile dressing or the cleanest cloth available over the wound.
• Apply direct pressure over the wound.
• *Do not* remove an impaled object.

No — Has the bleeding stopped? — Yes

Press harder and wider.

No — Has the bleeding stopped? — Yes

No — Is the bleeding from an arm or a leg? — Yes

Seek medical care.

Treat for shock.
Care for the wound.
Seek medical care if needed.

Bruises are a form of internal bleeding, but are not life threatening. To treat bruises:

1. Apply an ice pack over the injury for 20 minutes.
2. If an arm or a leg is involved, apply an elastic bandage for compression. Several layers of gauze pads or other cloth could be placed between the bandage and the injury to concentrate the compression to a specific location.

CAUTION

DO NOT give a victim anything to eat or drink. It could cause nausea and vomiting, which could result in aspiration. Food or liquids could also cause complications if surgery is needed.

▶ Emergency Care Wrap-up

Condition	What to Look For	What to Do
Bleeding	External bleeding	Protect against blood contact.
		Place sterile dressing over wound and apply pressure.
		Apply a pressure bandage.
	Internal bleeding	Minor internal bleeding (bruise):
		Use RICE procedures (see the chapter entitled Extremity Injuries):
		R = Rest
		I = Ice
		C = Compress the area with an elastic bandage.
		E = Elevate the injured extremity.
		Serious internal bleeding:
		Call 9-1-1.
		Treat for shock.
		If vomiting occurs, roll the victim onto his or her side.

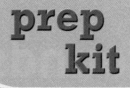

▶ Ready for Review

- Rapid blood loss of 1 quart or more can lead to shock and death.
- External bleeding can be classified into three types according to the type of blood vessel that is damaged: artery, vein, or capillary.
- Regardless of the type of bleeding or the type of wound, the first aid is the same. First, and most important, you must control the bleeding.

▶ Vital Vocabulary

arterial bleeding Bleeding from an artery; this type of bleeding tends to spurt with each heartbeat.

capillary bleeding Bleeding that oozes from a wound steadily but slowly.

hemorrhage A large amount of bleeding in a short time.

venous bleeding Bleeding from a vein; this type of bleeding tends to flow steadily.

▶ Assessment in Action

You are enjoying a bike ride on a paved trail with your friend. As she rounds the next bend, her bike tires slide out on the gravel and she falls to the ground. She gets up but has a large scrape on her knee and part of her lower leg. Blood is oozing from the wound.

Directions: Circle Yes if you agree with the statement; circle No if you disagree.

Yes　No　**1.** This victim is experiencing capillary bleeding.

Yes　No　**2.** This type of bleeding is the most common type.

Yes　No　**3.** This type of bleeding is difficult to control and usually does not clot and stop by itself.

Yes　No　**4.** Direct pressure will control this type of bleeding.

▶ Check Your Knowledge

Directions: Circle Yes if you agree with the statement; circle No if you disagree.

Yes　No　**1.** Most cases of bleeding require more than direct pressure to stop the bleeding.

Yes　No　**2.** Remove any blood-soaked dressings before applying additional ones.

Yes　No　**3.** Applying a pressure bandage over a wound can allow you to attend to another injury or another injured victim.

Yes　No　**4.** If a bleeding arm wound is not controlled through direct pressure, apply pressure to the brachial artery.

Yes　No　**5.** Dressings are placed directly on a wound.

Yes　No　**6.** Internal bleeding is normal.

Yes　No　**7.** Dressings should be sterile or as clean as possible.

Yes　No　**8.** Clotting is the body's way of stopping bleeding.

Yes　No　**9.** If the victim feels sick to the stomach and may vomit, roll him or her onto the left side.

Yes　No　**10.** It is important to remove impaled objects because they could be driven in deeper.

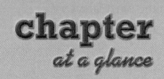

Wounds

▶ Open Wounds

An open wound is a break in the skin's surface resulting in external bleeding. It may allow bacteria to enter the body, causing an infection. There are several types of open wounds. Recognizing the type of wound helps you give proper first aid. With an **abrasion**, the top layer of skin is removed, with little or no blood loss **Figure 1**. Abrasions tend to be painful because the nerve endings often are abraded along with the skin. Ground-in debris may be present. This type of wound can be serious if it covers a large area or becomes embedded with foreign matter. Other names for an abrasion are scrape, road rash, and scuff.

A **laceration** is cut skin with jagged, irregular edges **Figure 2**. This type of wound is usually caused by a forceful tearing away of skin tissue. **Incisions** tend to have smooth edges and resemble a surgical or paper cut **Figure 3**. The amount of bleeding depends on the depth, the location, and the size of the wound. **Punctures** are usually deep, narrow wounds in the skin and underlying organs such as a stab wound from a nail or a knife **Figure 4**. The entrance is usually small, and the risk of infection is high. The object causing the injury may remain impaled in the wound.

With an **avulsion**, a piece of skin and/or underlying tissue is torn loose and is hanging from the body or completely removed. This type of wound can bleed heavily. If the flap is still attached, lay it flat and realign it into its normal position. Avulsions most often involve ears, fingers, and hands **Figure 5**. An **amputation** involves the cutting or

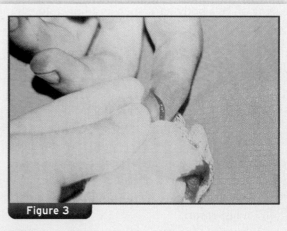

Figure 1

Abrasion.

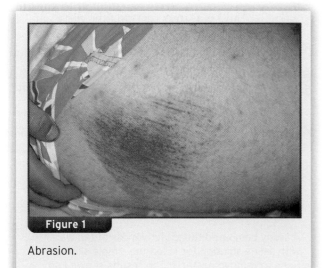

Figure 3

Incision.

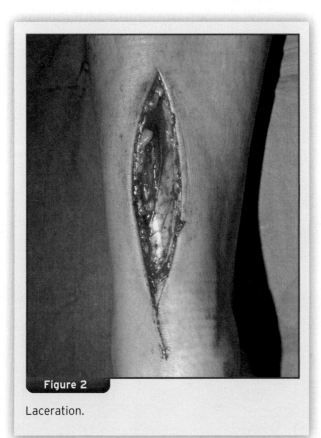

Figure 2

Laceration.

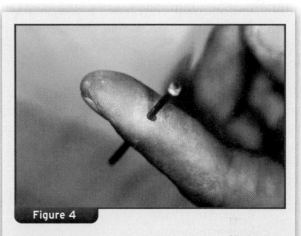

Figure 4

Puncture.

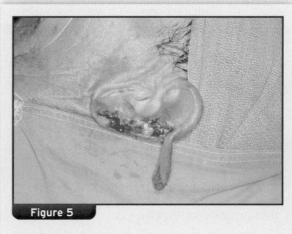

Figure 5

Avulsion.

tearing off of a body part, such as a finger, toe, hand, foot, arm, or leg.

Care for Open Wounds

1. Protect yourself against disease by wearing exam gloves. If they are not available, use several layers of gauze pads, clean cloths, plastic wrap or bags, or waterproof material. If none of these are available, you can have the victim apply pressure with his or her hand. Your bare hand should be used only as a last resort.
2. Expose the wound by removing or cutting away the clothing to find the source of the bleeding.
3. Control the bleeding by using direct pressure and, if needed, other methods described in the chapter entitled Bleeding.

Cleaning a Wound

A victim's wound should be cleaned to help prevent infection. Wound cleaning usually restarts the bleeding by disturbing the clot, but it should be done anyway for shallow wounds. For wounds with a high risk for infection, leave the pressure bandage in place because medical personnel will clean the wound.

1. Scrub your hands vigorously with soap and water. Put on exam gloves, if available.
2. Expose the wound.
3. Clean the wound.
   - *For a shallow wound:*
     - Wash inside the wound with soap and water.
     - Flush the wound with water (use water that is clean enough to drink) **Figure 6**. Run water directly into the wound and allow the water to run over the wound

and out, thus carrying the dirty particles away from the wound. Flushing with water needs pressure (at least 5 to 8 psi) to cleanse the tissue adequately. Water from a faucet provides sufficient pressure and quantity. Pouring water through the wound will not generate enough force for adequate cleaning. Irrigation with water is the most

---

FYI

A study compared the effectiveness of tap water with saline solution for irrigating simple skin lacerations to remove bacteria. The results showed no significant difference between bacterial counts in wounds irrigated with normal saline and those irrigated with tap water. The removal of bacteria from a wound depends more on the mechanical effects (speed and pressure) than on the type of solution. Tap water has these advantages over saline—it is readily available; it is more continuous and, therefore, takes less time; it is less expensive; and it does not require other materials such as sterile syringes or splash guards. Other irrigation solutions with antibacterial properties and detergents have an anticellular effect that impairs wound healing and/ or resistance to infection. Irrigation pressures more than the 20 to 30 psi range are discouraged because the higher pressure can damage tissue.

Source: Moscati R, Mayrose J, Fincher L, Jehle D. 1996. Comparison of normal saline with tap water for wound irrigation. *Am J Emerg Med* 164(4):379-381.

CAUTION

DO NOT clean large, extremely dirty, or life-threatening wounds. Let the hospital emergency department personnel do the cleaning.

DO NOT scrub a wound. The benefit of scrubbing a wound is debatable, and it can bruise the tissue.

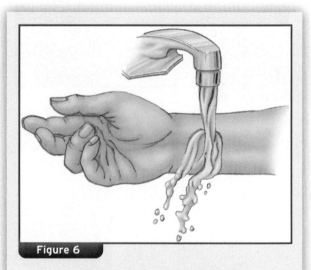

Figure 6

Irrigate a wound with water under pressure.

FYI

High-Risk Wounds

These types of wounds have a high potential for infection:

- Bite wounds
- Very dirty, contaminated wounds
- Crushing, ragged wounds
- Wounds over injured bone, joint, or tendon
- Puncture wounds

important factor in preventing infection.

- *For a wound with a high risk for infection* (such as an animal bite, a very dirty or ragged wound, or a puncture), clean the wound and then seek medical care for additional wound cleaning. If you are in a remote setting (more than 1 hour from medical care), clean the wound as best you can.

4. Remove small objects not flushed out with sterile tweezers, if available. A dirty abrasion or other wound that is not properly cleaned will leave a "tattoo" on the victim's skin.

5. If bleeding restarts, apply direct pressure over the wound.

FYI

Wound Care: What the Medical Literature Says

- Soaking wounds is not effective.
- The benefit of scrubbing wounds is debatable.
- Irrigating wounds requires a minimum pressure of 5 to 8 psi for tissue cleansing.
- Not closing a wound (for example, with butterfly bandages, elastic skin closures), especially a dirty wound, reduces the risk of infection.
- Applying antiseptic solutions such as Merthiolate, Mercurochrome, iodine, isopropyl alcohol, and hydrogen peroxide can injure wounded tissues.
- Applying an antibiotic ointment such as Neosporin or Polysporin reduces the risk of infection in shallow wounds or abrasions.

Source: Howell JM, Chisholm CD. 1992. Outpatient wound preparation and care: a national survey. *Ann Emerg Med* 21(8):976-981.

Covering a Wound

1. If the wound is small and does not require sutures, cover it with a thin layer of antibiotic ointment. These ointments can kill many bacteria and rarely cause allergic reactions. No physician prescription is needed.

2. Cover a small or large wound with a sterile dressing. Do not close gaping or dirty wounds with tape or butterfly bandages. Bacteria may remain, leading to a greater chance of infection. Large, deep, or contaminated wounds should be managed by a medical professional.

3. If a wound bleeds after a dressing has been applied and the dressing becomes stuck, leave it on as long as the wound is healing. Pulling the scab loose to change the dressing retards healing and increases the chance of infection. If you must remove a dressing that is sticking, soak it in warm water to help soften the scab and make removal easier.

4. If a dressing becomes wet or dirty, change it. Dirt and moisture are both breeding grounds for bacteria.

CAUTION

DO NOT irrigate a wound with full-strength iodine preparations such as povidone iodine (10%) or isopropyl alcohol (70%). They kill body cells as well as bacteria and are painful. Also, some people are allergic to iodine.

DO NOT use hydrogen peroxide. It does not kill bacteria well, it adversely affects capillary blood flow, and it extends wound healing.

DO NOT use antibiotic ointment on wounds that require sutures or on puncture wounds (the ointment may prevent drainage). Use an antibiotic ointment only on abrasions and shallow wounds.

DO NOT soak a wound to clean it. No evidence supports the effectiveness of soaking.

DO NOT close gaping wounds with tape such as butterfly tape. Infection is more likely when bacteria are trapped in the wound. If a wound requires closure, this should be done by medical personnel. Extremity wounds are best sutured within 6 hours of the injury.

DO NOT breathe or blow on a wound or the dressing.

Dressings and bandages are two different kinds of first aid supplies. A **dressing** is applied over a wound to control bleeding and prevent contamination. A **bandage** holds the dressing in place. Dressings should be sterile or as clean as possible; bandages need not be.

When to Seek Medical Care

High-risk wounds should receive medical care. Examples of high-risk wounds include those with embedded foreign material (such as gravel), animal and human bites, puncture wounds, and ragged wounds. Large or deep wounds should receive medical care. Any wound where edges do not come together spontaneously should receive medical care. Any wounds that have visible bone, joint, muscle, fat, or tendons and wounds that may have entered a joint or body cavity should receive medical care. A particularly high-risk wound is the "fight bite," a wound over the knuckle caused by punching a person in the teeth. Sutures, if needed, are best placed within 6 to 8 hours after the injury. Anyone who has not had a tetanus vaccination within 10 years (5 years in the case of a dirty wound) should seek medical attention within 72 hours to update his or her tetanus inoculation status.

Wound Infection

Any wound, large or small, can become infected. Once an infection begins, damage can be extensive, so prevention is the best way to avoid the problem. A wound should be cleaned using the procedures described earlier in this chapter.

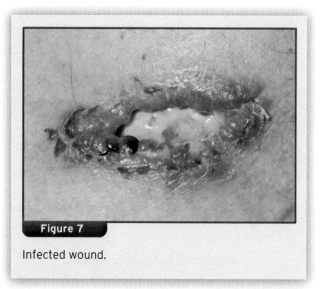

Figure 7

Infected wound.

It is important to know how to recognize and treat an infected wound . The signs and symptoms of infection include the following:

- Swelling and redness around the wound
- A sensation of warmth
- Throbbing pain
- Pus discharge
- Fever
- Swelling of lymph nodes
- One or more red streaks leading from the wound toward the heart

The appearance of one or more red streaks leading from the wound toward the heart is a serious sign

FYI

Using Topical Antibiotics to Improve Wound Healing

The use of topical triple-antibiotics significantly decreases infection rates in minor wounds that are contaminated. Topical antibiotics are effective for minor wounds, but not for major wounds.

Many studies support the use of topical antibiotics on wounds that are clean. Topical bacitracin zinc (Bacitracin); a triple ointment of neomycin sulfate, bacitracin zinc, and polymyxin B sulfate (Neosporin); and silver sulfadiazine (Silvadene) were compared with petrolatum as a control in patients with minor wounds. Wound infection rates were 17.6% for petrolatum, 5.5% for Bacitracin, 4.5% for Neosporin, and 12.1% for Silvadene.

Source: Diehr S, Hamp A, Jamieson B. 2007. *The Journal of Family Practice.* 56(2):140-144.

Q&A

When should wounds be closed by a physician?
Generally, a wound should be closed by one of several options (eg, sutures, staples, topical skin adhesives) when: (1) the edges of the skin do not fall together and/or (2) the cut is more than an inch long and is deep. Closing the wound speeds the healing process, lessens the risk of infection, and lessens scarring.

If sutures are needed, they should be made by a physician within 6 to 8 hours of the injury.

FYI

Myths About Wound Care

Myth: Wounds should be kept dry.

Fact: Healing is faster and infection rates are lower when wounds are kept moist. Keep them moist by applying an antibiotic ointment and a dressing.

Myth: Redness is a sign of an infected wound.

Fact: Although redness can signal an infected wound, it does indicate an inflammatory reaction. When you see it, check the other signs and symptoms of infection: fever and pus coming from the wound.

Myth: Saline solution should be used instead of tap water to irrigate a wound.

Fact: Saline solution is no more effective in preventing wound infections than tap water.

Myth: Don't cover a cut—let it "breathe."

Fact: If a cut is not covered, it dries out and scabs over. Scabs hinder healing. Keep a cut moist and prevent a scab from forming. Apply an antibiotic ointment and cover with a dressing.

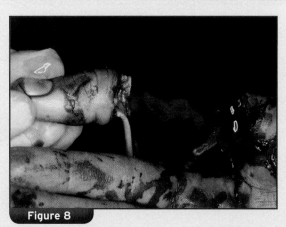

Figure 8

Guillotine amputation.

▶ Amputations

In many cases, an amputated extremity can be successfully replanted (reattached). It is generally attempted for only upper extremities. Amputations usually involve fingers, hands, and arms rather than legs **Figure 8** .

Care for Amputation

1. Control the bleeding with direct pressure. Apply a dry dressing or bulky cloths. Be sure to protect yourself against disease by following standard precautions. If bleeding cannot be controlled with direct pressure, a tourniquet may be required to prevent shock or death from blood loss.
2. Treat the victim for shock.
3. Recover the amputated part and, whenever possible, take it with the victim to the hospital. In multicasualty cases, in reduced lighting conditions, or when untrained people transport the victim, however, someone may be requested to locate and take the severed body part to the hospital after the victim's departure.
4. To care for the amputated body part **Figure 9** :
   - Do not clean the amputated portion.
   - Wrap the amputated part with dry, sterile gauze or other clean cloth.

that the infection is spreading and could cause death. If chills and fever develop, the infection has reached the circulatory system. Seek immediate medical care.

Factors that increase the likelihood for wound infection include the following:

- Dirty and foreign material left in the wound
- Ragged or crushed tissue
- Injury to an underlying bone, joint, or tendon
- Bite wounds (human or animal)
- Hand and foot wounds
- Puncture wounds or other wounds that cannot drain

In the early stages of an infection, a physician may allow a wound to be treated at home. Such home treatment would include the following:

- Keeping the area clean
- Soaking the wound in warm water or applying warm, wet packs
- Elevating the infected portion of the body
- Applying antibiotic ointment
- Changing the dressings daily
- Seeking medical care if the infection persists or becomes worse

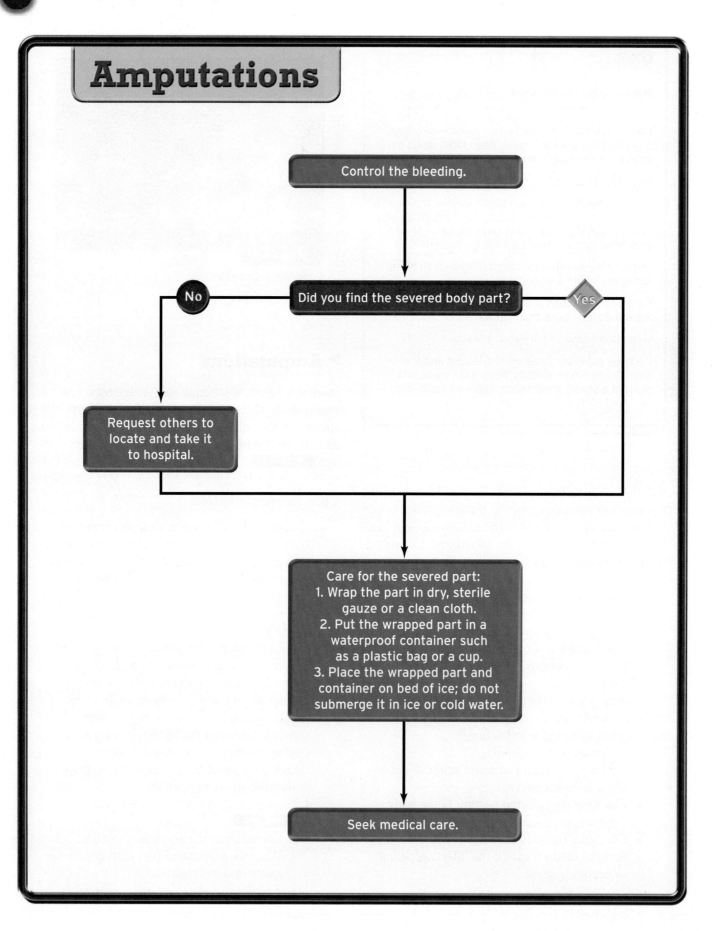

Amputations

Control the bleeding.

Did you find the severed body part?

No → Request others to locate and take it to hospital.

Yes →

Care for the severed part:
1. Wrap the part in dry, sterile gauze or a clean cloth.
2. Put the wrapped part in a waterproof container such as a plastic bag or a cup.
3. Place the wrapped part and container on bed of ice; do not submerge it in ice or cold water.

Seek medical care.

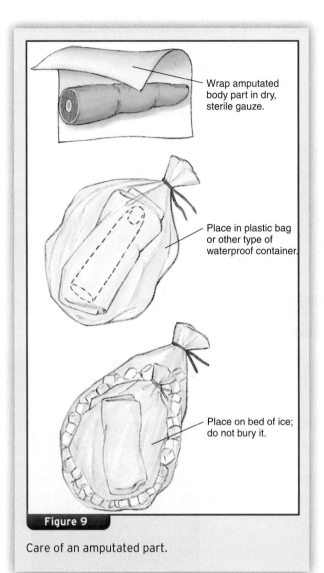

Wrap amputated body part in dry, sterile gauze.

Place in plastic bag or other type of waterproof container.

Place on bed of ice; do not bury it.

Figure 9

Care of an amputated part.

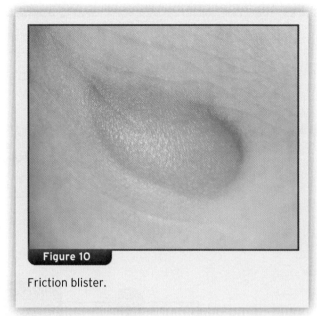

Figure 10

Friction blister.

Care for Blisters

When caring for a friction blister, try to (1) avoid the risk of infection, (2) minimize the victim's pain and discomfort, (3) limit the blister's development, and (4) promote a fast recovery. The best care for a particular blister is determined mainly by its size and location.

If an area on the skin becomes a "hot spot" (painful, red area), snugly apply a piece of tape (adhesive or duct). You could also cut a hole in several pieces of moleskin or molefoam in layered stacks around the blister, make a doughnut-shaped pad, and apply it over the blister.

If a blister on a foot is closed and not very painful, a conservative approach is to tape the blister with

- Put the wrapped amputated part in a plastic bag or other waterproof container.
- Place the bag or container with the wrapped part on a bed of ice. Keep the amputated part cool, but do not freeze.
5. Seek medical care immediately.

▶ Blisters

A blister is a collection of fluid in a "bubble" under the outer layer of skin. (Note: This section applies only to friction blisters and does not apply to blisters from burns, frostbite, drug reactions, insect or snake bites, or contact with a poisonous plant.)

Repeated rubbing of a small area of the skin will produce a blister **Figure 10**.

CAUTION

DO NOT try to decide whether a body part is salvageable or too small to save—leave that decision to a physician.

DO NOT wrap an amputated part in a wet dressing or cloth. Using a wet wrap on the part can cause waterlogging and tissue softening, which will make reattachment more difficult.

DO NOT bury an amputated part in ice—place it on ice. Reattaching frostbitten parts is usually unsuccessful.

DO NOT use dry ice.

DO NOT cut a skin "bridge," a tendon, or other structure that is connecting a partially attached part to the rest of the body. Instead, reposition the part in the normal position, wrap the part in a dry, sterile dressing or clean cloth, and place an ice pack on it.

Blisters

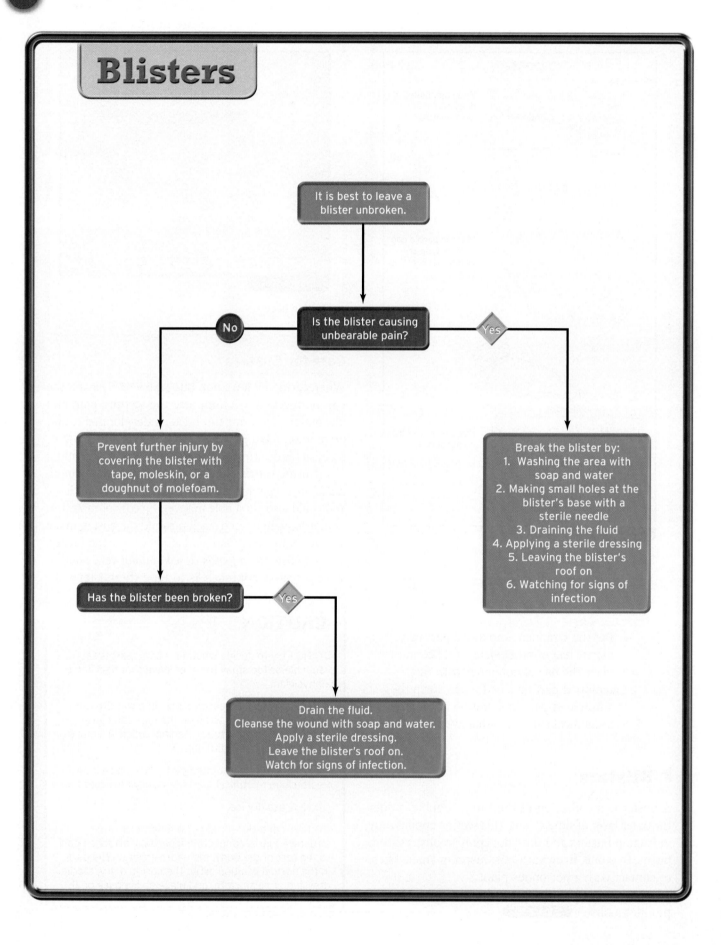

It is best to leave a blister unbroken.

Is the blister causing unbearable pain?

No — Prevent further injury by covering the blister with tape, moleskin, or a doughnut of molefoam.

Yes — Break the blister by:
1. Washing the area with soap and water
2. Making small holes at the blister's base with a sterile needle
3. Draining the fluid
4. Applying a sterile dressing
5. Leaving the blister's roof on
6. Watching for signs of infection

Has the blister been broken?

Yes — Drain the fluid. Cleanse the wound with soap and water. Apply a sterile dressing. Leave the blister's roof on. Watch for signs of infection.

duct tape or waterproof adhesive tape. The tape must remain on the blister for several days; removing it may tear off the blister's "roof" and expose unprotected skin. Unfortunately, the tape may become damp and contaminated and have to be replaced, risking a tear. Small blisters, especially on weight-bearing areas, generally respond better if left intact.

With a few exceptions, the blister's roof (which is the best and most comfortable "dressing") should be removed only when an infection is present. Once a blister has been opened, the area should be washed with soap to prevent further infection. For 10 to 14 days, or until new skin forms, a protective bandage or other cover should be used.

Even with no evidence of infection, consider removing the blister's roof when a partially torn blister roof may tear skin adjacent to the blister site, resulting in an even larger open wound. In such cases, use sterilized scissors to remove the loose skin of the blister's roof up to the edge of the normal tissue. Treat it the same as for an open blister. Rubbing alcohol is effective for sterilizing instruments such as needles or scissors.

If a blister on the foot is open or a very painful closed blister affects walking or running:

1. Clean the area with soap and water.
2. Drain all fluid out of the blister by making several small holes at the base of the blister with a sterilized needle. Press the fluid out. Do not remove the roof of a blister unless it is torn and it may tear adjacent skin, or if there is an infection.
3. Apply several layers of moleskin or molefoam cut in a doughnut shape on top of each other **Figure 11**. Another option is to apply a commercial callus or corn pad over the blister.
4. Apply antibiotic ointment in the hole and cover it securely with tape. The pressure dressing ensures that the blister's roof sticks to the underlying skin and that the blister does not refill with fluid after it has been drained.

▶ Impaled (Embedded) Objects

Impaled objects come in all shapes and sizes, from pencils and screwdrivers to knives, glass, steel rods, and fence posts **Figure 12**. Proper first aid requires that the impaled object be stabilized because there can be significant internal damage.

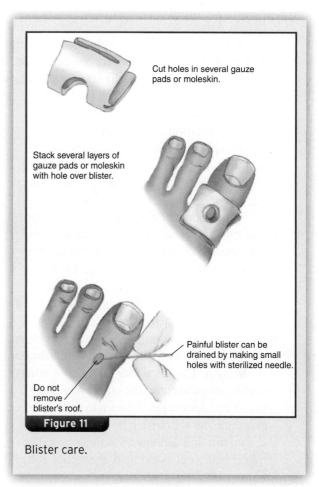

Cut holes in several gauze pads or moleskin.

Stack several layers of gauze pads or moleskin with hole over blister.

Painful blister can be drained by making small holes with sterilized needle.

Do not remove blister's roof.

Figure 11

Blister care.

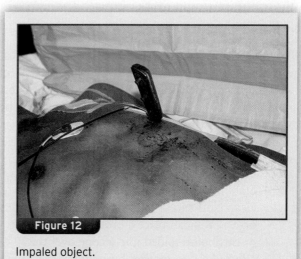

Figure 12

Impaled object.

Care for Impaled Objects

1. Expose the area. Remove or cut away any clothing surrounding the injury. If clothes cover the object, leave them in place; removing them could cause the object to move.

2. Do not remove or move the object. Movement of any kind could produce additional bleeding and tissue damage. Cheeks are one exception because the object or the bleeding could cause an airway obstruction. See the following section on impaled objects in the cheek for more information. Small objects such as slivers (splinters) can be safely removed.

3. Stabilize the object with bulky dressings or clean cloths around the object. Some experts suggest securing 75% of the object with bulky dressings or cloths to reduce motion.

4. Control any bleeding with pressure around the impaled object. Apply pressure on the dressing surrounding the object. Do not press directly on the object or along the wound next to the cutting edge, especially if the object has sharp edges.

5. Shorten the object only if necessary. In most cases, do not shorten the object by cutting or breaking it. There are times, however, when cutting or shortening the object allows for easier transportation. Be sure to stabilize the object before shortening it. Remember that the victim will feel any vibrations from the object being cut away; also, the injury could be worsened by this action.

Impaled Object in the Eye

If an object is impaled in the eye, it is vital that pressure not be put on the eye. The eyeball consists of two chambers, each filled with fluid. Do not exert any pressure against the eyeball because fluid can be forced out of it, worsening the injury.

Care for Impaled Object in the Eye

1. Stabilize the object. Use bulky dressings or clean cloths to stabilize a long, protruding object. You can place a protective paper cup or cardboard folded into a cone over the affected eye to prevent bumping of the object. For short objects, surround the eye—without touching the object—with a doughnut-shaped (ring) pad held in place with a roller bandage.

2. Cover the undamaged eye. Most experts suggest that the undamaged eye should be covered to prevent sympathetic eye movement (that is, the injured eye moves when the undamaged eye does, thus aggravating

the injury). Remember that the victim is unable to see when both eyes are covered and may be anxious. Make sure you explain to the victim everything you are doing.

3. Seek immediate medical care.

▶ Closed Wounds

A closed wound happens when a blunt object strikes the body. In other words, the skin is not broken, but tissue and blood vessels beneath the skin's surface are crushed, causing bleeding within a confined area.

Care for Closed Wounds

1. Control bleeding by applying an ice pack over the area for no more than 20 minutes. Place a cloth between the ice pack and the skin to prevent frostbite.

2. If the injury involves a limb, apply an elastic bandage for compression. A splint may help make the victim more comfortable.

3. Check for a possible fracture.

4. Elevate an injured extremity above the victim's heart level to decrease the pain and swelling.

▶ Wounds That Require Medical Care

At some point, you will probably have to decide whether medical care is needed for a wounded victim. As a guideline, seek medical care for the following conditions as offered by the American College of Emergency Physicians:

- Wounds that will not stop bleeding after 15 minutes of applying direct pressure
- Long or deep cuts that need stitches
- Cuts over a joint
- Cuts that may impair function of a body area such as an eyelid or lip
- Cuts that remove all of the layers of the skin; such as those from slicing off the tip of a finger
- Cuts from an animal or human bite
- Cuts that have damaged or may have damaged underlying nerves, tendons, or joints
- Cuts over a possible broken bone
- Cuts caused by a crushing injury
- Cuts with an object embedded in them
- Cuts caused by a metal object or a puncture wound

Call 9-1-1 immediately if:

- Bleeding from a cut does not slow during the first 15 minutes of steady pressure
- Signs of shock occur
- Breathing is difficult because of a cut to the neck or chest
- A deep cut to the abdomen causes moderate to severe pain
- A cut occurs to the eyeball
- A cut amputates or partially amputates an extremity

Sutures

If sutures (stitches) are needed, they usually should be placed by a physician within 6 to 8 hours of the injury. Suturing wounds allows faster healing, reduces infection, and lessens scarring. Some wounds do not usually require sutures:

- Wounds in which the skin's cut edges tend to fall together
- Shallow cuts less than 1 inch long

Rather than close a gaping wound with butterfly bandages or elastic skin closures, cover the wound with sterile gauze. Closing the wound might trap bacteria inside, resulting in an infection. In most cases, a physician can be reached in time for sutures to be placed; if not, a wound without sutures will still heal but with scars. Scar tissue can be attended to later by a plastic surgeon.

▶ Dressings and Bandages

First aid kits include dressings and bandages to be used when controlling bleeding and caring for wounds. Wounds heal better with less infection if they are covered with a clean dressing. A dressing is a covering that is placed directly over a wound to help absorb blood, prevent infection, and protect the wound from further injury. Dressings come in different shapes, sizes, and types. Dressings can be gauze pads (eg, 2- or 4-inch square or larger) used to cover larger wounds, or adhesive strips, such as Band-Aids, which are dressings combined with a bandage for small cuts or scrapes **Figure 13**.

A bandage, such as a roll of gauze, is often used to cover a dressing, to keep it in place on the wound and to apply pressure to help control the bleeding. Like dressings, bandages also come in different shapes, sizes, and material **Figure 14**. Elastic bandages can be used to provide support and stability for a extremity or joint and to decrease swelling, but they are not usually used to cover wounds.

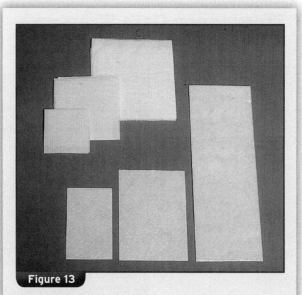

Figure 13

Gauze pads.

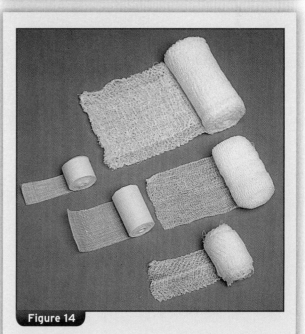

Figure 14

Self-adhering conforming bandages and gauze bandages of various sizes.

When commercial bandages are unavailable, improvise bandages from neckties, bandannas, or strips of cloth torn from a sheet or other similar material.

When applying a bandage, do not apply it so tightly that it restricts blood circulation. The signs that a bandage is too tight include:

- Blue tinge to the fingernails or toenails
- Blue or pale skin
- Tingling or loss of sensation
- Coldness of the arm or leg

▶ Emergency Care Wrap-up

Condition	What to Look For	What to Do
Open wound	Break in the skin's surface External bleeding	Wash with soap and water. Flush with running water under pressure. Remove remaining small object(s). If the bleeding restarts, apply pressure on the wound. Apply antibiotic ointment if wound is shallow. Cover with sterile or clean dressing. For wounds with a high risk for infection, seek medical care for cleaning, possible tetanus booster, and closing.
Amputation	Body part (eg, finger, toe, hand, foot, arm, leg) completely cut or torn off the body	Call 9-1-1. Control bleeding. Care for shock. Recover amputated part(s) and wrap in sterile or clean dressing. Place wrapped part(s) in a plastic bag or waterproof container. Keep part(s) cool.
Embedded (impaled) object	Foreign object penetrating a body part	Do not remove object. Stabilize the object with bulky dressings or clean cloths. Control bleeding with pressure around the object.

▶ Ready for Review

- An open wound is a break in the skin's surface resulting in external bleeding.
- Knowing what type of open wound the victim has will help you in providing first aid.
- In many cases, an amputated extremity can be successfully replanted.
- A blister is a collection of fluid in a bubble under the outer layer of skin.
- Proper first aid of an impaled object requires that the object be stabilized because significant internal damage can occur.
- A closed wound happens when a blunt object strikes the body. Although the skin remains unbroken, the tissue and blood vessels beneath the skin's surface are crushed, causing bleeding within a confined area.
- Wounds that require medical care include:
  - Wounds that will not stop bleeding after 15 minutes of applying direct pressure
  - Long or deep cuts that need stitches
  - Cuts over a joint
  - Cuts that may impair function of a body area such as an eyelid or lip
  - Cuts that remove all of the layers of the skin such as those from slicing off the tip of a finger
  - Cuts from an animal or human bite
  - Cuts that have damaged or may have damaged underlying nerves, tendons, or joints
  - Cuts over a possible broken bone
  - Cuts caused by a crushing injury
  - Cuts with an object embedded in them
  - Cuts caused by a metal object or a puncture wound
- Call 9-1-1 immediately if:
  - Bleeding from a cut does not slow during the first 15 minutes of steady pressure
  - Signs of shock occur
    - Breathing is difficult because of a cut to the neck or chest
    - A deep cut to the abdomen causes moderate to severe pain
  - A cut occurs to the eyeball
  - A cut amputates or partially amputates an extremity

▶ Vital Vocabulary

abrasion An injury consisting of the loss of the partial thickness of skin from rubbing or scraping on a hard, rough surface.

amputation Complete removal of an appendage.

avulsion An injury that leaves a piece of skin or other tissue either partially or completely torn away from the body.

bandage Used to cover a dressing to keep it in place on the wound and to apply pressure to help control bleeding.

dressing A sterile gauze pad or clean cloth covering that is placed over an open wound.

incisions Wounds usually made deliberately in connection with surgery; clean-cut as opposed to a laceration.

laceration A wound made by the tearing or cutting of body tissues.

punctures Deep, narrow wounds in the skin and underlying organs.

prep kit

▶ Assessment in Action

You are helping your mother prepare for a barbeque on a Saturday afternoon. She is slicing tomatoes with a very dull kitchen knife. She is startled by something and cuts into her finger. The wound is bleeding and you can see the bone in the wound.

Directions: Circle Yes if you agree with the statement; circle No if you disagree.

Yes   No   **1.** This type of wound is called an avulsion.

Yes   No   **2.** You should not be concerned about infection because she was using a clean knife.

Yes   No   **3.** You should cover the wound with a sterile dressing but do not close the wound with tape or butterfly bandages.

Yes   No   **4.** You decide to take her to the emergency department for possible sutures. However, both you and your mother want to wait until the next day because you don't want to miss the barbeque.

▶ Check Your Knowledge

Directions: Circle Yes if you agree with the statement; circle No if you disagree.

Yes   No   **1.** An open wound may allow bacteria to enter the body, causing an infection.

Yes   No   **2.** A laceration is cut skin with smooth, straight edges.

Yes   No   **3.** A dressing is applied over a wound to control bleeding and prevent contamination.

Yes   No   **4.** A bandage is also applied over a wound to hold a dressing in place.

Yes   No   **5.** Any wound can become infected.

Yes   No   **6.** The signs and symptoms of an infection include swelling and redness around the wound, throbbing pain, and a lack of fever.

Yes   No   **7.** A bite wound is more likely to become infected.

Yes   No   **8.** Impaled objects should be removed immediately.

Yes   No   **9.** Tetanus is communicable from one person to another.

Yes   No   **10.** In many cases, an amputated extremity can be successfully reattached.

Burns

▶ Types of Burns

Burn injuries can be classified as thermal (heat), chemical, or electrical.

- Not all **thermal (heat) burns** are caused by flames. Contact with hot objects, flammable vapor that ignites and causes a flash or an explosion, and steam and hot liquid are other common causes of burns. Just 3 seconds of exposure to water at 140°F can cause a full-thickness (third-degree) burn in an adult. At 156°F, the same burn occurs in 1 second.
- **Chemical burns**. A wide range of chemical agents can cause tissue damage and death on contact with the skin. As with thermal burns, the amount of tissue damage depends on the duration of contact, the skin thickness in the area of exposure, and the strength of the chemical agent. Chemicals will continue to cause tissue destruction until the chemical agent is removed. Three types of chemicals—acids, alkalis, and organic compounds—are responsible for most chemical burns. Alkalis produce deeper, more extensive burns than acids.
- **Electrical burns**. The injury severity from contact with electric current depends on the type of current (direct or alternating), the voltage, the area of the body exposed, and the duration of contact. Electricity can induce ventricular fibrillation (a type of cardiac arrest), cause respiratory arrest, or "freeze" the victim to the electrical contact point with

powerful muscle spasms that increase the length of exposure. Victims of low-voltage electrical injuries may have no skin burns at all but might still have cardiac or respiratory arrest.

Thermal Burns

Evaluate a thermal burn using the following steps. These steps form the basis for treatment of thermal burns.

1. **Determine the depth (degree) of the burn**. Historically, burns have been described as first-degree, second-degree, and third-degree injuries. The terms *superficial*, *partial thickness*, and *full thickness* are often used by burn-care professionals because they are more descriptive of the tissue damage.

   - **First-degree (superficial) burns** affect the skin's outer layer (epidermis) 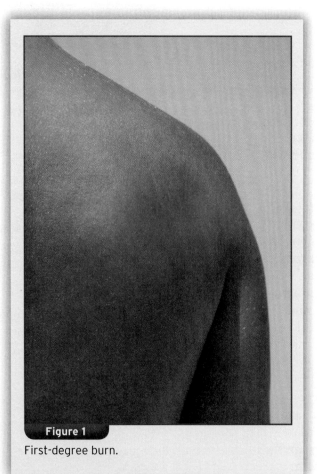. Signs and symptoms include: redness, mild swelling, tenderness, and pain. Healing occurs without scarring,

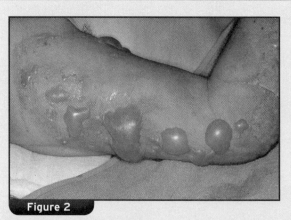
Figure 2
Second-degree burn blisters.

usually within a week. The outer edges of deeper burns often are first-degree burns.

   - **Second-degree (partial-thickness) burns** extend through the entire outer layer and into the inner skin layer **Figure 2**. Signs and symptoms include: blisters, swelling, weeping of fluids, and severe pain. The signs occur because the capillary blood vessels in the dermis are damaged and give up fluid into surrounding tissues. Intact blisters provide a sterile, waterproof covering. Once a blister breaks, a weeping wound results, and the risk of infection increases.

   - **Third-degree (full-thickness) burns** are severe burns that penetrate all the skin layers into the underlying fat and muscle **Figure 3**. Signs and symptoms include: leathery, waxy, or pearly gray skin that is sometimes charred. It has a dry appearance because capillary blood vessels have been destroyed and no more fluid is brought to the area. The skin does not blanch after being pressed because the area is dead. The victim feels no pain from a third-degree burn because the nerve endings have been damaged or destroyed. Any pain felt is from surrounding burns of lesser degrees. A third-degree burn requires medical care and the removal of dead tissue and often a skin graft to heal properly.

2. **Determine the extent of the burn.** Skin will not ignite unless heated to thousands of

Figure 1
First-degree burn.

degrees. However, if clothing ignites or skin is kept in contact with a heat source, such as scalding water, large areas of the skin will be injured. Determining the extent of a burn means estimating how much body surface area the burn covers. A rough guide known as the rule of nines assigns a percentage value of total body surface area (BSA) to each part of an adult's body **Figure 4**. The entire head is 9%, one complete arm is 9%, the front torso is 18%, the complete back is 18%, and each leg is 18%. The rule of nines must be modified to take into account the different proportions of a small child. In small children and infants, the head accounts for 18% and each leg is 14%. For small or scattered burns, use the rule of the hand **Figure 5**. The victim's hand, including the fingers and the thumb held together, represents about 1% of his or her total body surface. For a very large burn, estimate the unburned area in number of hands and subtract from 100%.

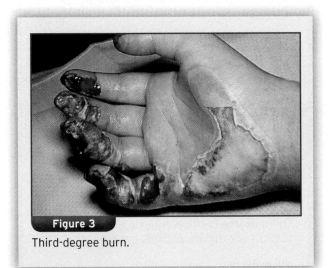

Figure 3
Third-degree burn.

3. **Determine which parts of the body are burned**. Burns on the face, hands, feet, and genitals are more severe than those on other body parts. A circumferential burn (one that goes around a finger, toe, arm, leg, neck, or chest) is considered more severe than a noncircumferential one because of the possible constriction and tourniquet effect on circulation and, in some cases, breathing. All of these burns require medical care.

4. **Determine respiratory involvement**. Respiratory tract damage caused by heat associated with a burn can cause death after a victim is hospitalized. Respiratory damage may result from breathing heat or the products of combustion, from being burned by a flame while in a closed space, or from being in an explosion. In these

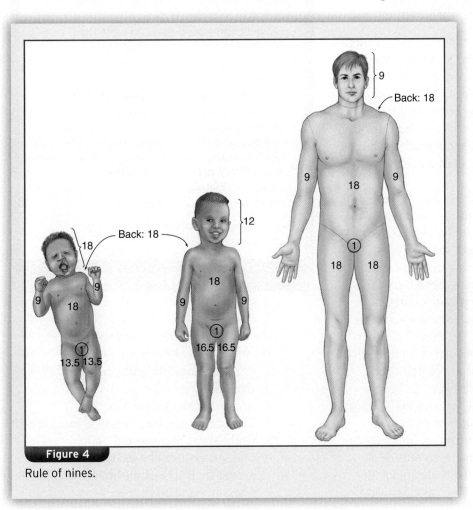

Figure 4
Rule of nines.

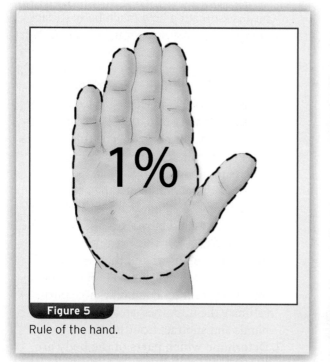

Figure 5
Rule of the hand.

Table 1: Burn Severity

Minor Burns

- First-degree burn covering less than 50% BSA in adults (face, hands, feet, and genitals not burned)*
- Second-degree burn covering less than 10% BSA in adults
- Second-degree burn covering less than 10% BSA in children and elderly persons

Moderate Burns

- First-degree burn covering more than 50% BSA in adults
- Second-degree burn covering 15% to 30% BSA in adults*
- Second-degree burn covering 10% to 20% BSA in children and elderly persons
- Third-degree burn covering up to 10% BSA in adults (face, hands, and feet not burned)

Critical Burns

- Second-degree burn covering more than 30% BSA in adults
- Second-degree burn covering more than 20% BSA in children and elderly persons
- Third-degree burn covering more than 10% BSA in adults
- Third-degree burn covering more than 2% BSA in children and elderly persons
- Third-degree burn of hands, face, eyes, feet, or genitalia; also most inhalation injuries, electrical injuries, and burns accompanied by major trauma or significant preexisting conditions

*Criteria for children have not been established. If in doubt, consult a medical professional.

Source: Adapted from the American Burn Association.

cases, even with no skin burn injury, there may be respiratory damage. Super-heated air is absorbed by the upper respiratory tract (the area from the nose to the trachea), resulting in inflammation. Swelling occurs in 2 to 24 hours, restricting or completely shutting off the airway so that air cannot reach the lungs. All respiratory injuries must receive medical care.

5. **Determine whether other injuries or preexisting medical problems exist or if the victim is elderly (older than 55 years) or very young (younger than 5 years).** A medical problem or being in one of the sensitive age groups increases a burn's severity. Burns can aggravate existing medical conditions such as diabetes, heart disease, and lung disease, as well as other medical problems. Concurrent injuries such as fractures, internal injuries, and open wounds increase the severity of a burn.

6. **Determine the burn's severity** `Table 1`. This forms the basis for how to treat the burned victim. Most burns are minor, occur at home, and can be managed outside a medical setting. Seek medical care for all moderate and severe burns, as classified by the American Burn Association, or if any of the following conditions applies:

- The victim has difficulty breathing
- Other injuries exist
- An electrical injury exists
- The face, hands, feet, or genitals are burned
- Child abuse is suspected
- The surface area of a second-degree burn is greater than 10% of the body surface area
- The burn is third degree

Table 2 First Aid for Burns

Type of Burn	Do . . .	Don't . . .
First-degree burn (redness, mild swelling, and pain)	Apply cold water and, after cooled, apply aloe vera gel or a body lotion.	Apply butter, oleomargarine, or similar substances.
Second-degree burn (deeper injury; blisters develop)	Apply cold water. After cooled, apply antibiotic ointment. Treat for shock.	Break blisters. Remove shreds of tissue. Use a home remedy.
Third-degree burn (deeper destruction; skin layers destroyed)	Cover the burn with a sterile cloth to protect it. Treat the victim for shock. Watch for breathing difficulty. Obtain medical attention quickly.	Remove charred clothing that is stuck to the burn. Apply ice. Use a home medication.
Chemical burn	Remove chemical by flushing with large quantities of water for at least 20 minutes. Remove surrounding clothing. Quickly obtain medical care.	Apply water under high pressure. Try to neutralize with other chemicals.

Q&A

What is the rule of the palm?
The rule of the palm says that a person's palm surface represents 1% of the BSA, but in actuality, it represents about 0.4%. The entire hand including the closed fingers and thumb represents about 0.8%. This textbook suggests using the rule of the hand–using the entire hand, including the closed fingers and thumb–as an easy method to estimate the extent of a burned area. The extent of a burn is calculated only on people with partial-thickness or full-thickness burns.

CAUTION

DO NOT remove clothing stuck to the skin. Cut around the areas where clothing sticks to the skin.

DO NOT pull on stuck clothing; pulling will further damage the skin.

Care for Thermal Burns

Burn care aims to reduce pain, to provide physical protection, and to provide a favorable environment for healing that minimizes the chances of scarring and infection Table 2 . Because burns can continue to injure tissue for a surprisingly long time, it is critical to stop the burning. If clothing is burning, have the victim roll on the ground using the "stop, drop, and roll" method. Smother the flames with a blanket or douse the victim with water. Stop a person whose clothes are on fire from running, which only fans the flames. The victim should not remain standing, because he or she is more apt to inhale flames. Once the fire is extinguished, remove all hot or smoldering clothing because the burning may continue if the clothing is left on. If possible, remove jewelry because heat may be held near the skin and cause more damage. Swelling could make jewelry difficult to remove later. Monitor the victim's breathing.

Care for First-Degree Burns
1. Run cold tap water (60° to 77°F [15° to 25°C]) over the area as soon as possible Figure 6 or apply a wet, cold cloth to reduce pain. Apply cold until the part is pain free while in and out of the water (usually in 10 minutes, but it may take up to 45 minutes). Cold stops the progression of the burn into deeper tissue. If cold water is unavailable, use any cold, drinkable liquid to reduce the temperature of the burned skin.
2. Give ibuprofen to relieve pain and inflammation.

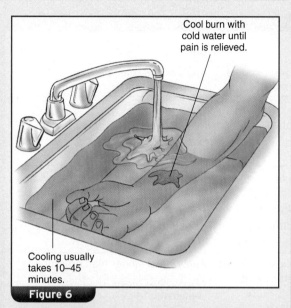

Cool burn with cold water until pain is relieved.

Cooling usually takes 10–45 minutes.

Figure 6

Immerse the burn. Cool burn with cold water until pain is relieved. Cooling usually takes 10-45 minutes.

Q&A

When cooling a burn, how cold should the water be and how long should cooling last?

Immediately cool the burn with cold—but not ice-cold—water. Cooling of burns has many beneficial effects, including pain relief, reduced swelling, reduced depth of the burn, and more rapid healing. Although cooling should begin as soon as possible, delayed cooling may still be beneficial. Studies recommend various temperatures and durations. Optimal healing involves temperatures of 60°F to 77°F (20°C to 25°C). Other studies have water temperature ranging from 50°F to 59°F (10°C to 15°C). Typical cold water available in North American homes ranges from 50°F to 59°F (10°C to 15°C).

The duration of cooling is controversial, but cooling should continue at least until the pain is relieved and probably for a total duration of 15 to 30 minutes. Whenever using any cold water for a burn, monitor for hypothermia (ie, shivering and cold skin on unburned areas). Although brief exposure to ice or ice water may be beneficial, prolonged cooling may cause additional injury.

3. Have the victim drink as much water as possible without becoming nauseous.

4. After the burn has been cooled, apply an aloe vera gel or an inexpensive skin moisturizer lotion to keep the skin moistened and to reduce itching and peeling. Use a lotion that does not have alcohols or strong fragrances. Lotions with glycerin and mineral oil are best. Aloe vera has antimicrobial and anti-inflammatory properties and is a mild analgesic.

5. Keep a burned arm or leg raised to reduce swelling and pain.

Care for Small Second-Degree Burns (<20% BSA)

1. Run cold tap water (60° to 77°F [15° to 25°C]) over the area as soon as possible or apply a wet, cold cloth to reduce pain. Apply cold until the part is pain free while in and out of the water (usually in 10 minutes, but it may take up to 45 minutes). Cold stops the progression of the burn into deeper tissue. If cold water is unavailable, use any cold, drinkable liquid to reduce the temperature of the burned skin.

2. Give ibuprofen to relieve pain and inflammation.

3. Have the victim drink as much water as possible without becoming nauseated.

4. After a burn has been cooled, apply a thin layer of an antibiotic ointment. Topical antibiotic therapy does not sterilize a wound, but it decreases the number of bacteria to a level that can be controlled by the body's defense mechanisms and prevents the entrance of bacteria. Physicians may prescribe a silver-based antibiotic, which is the agent of choice for burn wounds.

5. Cover the burn with a dry, nonstick, sterile dressing or a clean cloth. Covering the burn reduces the amount of pain by keeping air from the exposed nerve endings. The main

CAUTION

DO NOT apply cold over a large burn for a prolonged time because it can produce hypothermia.

DO NOT use an ice pack or ice water unless it is the only source of cold available. If you must use it, apply it for only 10 to 15 minutes.

DO NOT apply grease, butter, cream, or a home remedy. Such coatings are unsterile and can lead to infection. They also can seal in heat, causing further damage.

DO NOT cover a first-degree burn.

purpose of a dressing over a burn is to keep the burn clean, prevent evaporative moisture loss, and reduce pain. If fingers or toes have been burned, place dry dressings between them and seek medical care.

6. Seek medical care for second-degree burns covering more than 10% of the BSA.

Care for Large Second-Degree Burns (>20% BSA)
1. Cold can be applied if you monitor the victim for hypothermia (eg, shivering, cold skin on unburned areas).
2. Follow steps 2 and 3 for first-degree and small second-degree burn care.
3. Cover the burn with a dry, nonstick, sterile, or clean dressing.
4. Treat for shock.
5. Seek medical care.

Care for Third-Degree Burns
1. Cover the burn with a dry, nonstick, sterile dressing or a clean cloth.
2. Treat the victim for shock and keep the victim warm with a clean sheet or blanket.
3. Seek medical care.

Later Thermal Burn Care

For after-thermal burn care, follow a physician's recommendations, if a physician has been consulted (many burns are never seen by a doctor). The following suggestions may apply:
- Wash hands thoroughly before changing any dressing.
- Leave unbroken blisters intact.
- Change dressings once or twice a day unless a physician instructs otherwise.

To change a dressing:
1. Remove the old dressing. If a dressing sticks, soak it off with cool, clean water.
2. Cleanse the area gently with mild soap and water.
3. Pat the area dry with a clean cloth.
4. Apply a thin layer of antibiotic ointment to the burn.

CAUTION

DO NOT cool more than 20% of an adult's body surface area (10% for a child) except to extinguish flames.

CAUTION

DO NOT break any blisters. Intact blisters serve as excellent burn dressings. Cover a ruptured blister with an antibiotic ointment and a dry, sterile dressing.

DO NOT use plastic as a dressing because it will trap moisture and provide a good place for bacteria to grow (its only advantage is that it will not stick to the burn).

5. Apply a nonstick sterile dressing.

Watch for signs of infection. Call a physician if any of these appear:
- Increased redness, pain, tenderness, swelling, or red streaks near the burn
- Pus
- Elevated temperature (fever)

Keep the area and dressing as clean and dry as possible. Elevate the burned area, if possible, for the first 24 hours. Give pain medication, if necessary.

Chemical Burns

A *chemical burn* is the result of an acid or an alkali substance touching the skin **Figure 7**. Because chemicals continue to "burn" as long as they are in contact with the skin, they should be removed from the victim as rapidly as possible.

First aid is the same for all chemical burns. Alkalis such as drain cleaners cause more serious burns than acids such as battery acid because they penetrate deeper and remain active longer. Organic compounds such as petroleum products are also capable of burning.

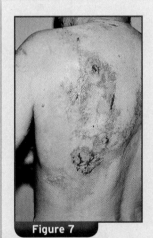

Figure 7

Chemical burn from sulfuric acid.

Care for Chemical Burns
1. Immediately remove the chemical by flushing the body portion with water **Figure 8**. If available, use a hose or a shower. Brush dry powder chemicals from the skin before

Thermal Burns

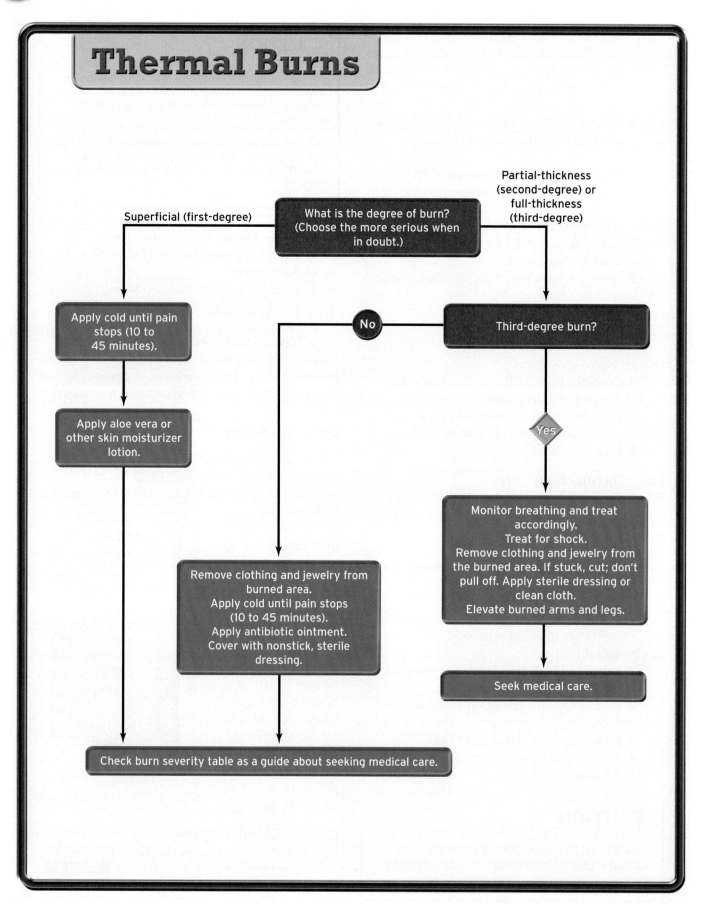

What is the degree of burn? (Choose the more serious when in doubt.)

Superficial (first-degree)

Partial-thickness (second-degree) or full-thickness (third-degree)

Apply cold until pain stops (10 to 45 minutes).

Apply aloe vera or other skin moisturizer lotion.

No — Third-degree burn?

Yes

Monitor breathing and treat accordingly.
Treat for shock.
Remove clothing and jewelry from the burned area. If stuck, cut; don't pull off. Apply sterile dressing or clean cloth.
Elevate burned arms and legs.

Remove clothing and jewelry from burned area.
Apply cold until pain stops (10 to 45 minutes).
Apply antibiotic ointment.
Cover with nonstick, sterile dressing.

Seek medical care.

Check burn severity table as a guide about seeking medical care.

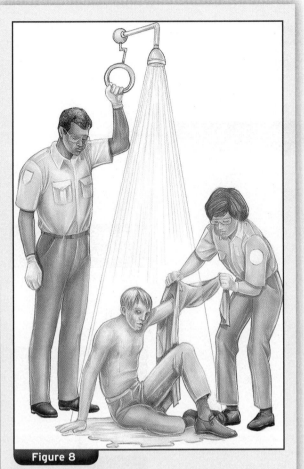

Figure 8

Flushing a chemical burn.

CAUTION

DO NOT use topical OTC burn ointments or sprays or anesthetic sprays because:

- Some products may cause allergic reactions.
- Most do not contain enough benzocaine or lidocaine to suppress pain.
- The duration of any possible relief is relatively short (30 to 40 minutes). More than three or four applications per day of products containing local anesthetics is discouraged because toxic effects can occur if the agents are used too frequently.
- They seal in the heat.
- They are expensive.

flushing. Water may activate a dry chemical and cause more damage to the skin. Take standard precautions to protect yourself from exposure to the chemical.

CAUTION

DO NOT waste time! A chemical burn is an emergency!

DO NOT apply water under high pressure; it will drive the chemical deeper into the tissue.

DO NOT try to neutralize a chemical even if you know which chemical is involved; heat may be produced, resulting in more damage. Some product labels for neutralizing may be wrong. Save the container or the label for the chemical's name.

2. Remove the victim's contaminated clothing and jewelry while flushing with water. Clothing can hold chemicals, allowing them to continue to burn as long as they are in contact with the skin.
3. Flush for 20 minutes or longer. Let the victim wash with a mild soap before a final rinse. Washing with large amounts of water dilutes the chemical concentration and washes it away.
4. Cover the burned area with a dry, sterile dressing or, for large areas, a clean lint-free cloth, such as a pillowcase.
5. If the chemical is in an eye, flood it for at least 20 minutes, using a gentle stream of water.
6. Seek medical care immediately for all chemical burns.

Electrical Burns

Even a mild electrical shock can cause serious internal injuries **Figure 9** . A current of 1,000 volts or more is considered high voltage, but even the 110 volts found in ordinary household current can be deadly. There are three types of electrical injuries: *thermal burn* (flame), arc burn (flash), and true electrical injury (contact). A thermal burn (flame) results when clothing or objects in direct contact with the skin are ignited by an electric current. These injuries are caused by the flames produced by the electric current and not by the passage of the electric current or arc.

An *arc burn* (flash) occurs when electricity jumps, or arcs, from one spot to another and not from the passage of an electric current through the body. Although the duration of the flash may be brief, it usually causes extensive superficial injuries.

Chemical Burns

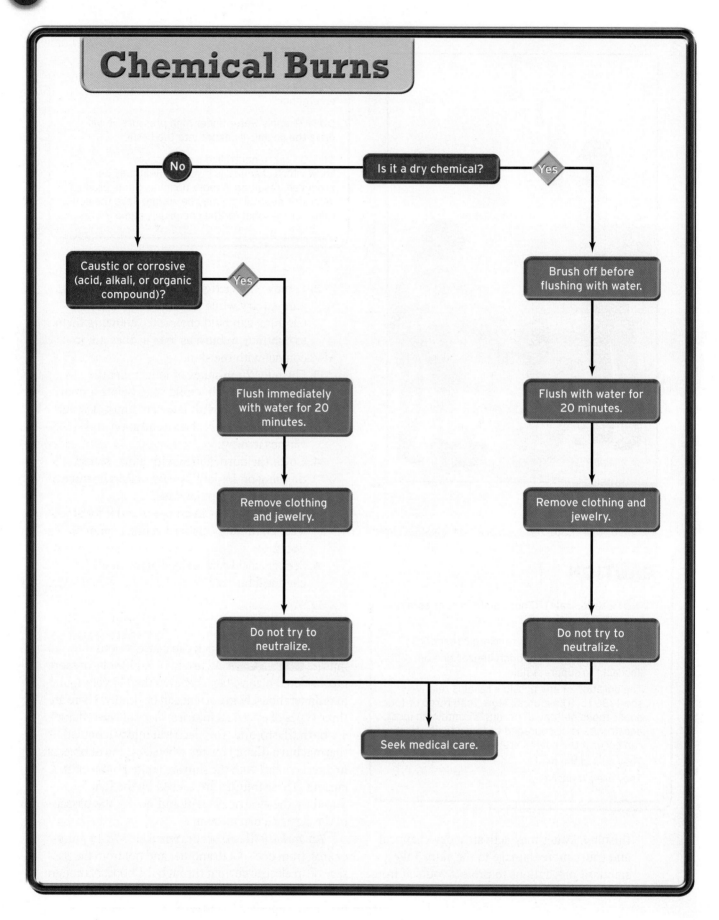

Is it a dry chemical?

No → Caustic or corrosive (acid, alkali, or organic compound)?

Yes → Flush immediately with water for 20 minutes. → Remove clothing and jewelry. → Do not try to neutralize.

Yes → Brush off before flushing with water. → Flush with water for 20 minutes. → Remove clothing and jewelry. → Do not try to neutralize.

Seek medical care.

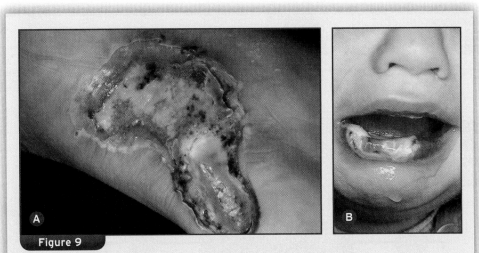

Figure 9

Electrical burns. **A.** Exit wound on a foot. **B.** Electrical burn caused by chewing through an electrical cord.

A true *electrical injury* (contact) happens when an electric current passes directly through the body. This type of injury is characterized by an entrance wound and an exit wound. The important factor with this type of injury is that the surface injury may be just the tip of the iceberg. High-voltage electric currents passing through the body may disrupt the normal heart rhythm and cause cardiac arrest, internal burns, and other injuries.

During an electrical shock, electricity enters the body at the point of contact and travels along the path of least resistance (nerves and blood vessels). The major damage occurs inside the body—the entrance burn may appear small. Usually, the electricity exits where the body is touching a surface or is in contact with a ground (for example, a metal object). The exit wound can be extensive. Sometimes, a victim has more than one exit site.

Care for Electrical Burns

1. Make sure the area is safe. Unplug, disconnect, or turn off the power. If that is impossible, call 9-1-1 for help. Never touch an energized wire, object, or victim yourself.
2. Check breathing and, if absent, begin CPR.
3. If the victim fell, check for a spinal injury.
4. Treat the victim for shock.
5. Place dry, sterile dressings on all burn wounds.
6. Place blankets under and over the victim.
7. Seek medical care immediately. Electrical injuries may require treatment in a burn center.

Contact With an Outdoor Power Line

If the electrical shock is from contact with a downed power line, the power must be turned off before a rescuer approaches anyone who may be in contact with the wire. If a power line falls across a car containing a person, tell the person to stay in the car until the power can be shut off. The only exception is if fire threatens the car. In that case, tell the victim to jump out of the car without making contact with the car or the wire.

If you feel a tingling sensation in your legs and lower body as you approach a victim, stop. The sensation signals that you are on energized ground and that an electric current is entering through one foot, passing through your lower body, and leaving through the other foot. Raise one foot off the ground, turn around, and hop to a safe place.

If you can safely reach the victim, do not attempt to move any wires, even with wooden poles, tools with wood handles, or tree branches. Wood can conduct electricity and the rescuer will be electrocuted. Do not attempt to move downed wires unless you are trained and equipped with tools able to handle the high voltage. Wait until trained personnel with the proper equipment can cut the wires or disconnect them. Prevent bystanders from entering the danger area.

Contact Inside Buildings

Most electrical burns that occur indoors are caused by faulty electrical equipment or careless use of electrical appliances. Turn off the electricity at the circuit breaker, fuse box, or outside switch box, or unplug the appliance if the plug is undamaged. Do not touch the appliance or the victim until the current is off.

Once there is no danger to rescuers, first aid can begin. Electric current flows quickly into the body's tissues and then exits. The surface injuries of the skin involve small surface areas (entrance and exit points); the major damage occurs deep under the skin **Figure 10** .

Electrical Burns

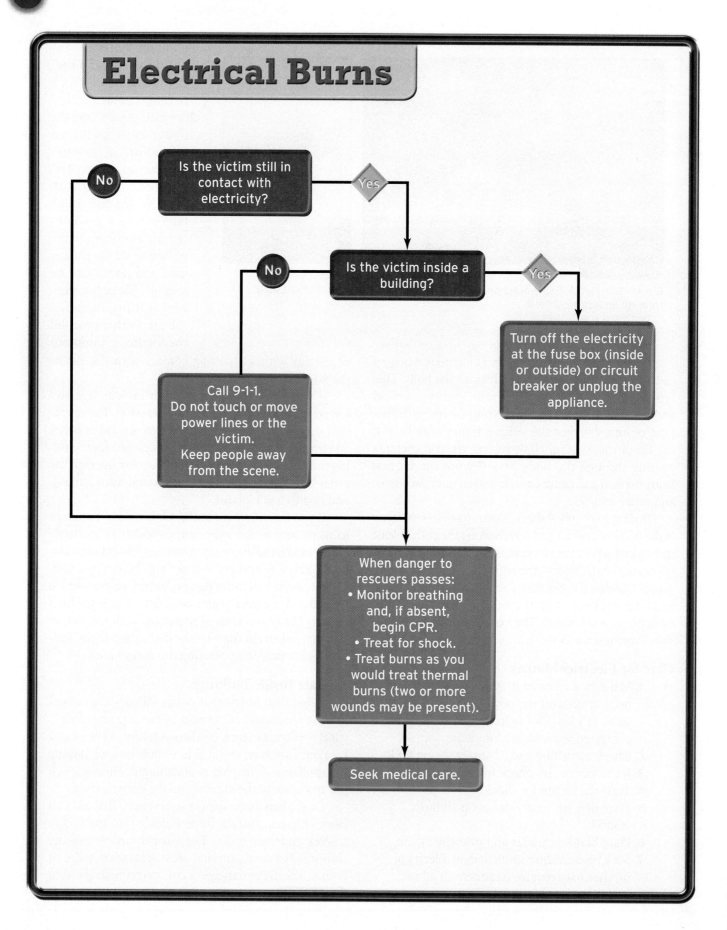

No ← Is the victim still in contact with electricity? → **Yes**

No ← Is the victim inside a building? → **Yes**

Turn off the electricity at the fuse box (inside or outside) or circuit breaker or unplug the appliance.

Call 9-1-1.
Do not touch or move power lines or the victim.
Keep people away from the scene.

When danger to rescuers passes:
• Monitor breathing and, if absent, begin CPR.
• Treat for shock.
• Treat burns as you would treat thermal burns (two or more wounds may be present).

Seek medical care.

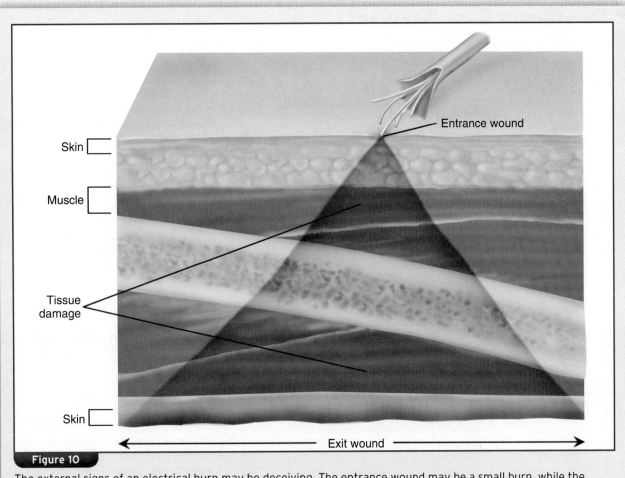

Skin

Muscle

Tissue damage

Entrance wound

Skin

Exit wound

Figure 10

The external signs of an electrical burn may be deceiving. The entrance wound may be a small burn, while the damage to deeper tissue may be massive.

▶ Emergency Care Wrap-up

Condition	What to Look For	What to Do
Thermal (Heat) Burns	First-degree burn (superficial) Redness Mild swelling Pain	Cool the burn with cold water. Apply aloe vera gel or a skin moisturizer. If available, give an OTC medication to reduce pain and swelling.
	Second-degree burn (partial thickness) Blisters Swelling Pain Weeping of fluid	Cool burn with cold water and monitor victims with large, second-degree burns for hypothermia. Apply antibiotic ointment. Cover with a dry, nonstick sterile dressing. If available, give an OTC medication to reduce pain and swelling. Seek medical care.
	Third-degree burn (full thickness) Dry, leathery skin Gray or charred skin	Monitor breathing and provide care as needed. Cover burn with a dry, nonstick sterile, or clean dressing. Treat for shock. Seek medical care.
Chemical Burns	Stinging pain	Brush dry chemicals off skin. Flush with a large amount of water for 20 minutes (gentle water flow). Remove the victim's contaminated clothing and jewelry while flushing. Cover the area with a dry, sterile, or clean dressing. Seek medical care.
Electrical Burns	Possible third-degree burn with entrance and exit wounds	Safety first! Unplug, disconnect, or turn off the electricity. Open the airway, check breathing, and provide care as needed. Care for burns as you would a third-degree burn. Seek medical care.

▶ Ready for Review

- Burns occur in every age group; across all socioeconomic levels; at home and in the workplace; and in urban, suburban, and rural settings.
- Burn injuries can be classified as thermal, chemical, or electrical.
- Treatment depends on the depth of burns.
- A chemical burn is the result of a caustic or corrosive substance touching the skin.
- There are three types of electrical injuries: thermal burn (flame), arc burn (flash), and true electrical injury (contact).

▶ Vital Vocabulary

chemical burns Damage caused to the skin by chemicals.

electrical burns Injury caused from contact with electric current.

first-degree (superficial) burns Burns affecting only the epidermis. Characterized by skin that is red but not blistered or burned through.

second-degree (partial-thickness) burns Burns affecting the epidermis and some portion of the dermis but not the subcutaneous tissue. Characterized by blisters and skin that is white to red and moist.

thermal (heat) burns Damage to the skin caused by contact with hot objects, flammable vapor, steam, hot liquid, or flames.

third-degree (full-thickness) burns Burns that affect all skin layers and may affect the subcutaneous layers, muscle, bone, and internal organs, leaving the area dry, leathery, and white, dark brown, or charred.

▶ Assessment in Action

After a long, hot day at the water park, your friend complains of severe sunburn on his back and shoulders. He failed to apply sunscreen while at the water park. Blisters have formed, and your friend refuses to sit up in a chair and complains of severe pain.

Directions: Circle Yes if you agree with the statement; circle No if you disagree.

Yes No 1. The blisters and pain are signs that this is a first-degree burn.

Yes No 2. You should break the blisters to relieve pressure and clean the burn.

Yes No 3. Cool compresses can be used to relieve pain.

Yes No 4. You can apply antibiotic ointment and aloe vera to keep the skin moist.

Yes No 5. This person does not need medical care.

▶ Check Your Knowledge

Directions: Circle Yes if you agree with the statement; circle No if you disagree.

Yes No 1. Victims of a burn should immediately drink water.

Yes No 2. Petroleum jelly can be applied over a burn.

Yes No 3. The rule of the hand can help determine the size of a burned area.

Yes No 4. Neutralize an acid on the skin by using baking soda.

Yes No 5. Use a large amount of water to flush chemicals off the body.

Yes No 6. Brush a dry chemical off the skin before flushing with water.

Yes No 7. When someone gets electrocuted, there can be two burn wounds: entrance and exit.

Yes No 8. When a victim is in contact with a power line, use a tree branch to remove the wires.

Yes No 9. Ibuprofen helps relieve pain and swelling.

Yes No 10. Cold water can be used, in moderation, on any burn of any size.

Head and Spinal Injuries

chapter
at a glance

Head Injuries

Any head injury is potentially serious. If not properly treated, injuries that seem minor could become life threatening. Head injuries include scalp wounds, skull fractures, and brain injuries. Spinal injuries (that is, neck and back injuries) can also be present in head-injured victims.

▶ Scalp Wounds

Scalp wounds bleed profusely because the scalp has many blood vessels. A bleeding scalp wound does not affect the blood supply to the brain. The brain obtains its blood supply from arteries in the neck, not the scalp. A severe scalp wound may have an accompanying concussion, skull fracture, an impaled object, a brain injury or a spinal injury.

Care for Scalp Wounds

1. Control the bleeding by applying direct pressure with a dry, sterile or clean dressing. If the dressing becomes blood filled, do not remove it. Add another dressing on top of the first one **Figure 1** .
2. If you suspect a skull fracture, apply pressure around the edges of the wound and over a broad area rather than on the center of the wound **Figure 2** .

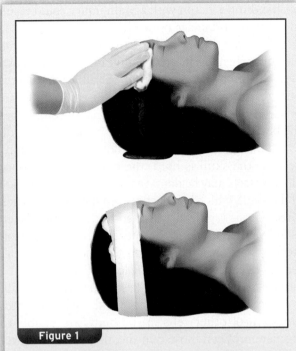

Figure 1

Apply direct pressure with a dry, sterile dressing to control the bleeding.

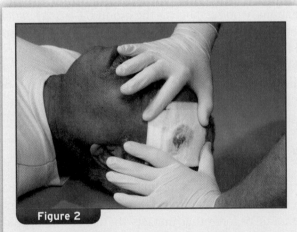

Figure 2

Apply pressure around the edges of the wound to control bleeding from a suspected skull fracture.

3. Keep the head and shoulders slightly elevated to help control the bleeding if no spinal injury is suspected.
4. Seek medical care.

▶ Skull Fracture

A **skull fracture** is a break or a crack in the cranium (bony case surrounding the brain). Skull fractures may be open (with an accompanying scalp laceration) or closed (without an accompanying scalp laceration).

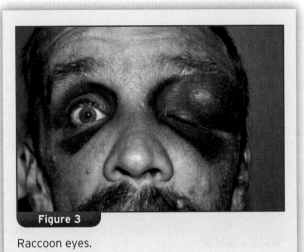

Figure 3

Raccoon eyes.

Recognizing Skull Fracture

It is difficult to determine a skull fracture except by X-ray or a CT scan unless the skull deformity is severe. Signs and symptoms of a skull fracture include the following:

- Pain at the point of injury
- Deformity of the skull
- Bleeding from the ears or nose
- Clear, pink, watery cerebrospinal fluid (CSF) leaking from an ear or the nose. A drop of CSF on a handkerchief, pillowcase, or other white or light-colored cloth will form a pink ring around a slightly blood-tinged center, resembling a target; this is called the halo sign (ring sign).
- Discoloration around the eyes ("raccoon eyes") appearing several hours after the injury **Figure 3** .
- Discoloration behind an ear (known as **Battle's sign**), appearing several hours after the injury **Figure 4** .
- Heavy scalp bleeding if the skin is broken. A scalp wound may expose the skull or brain tissue.
- Penetrating wound such as from a bullet or an impaled object.

Care for Skull Fracture

1. Monitor the victim's breathing and, if absent, begin CPR.
2. Stabilize the victim's neck to prevent movement.
3. Keep the head and shoulders slightly elevated if no spinal injury is suspected.

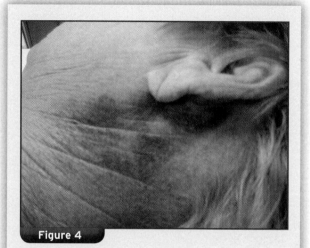

Figure 4

Battle's sign.

| **CAUTION** |

DO NOT stop the flow of blood or CSF from an ear or nose. Blocking the flow could increase pressure within the skull.

DO NOT remove an impaled object from the head. Stabilize it in place with bulky dressings.

DO NOT clean an open skull fracture; infection of the brain could result.

DO NOT press on the fractured area.

4. Cover the wounds with a sterile dressing.
5. To control bleeding, apply pressure around the edges of the wound, not directly on it.

▶ Brain Injuries

It is not injury specifically to the head that causes most short- and long-term problems, but injuries to the brain itself. Most head injuries are a result of motor vehicle crashes and falls. Many of these injuries are minor—shallow lacerations or localized bruising and swelling. However, about 50,000 people die each year in the United States of head trauma, and twice that many have brain injuries that leave them with permanent damage.

The brain is a delicate organ. When the head is struck with sufficient force, the brain bounces against the inside of the skull. Brain injuries can be serious and difficult first aid emergencies to handle. The victim is often confused or unresponsive, making assessment difficult. Many brain injuries are life threatening.

Mishandling a victim with a brain injury could result in permanent damage or death.

The brain, like other body tissues, will swell from bleeding when it is injured. Unlike other tissues, however, the brain is confined in the skull where there is little room for swelling. Any swelling of brain tissue or accumulation of blood inside the skull compresses the brain and increases the pressure inside the skull, which interferes with brain functioning. Furthermore, because the skull is hard, the brain and its surface blood vessels may be damaged if they strike the inside of the skull, which can occur when the head is struck directly or is rapidly accelerated or decelerated (such as in a vehicle accident). The phenomenon of a person "seeing stars" when struck on the back of the head results because the occipital lobe of the brain (the part that controls vision) strikes the back of the skull.

The nerve cells of the brain and the spinal cord, unlike most other cells in the body, are unable to regenerate. When those cells die, they are lost forever and cannot be replaced. Injuries to the brain can be caused by a penetrating foreign object, by bony fragments from a skull fracture, or by the brain striking the inside of the skull after a person's head has hit a stationary object (such as the ground)—a *deceleration* injury—or has been hit by something like a baseball bat or a teammate's knee—an *acceleration* injury. Sometimes there will be two points of injury: one at the point of impact and one where the brain rebounds off the skull on the opposite side.

▶ Types of Brain Injury

All brain injuries are unique. The brain can receive several types of injuries depending on the type and amount of force that impacts the head. The type of injury the brain receives may affect just one functional area of the brain, various areas, or even the entire brain. Two types of brain injury are traumatic brain injury and acquired brain injury.

Traumatic Brain Injury

The following sections on traumatic brain injury are adapted from Centers for Disease Control and Prevention, National Injury and Violence Prevention.

Concussion

A **concussion** is considered a mild traumatic brain injury (MTBI) and occurs when a blow to the head alters the function of the brain Table 1 .

Table 1 Symptoms of MTBI

Thinking/Remembering

- Difficulty thinking clearly
- Feeling slowed down
- Difficulty concentrating
- Difficulty remembering new information

Physical

- Headache
- Nausea or vomiting (early on)
- Balance problems
- Dizziness
- Fuzzy or blurry vision
- Feeling tired, having no energy
- Sensitivity to noise or light

Emotional/Mood

- Irritability
- Sadness
- More emotional
- Nervousness or anxiety

Sleep Disturbance

- Sleeping more than usual
- Sleeping less than usual
- Trouble falling asleep

Source: Centers for Disease Control and Prevention, National Center for Injury Prevention and Control

FYI

Suspect a Concussion (MTBI)

- High-speed activities (motor vehicle crashes, bicycle riding, skateboarding)
- Sports and recreation activities
- Falls (including those among older adults), especially from a significant distance (eg, off a ladder, from a tree)
- Suspected child maltreatment (eg, shaking, hitting, throwing)
- Exposure to blasts (including military personnel returning from war zones)
- Injuries to the external parts of the head and/or scalp (eg, lacerations) and orthopaedic injuries (eg, fractures, dislocations)

Source: Centers for Disease Control and Prevention, U.S. Department of Health and Human Services. Heads Up: Facts for Physicians about Mild Traumatic Brain Injury (MTBI). (5) (Accessed January 14, 2011: http://www.cdc.gov/concussion/headsup/pdf/Facts_for_Physicians_booklet-a.pdf)

Recovery from a concussion can last anywhere from several minutes to days, weeks, months, or even longer. Children, adolescents, and older adults tend to take longer to recover than adults. Concussion victims who have already experienced previous concussions may need increased recovery time as well. Although most concussion victims make a full recovery, it is possible for victims to experience post-concussion syndrome, in which concussion symptoms last longer than 3 months.

Sometimes additional problems can occur in a concussion victim. A concussion victim experiencing any of the following signs and symptoms may have a blood clot that is pushing the brain against the skull:

- Loss of consciousness, even if brief
- Persistent, worsening headache
- Weakness, numbness, or decreased coordination
- Vomiting or nausea
- Slurred speech
- Very drowsy or cannot be awakened
- Increasingly confused, restless, or agitated
- Unusual behavior
- One pupil larger than the other
- Convulsions or seizures
- Inability to recognize people or places
- Will not stop crying and cannot be consoled (child)
- Will not nurse or eat (child)

Victims experiencing any of these signs and symptoms should seek immediate medical care.

If the victim is wearing a helmet, such as a motorcycle or football helmet, it should not be removed by a first aider unless:

- You suspect an obstructed airway.
- The helmet is so loose that you cannot stabilize the spine.

If the helmet must be removed to provide lifesaving care of an airway problem, make sure to stabilize the head and neck as the helmet is carefully removed.

Other Traumatic Brain Injuries

Other types of traumatic brain injuries include the following:

- <u>Contusion</u>: A direct blow to the head can cause a bruise to the brain.
- Coup-contrecoup: A blow to the head is strong enough to cause a contusion at the site of impact, as well as move the brain, causing it to hit the opposite side of the skull. This second hit causes a second contusion.
- Diffuse axonal: Shaking or strong rotation of the head causes this tearing injury. One example of diffuse axonal injury is Shaken Baby Syndrome.
- Penetration: Objects such as a bullet, knife, or other sharp object enters the brain. The wound is then contaminated by hair, skin, bone, and pieces of the penetrating object. These contaminants may not be retrievable.

Acquired Brain Injuries

Acquired brain injuries are injuries that develop during or after birth and are not due to injuries. This is in contrast to congenital problems, which are due to abnormal brain development before birth. Acquired injuries include infection, stroke, tumors, and anoxia (lack of oxygen). Anoxia can be due to conditions such as respiratory arrest, problems during birth, or drowning. Acquired brain injuries can cause signs and symptoms that are similar to traumatic brain injuries. Care is mainly supportive and requires immediate medical attention.

Further Care

Several signs appearing within 48 hours of a head injury indicate a need to seek medical care.

- **Headache**: Expect a headache. If it lasts more than 1 or 2 days or increases in severity, seek medical advice.
- **Nausea, vomiting**: If nausea lasts more than 2 hours, seek medical advice. Vomiting once or twice, especially in children, may be expected after a head injury. Vomiting does not indicate the severity of the injury. However, if vomiting begins again hours after the initial episodes have ceased, seek medical care.
- **Drowsiness**: Allow a victim to sleep, but wake the victim at least every 2 hours to check the

state of consciousness and sense of orientation by asking his or her name and to use information-processing skills (for example, "Recite the months of the year backward"). If the victim cannot respond or appears confused or disoriented, seek medical advice.

- **Vision problems**: If the victim "sees double," if the eyes do not move together, or if one pupil appears to be larger than the other, seek medical advice.
- **Mobility**: If the victim cannot use his or her arms or legs as well as previously or is unsteady when walking, seek medical care.
- **Speech**: If the victim has slurred speech or is unable to talk, seek medical care.
- **Seizures (convulsions)**: If the victim has a violent involuntary contraction (spasm) or series of contractions of the skeletal muscles, seek medical care.

Eye Injuries

Of all the parts of the human body, an injured eye probably causes the most anxiety and concern in a victim. The eyes—arguably the most important human sense organs—are easily damaged by trauma. A very slight penetration by a metal fragment, for example, means hospitalization. Medical care may include surgery; despite technical advances, blindness or the loss of an eye remains a possibility whenever there is an eye injury. Have an opthamologist or other physician examine the eye as soon as possible, even if an injury seems minor at first.

▶ Penetrating Eye Injuries

Penetrating eye injuries are severe injuries that result when a sharp object, such as a knife or a needle, penetrates the eye. Most penetrating injuries, although not all, are obvious. Suspect penetration any time you see a lid laceration or cut.

Care for Penetrating Eye Injuries

1. Seek immediate medical care. Any penetrating eye injury should be managed in the hospital.
2. Stabilize the object. Stabilize a long, protruding object with bulky dressings or clean

Head Injuries

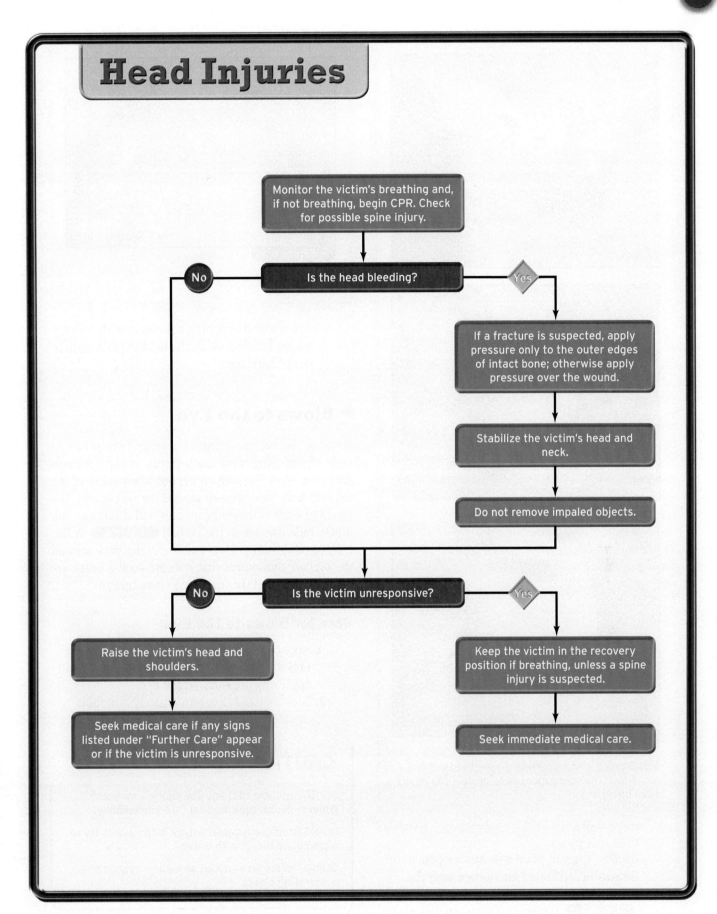

Monitor the victim's breathing and, if not breathing, begin CPR. Check for possible spine injury.

Is the head bleeding?

No

Yes

If a fracture is suspected, apply pressure only to the outer edges of intact bone; otherwise apply pressure over the wound.

Stabilize the victim's head and neck.

Do not remove impaled objects.

Is the victim unresponsive?

No

Yes

Raise the victim's head and shoulders.

Keep the victim in the recovery position if breathing, unless a spine injury is suspected.

Seek medical care if any signs listed under "Further Care" appear or if the victim is unresponsive.

Seek immediate medical care.

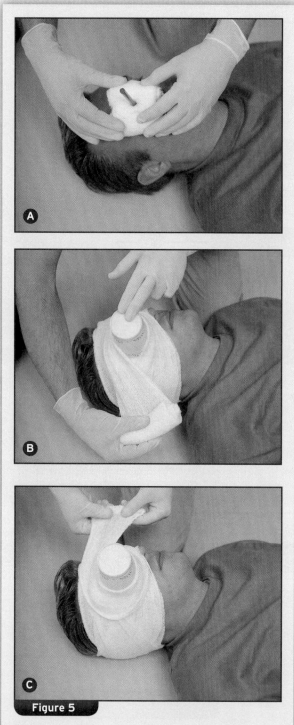

Figure 5

Stabilizing a long, penetrating object against movement (using a paper cup to protect the object from being hit).

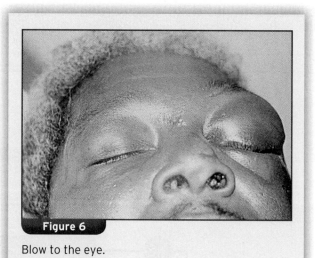

Figure 6

Blow to the eye.

eye without touching the object with roller gauze bandage or cloths held in place with a roller bandage.

▶ Blows to the Eye

Blows to the eye can range in severity from minor to sight threatening. One such injury is the common shiner or black eye, which occurs when some of the many delicate blood vessels around the eye rupture. The bleeding itself is insignificant and will disappear, but it may hide damage to the eyeball **Figure 6**. A fist, ball, or other blunt object can break the bone around the eyeball. Symptoms that indicate such a break are double vision and the inability to look upward.

Care for Blows to the Eye

1. Apply an ice or cold pack for about 15 minutes to reduce the pain and swelling. Do not apply any pressure on the eye.
2. Seek medical care immediately if there is double vision, pain, or reduced vision.

CAUTION

DO NOT assume that any eye injury is innocent. When in doubt, seek medical care immediately.

DO NOT remove an object stuck in the eye or try to wash out an object with water.

DO NOT exert pressure on an injured eyeball or a penetrating object.

cloths. You can place a protective paper cup or cardboard folded into a cone over the affected eye to prevent bumping of the object **Figure 5**. For short objects, surround the

Eyes move in the same direction together, focusing on the same object. This is known as sympathetic eye movement. Therefore, when the uninjured eye moves, the injured eye moves as well. This may aggravate an injury.

To lessen movement in an injured eye:

- Tell the victim to keep the uninjured eye closed.
- Cover the undamaged eye with a cravat or roller bandage.

The victim may become anxious if both eyes are covered and he cannot see. Help overcome anxiety by:

- Explaining everything that you are doing.
- Leaving a small peephole at the bottom of the bandage for the uninjured eye to see through. This keeps the victim's eyes still by allowing the eyes to look in only one direction.

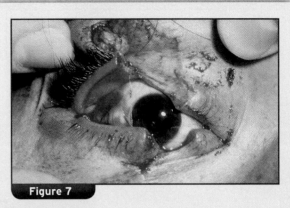

Figure 7

Lacerated eyelid.

▶ Cuts of the Eye or Lid

The signs of a cut eyeball or lid include the following **Figure 7**:

- "Cut" appearance of the cornea (clear part of the eye) or sclera (white part of eye).
- Inner liquid filling of the eye may come out through the wound.
- Lid is cut.

Care for Cuts of the Eye or Lid

1. If the eyeball is cut, do not apply pressure. If only the eyelid is cut, apply a sterile or clean dressing with gentle pressure.
2. Bandage both eyes lightly.
3. Seek medical care immediately.

▶ Chemical in the Eyes

Chemicals in the eyes can threaten sight. First aid may determine the fate of the eye and vision. Alkalis cause greater damage than acids because they penetrate deeper and continue to burn longer. Common alkalis include drain cleaners, cleaning agents, ammonia, cement, plaster, and caustic soda. Common acids include hydrochloric acid, nitric acid, sulfuric (battery) acid, and acetic acid. Because damage can occur in 1 to 5 minutes, the chemical must be removed immediately **Figure 8**.

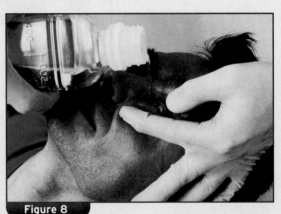

Figure 8

Flushing the eye to treat a chemical burn.

Care for Chemical in the Eye

1. Use your fingers to keep the eye open as widely as possible.
2. Flush the eye with water immediately. If possible, use warm water. If water is not available, use any nonirritating liquid.
   - Hold the victim's head under a faucet or pour water into the eye from any clean container for at least 20 minutes, continuously and gently. It is impossible to use too much water on these injuries.
   - Irrigate from the nose side of the eye toward the outside to avoid flushing the material into the other eye.
   - Tell the victim to roll the eyeball as much as possible to help wash out the eye.
3. Loosely bandage both eyes with cold, wet dressings.
4. Seek immediate medical care.

Eye Injuries

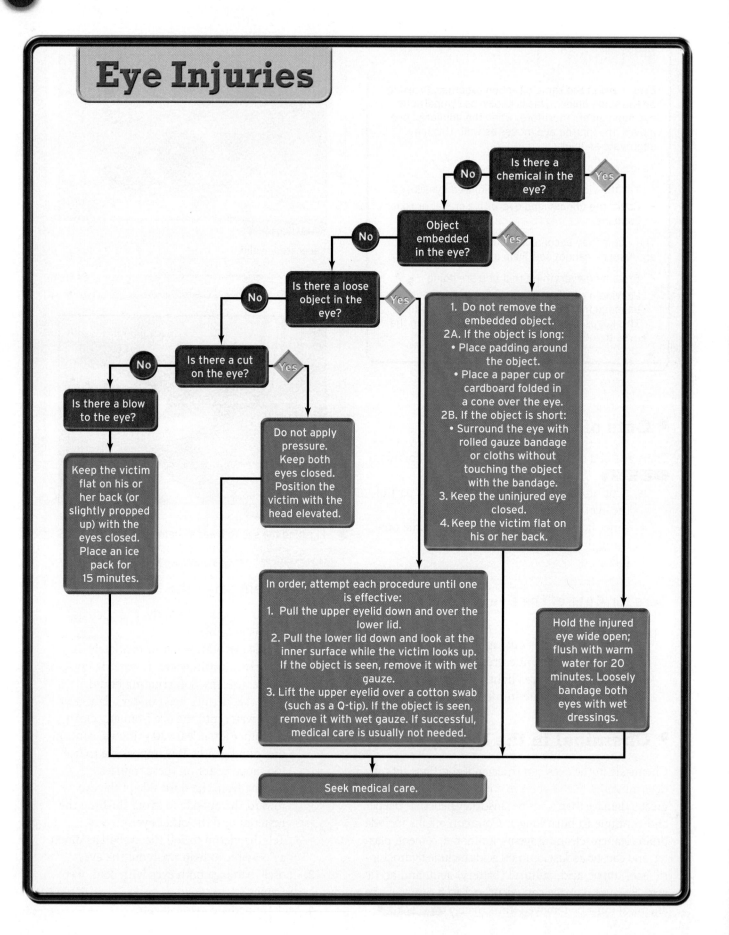

Is there a chemical in the eye?
No → Object embedded in the eye?
Yes →

Object embedded in the eye?
No → Is there a loose object in the eye?
Yes →
1. Do not remove the embedded object.
2A. If the object is long:
 • Place padding around the object.
 • Place a paper cup or cardboard folded in a cone over the eye.
2B. If the object is short:
 • Surround the eye with rolled gauze bandage or cloths without touching the object with the bandage.
3. Keep the uninjured eye closed.
4. Keep the victim flat on his or her back.

Is there a loose object in the eye?
No → Is there a cut on the eye?
Yes →

Is there a cut on the eye?
No → Is there a blow to the eye?
Yes →
Do not apply pressure. Keep both eyes closed. Position the victim with the head elevated.

Is there a blow to the eye?
Keep the victim flat on his or her back (or slightly propped up) with the eyes closed. Place an ice pack for 15 minutes.

In order, attempt each procedure until one is effective:
1. Pull the upper eyelid down and over the lower lid.
2. Pull the lower lid down and look at the inner surface while the victim looks up. If the object is seen, remove it with wet gauze.
3. Lift the upper eyelid over a cotton swab (such as a Q-tip). If the object is seen, remove it with wet gauze. If successful, medical care is usually not needed.

Hold the injured eye wide open; flush with warm water for 20 minutes. Loosely bandage both eyes with wet dressings.

Seek medical care.

CAUTION

DO NOT try to neutralize the chemical. Water usually is readily available for eye irrigation.

DO NOT use an eye cup for a chemical burn.

DO NOT bandage the eye tightly.

CAUTION

DO NOT allow the victim to rub the eye.

DO NOT try to remove an embedded foreign object.

DO NOT use dry cotton (cotton balls or cotton-tipped swabs) or instruments such as tweezers to remove an object from an eye.

▶ Eye Avulsion

A blow to the eye can *avulse* it (knock it out) from its socket. This is a serious injury.

Care for Eye Avulsion

1. Cover the eye loosely with a sterile or clean dressing that has been moistened with clean water. Do not try to push the eyeball back into the socket.
2. Protect the injured eye with a paper cup, a piece of cardboard folded into a cone, or a doughnut-shaped pad made from a roller gauze bandage or a cravat bandage.
3. Cover the undamaged eye with a patch to stop movement of the damaged eye.
4. Seek medical care immediately.

▶ Loose Objects in the Eye

Loose objects in the eye are the most frequent eye injury and can be very painful. Tearing is common because it is the body's way of trying to remove the object.

Care for Objects in the Eye

Try one or more of the following methods to remove the object:

1. Lift the upper lid over the lower lid so that the lower lashes can brush the object off the inside of the upper lid. Have the victim blink a few times and let the eye move the object out. If the object remains, keep the eye closed.
2. Try flushing the object out by rinsing the eye gently with warm water. Hold the eyelid open

CAUTION

DO NOT try to remove an object stuck in the eye.

and tell the victim to move the eye as it is rinsed.

3. Examine the lower lid by pulling it down gently. If you can see the object, remove it with moistened sterile gauze or a clean cloth **Figure 9**.
4. Many foreign bodies lodge under the upper eyelid; however, expertise is required to invert the lid and remove the object. Examine the underside of the upper lid by grasping the lashes of the upper lid, placing a matchstick or cotton-tipped swab across the upper lid, and rolling the lid upward over the stick or swab. If you can see the object, remove it with moistened sterile gauze or a clean cloth.

FYI

An Unresponsive Victim's Eyes
An unconscious victim may lose the reflexes such as blinking that protect the eye. If the eyes do not stay closed, keep them closed by covering them with moist dressings.

▶ Light Burns to the Eye

Burns can result if a person looks at a source of ultraviolet light such as sunlight, arc welding, bright snow, or tanning lamps. Severe pain occurs 1 to 6 hours after exposure.

Care for Light Burns

1. Cover both eyes with cold, wet packs. Tell the victim not to rub the eyes.
2. Have the victim rest in a darkened room. Do not allow light to reach the victim's eyes.
3. Give pain medication, if needed.
4. Seek medical care.

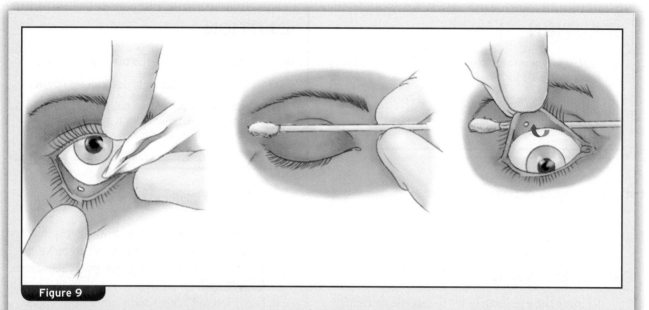

Figure 9

Removing loose objects from the eye. Lower lid: If tears or gentle flushing do not remove the object, gently pull down the lower lid. Remove an object by gently flushing with lukewarm water or by using wet, sterile gauze. Upper lid 1: Tell the person to look down. Pull gently downward on the upper eyelashes. Lay a swab or matchstick across the top of the lid. Upper lid 2: Fold the lid over the swab or matchstick. Remove an object by gently flushing with lukewarm water or by using wet, sterile gauze.

FYI

Contact Lenses
Determine whether a victim is wearing contact lenses by asking, by checking a driver's license, or by looking for them on the eyeball, using a light shining on the eye from the side. In cases of chemicals in the eye, lenses should be removed immediately. Usually the victim can remove the lenses.

Ear Injuries

Most ear problems are not life threatening. Fast action may be needed, however, to relieve pain and to prevent or reverse hearing loss. Head trauma may involve the ear. Foreign bodies in the ear canal usually produce overzealous removal attempts. Except for disk batteries (which damage moist tissue by creating a current) and live insects, few foreign bodies must be extracted immediately. First aiders should seek medical care for the victim because attempts to remove a foreign body from the ear can rupture the eardrum or lacerate the ear canal.

A live insect crawling around in the ear canal can be very uncomfortable for the victim. Shine a small light into the ear. Sometimes the insect will crawl out toward the light. If it will not leave the ear, drown the insect by placing several drops of light mineral oil or vegetable oil (not motor oil) into the ear. Often the insect will crawl out before it dies. When it stops moving and the insect is near the opening, carefully irrigate the ear with warm water. The insect should wash out. If that is unsuccessful, use a bulb syringe to suck the insect out. If the insect cannot be removed, seek medical care.

Children insert all sorts of things into their ears that may be impossible for you to remove safely. If the object is visible near the ear canal opening and you feel it is safe, cautiously try to remove the object with tweezers. Small objects can sometimes be removed by irrigating the ear with warm water. Do not try irrigation if the object blocks the entire ear canal or if the object is vegetable matter such as a kernel of corn or a bean, which will swell when wet.

Nose Injuries

▶ Nosebleeds

A severe nosebleed frightens the victim and often challenges the first aider's skill. Most nosebleeds are self-limiting and seldom require medical attention. In cases of accompanying head or neck injuries, stabilize the head and neck for protection. In some cases, loss of blood could cause shock.

There are two types of nosebleeds:

- **Anterior nosebleed** (front of nose) is the most common type (90%). Blood flows from the nose through one nostril.
- The **posterior nosebleed** (back of nose) involves massive bleeding, usually backward into the mouth or down the back of the throat. A posterior nosebleed is serious and requires medical care.

Care for Nosebleeds

To care for an anterior nosebleed, follow these guidelines from the American Academy of Otolaryngology:

1. Keep the head higher than the level of the heart. Have the victim sit and lean slightly forward to prevent blood draining into the throat.
2. Pinch the soft parts of the nose together between your thumb and two fingers **Figure 10**.
3. Continue compressing the pinched parts for 5 to 10 minutes.
4. Apply ice (crushed in a plastic bag or washcloth) to the nose and cheeks.

If bleeding continues:

1. Clear the nose of all blood clots by gently blowing the nose.
2. If available, spray a decongestant spray (such as Afrin or Neo-Synephrin) into the nostril.
3. Pinch the nose again for 10 minutes.
4. If the nosebleed continues, seek medical care.

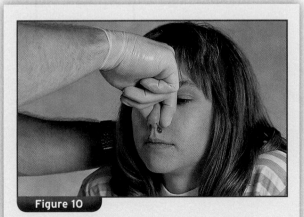

Figure 10

Control bleeding from the nose by pinching the nostrils together.

> **CAUTION**
>
> DO NOT allow the victim to tilt the head backward.
>
> DO NOT probe the nose with a cotton-tipped swab.
>
> DO NOT move the victim's head and neck if a spinal injury is suspected.

Seek professional medical help if:

- Bleeding cannot be stopped or keeps reappearing.
- Bleeding is rapid or blood loss is large.
- Weakness or fainting is present.
- Blood begins to go down the back of the throat rather than out the front of the nose.

Care After a Nosebleed

After a nosebleed has stopped, suggest that the victim:

- Sneeze through an open mouth, if he or she needs to sneeze.
- Avoid bending over and participating in too much physical exertion.
- Elevate the head with two pillows when lying down.
- Keep the nostrils moist by applying a little petroleum jelly just inside the nostril for 1 week; increase the humidity in the bedroom during the winter months by using a cold-mist humidifier.
- Avoid picking or rubbing the nose.

▶ Broken Nose

The signs of a broken nose include the following:

- Pain, swelling, and a possible crooked appearance
- Bleeding and difficulty breathing through the nostrils
- Black eyes appearing 1 to 2 days after the injury

Care for a Broken Nose

1. Seek medical care.
2. If bleeding is present, give care as for a nosebleed.
3. Apply an ice pack to the nose for 15 minutes at a time throughout the day.
4. Do not try to straighten a crooked nose.

Nosebleeds

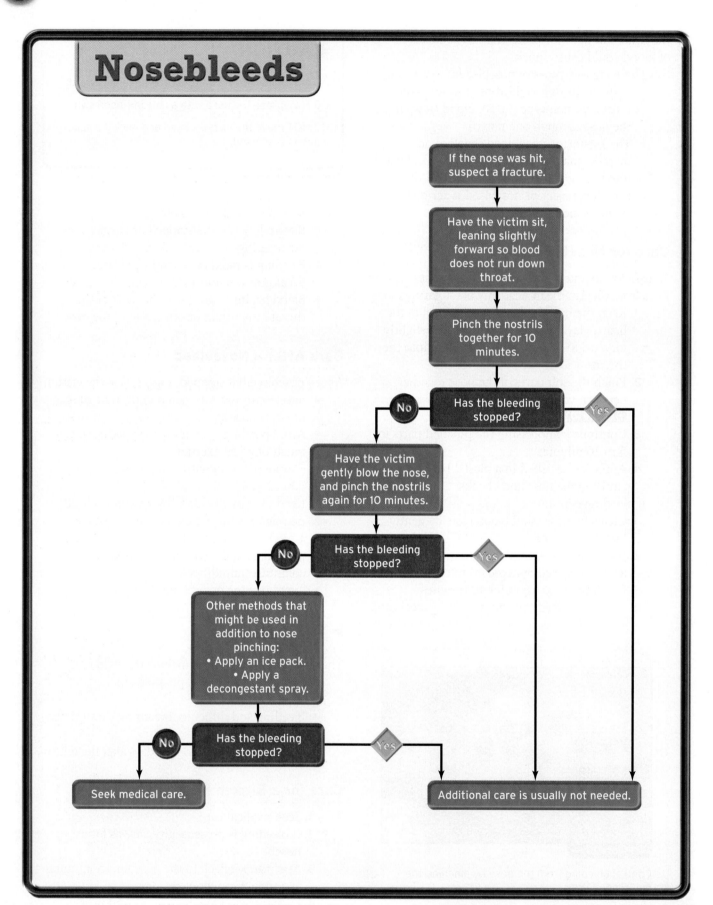

If the nose was hit, suspect a fracture.

Have the victim sit, leaning slightly forward so blood does not run down throat.

Pinch the nostrils together for 10 minutes.

Has the bleeding stopped?

No →

Yes →

Have the victim gently blow the nose, and pinch the nostrils again for 10 minutes.

Has the bleeding stopped?

No →

Yes →

Other methods that might be used in addition to nose pinching:
• Apply an ice pack.
• Apply a decongestant spray.

Has the bleeding stopped?

No →

Yes →

Seek medical care.

Additional care is usually not needed.

▶ Objects in the Nose

A foreign object in the nose is a problem mainly among small children, who seem to gain satisfaction from putting peanuts, beans, raisins, and other similar objects into their nostrils.

Care for Objects in the Nose

To remove objects from the nose, try one or more of the following methods:

1. Induce sneezing by having the victim sniff pepper or by tickling the opposite nostril.
2. Have the victim blow gently while you put compression on the opposite nostril.
3. Use tweezers to pull out an object that is visible. Do not probe or push an object deeper.
4. Seek medical care if the object cannot be removed.

Dental Injuries

Because dental emergencies generally cause considerable pain and anxiety, managing them promptly can provide great relief to the victim.

▶ Objects Caught Between the Teeth

The signs of an object caught between teeth include the following:

- Victim says that something is caught between his or her teeth. This is the main method of detecting the problem.
- The object may or may not be seen. Even with the use of a flashlight, it is still difficult to see a small object.

Care for Objects Caught Between the Teeth

1. Try to remove the object with dental floss. Guide the floss carefully to avoid cutting the gums. Do not try to remove the object with a sharp or pointed instrument.
2. If unsuccessful, seek dental care.

▶ Bitten Lip or Tongue

The signs of a bitten lip or tongue include the following:

- Immediate pain when it happens.
- Blood may be seen.

Care for a Bitten Lip or Tongue

1. Apply direct pressure to the bleeding area with sterile gauze or a clean cloth.
2. Clean the area with a cloth.
3. If swelling is present, apply an ice pack or have the victim suck on a popsicle or ice chips.
4. If the bleeding does not stop, seek medical care.

▶ Loosened Tooth

Trauma can cause teeth to become loosened in their sockets. Applying pressure on either side of each tooth with the fingers can determine looseness. Any tooth movement, even if it is barely felt, indicates a possibly loose tooth.

Care for a Loosened Tooth

1. Have the victim bite down on a piece of gauze to keep the tooth in place.
2. Consult a dentist or an oral surgeon

▶ Knocked-Out Tooth

A knocked-out tooth is a dental emergency but it is also a common one. A majority of the teeth knocked out each year in the United States could be saved with proper treatment Figure 11 . Emergency care for knocked-out teeth has changed dramatically in recent years. The first question you want to ask when a tooth has been knocked out is, "Where is the tooth?" Time is crucial for successful

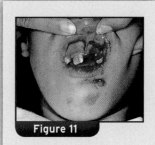

Figure 11
Knocked-out tooth.

reimplantation. After a tooth is knocked out, ligament fiber fragments remain attached to the tooth and to the bone in the socket. These ligament fibers begin to die soon after the injury. Therefore, it is important to prevent the tooth from drying and to protect the ligament fibers from damage. Moisture alone is not sufficient to preserve the tooth's ligament fibers. Steps must be taken to prevent the tooth from becoming dehydrated and to protect the ligament fibers from damage

Care for a Knocked-Out Tooth

1. Have the victim rinse his or her mouth, and, if bleeding, put a rolled gauze pad in the socket to control the bleeding.
2. Find the tooth and handle it by the crown, not the root, to minimize damage to the ligament fibers.
3. A tooth often can be successfully reimplanted if it is replaced in its socket within 30 minutes after the injury; the odds of successful reimplantation decrease about 1% for every minute the tooth is absent from the socket.
   - One of the worst things you can do to a knocked-out tooth is to transport it dry. Consider using the victim's own saliva for the short term (less than 1 hour). Whole milk is much better because it maintains the vitality of the ligaments for 3 hours. Ideally, the milk should be kept cold to minimize bacterial growth. Do not use reconstituted powdered milk or milk by-products such as yogurt; they can damage the ligaments.
   - The best transport medium is Hank's solution, a balanced-pH cell-culture medium that helps restore the ligament fibers. The use of Hank's solution extends the viability of the ligament fibers for 6 to 12 hours. The solution, which is available commercially as the Save-a-Tooth kit, has been approved by the US Food and Drug Administration for use up to 24 hours after an injury, and there is some evidence that using it enables successful reimplantation, even after 96 hours. A tooth-saving kit is available in drugstores or online and deserves consideration as a standard item at schools, sporting events, and summer camps.

CAUTION

DO NOT handle a knocked-out tooth roughly.

DO NOT put a knocked-out tooth in water, mouthwash, alcohol, or povidone iodine (Betadine).

DO NOT put a knocked-out tooth in skim milk, reconstituted powdered milk, or milk by-products such as yogurt.

DO NOT rinse a knocked-out tooth unless you are reinserting it in the socket.

DO NOT place a knocked-out tooth in anything that can dry or crush the outside of the tooth.

DO NOT scrub a knocked-out tooth or remove any attached tissue fragments.

DO NOT remove a partially extracted tooth. Push it back into place and seek a dentist so the loose tooth can be stabilized.

FYI

First Aid
If you are in a remote area with no dentist nearby, you can make a temporary cap from melted candle wax or paraffin and a few strands of cotton. When the wax begins to harden but can still be molded, press a wad of it onto the tooth. Other improvisations include using ski wax or chewing gum (preferably sugarless).

   - Some experts recommend that the tooth be placed in the victim's mouth to keep it moist until dental treatment is available. Do not use this method for children or others who may swallow the tooth.
4. Take the victim and the tooth immediately to a dentist.
5. If you are in a remote location, try to replace the tooth into the socket, using adjacent teeth as a guide. Apply pressure on the tooth so the top is even with the adjacent teeth. Asking the victim to bite down gently on gauze is helpful. Immediate reinsertion is not always possible, however. The victim may be reluctant to put the knocked-out tooth back into its socket, especially if it has fallen on the ground and is covered with debris—or the tooth may

Dental Injuries

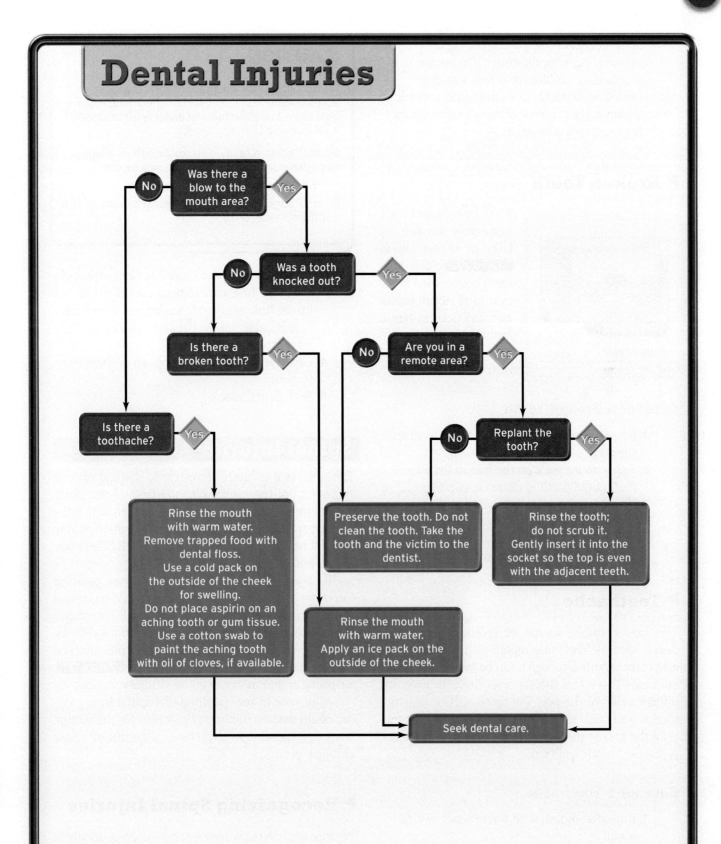

repeatedly fall out, putting the victim at risk of inhaling or swallowing it. Do not use this method for children or others who may swallow the tooth. In victims with multiple trauma, the presence of more serious injuries may prevent reinsertion.

▶ Broken Tooth

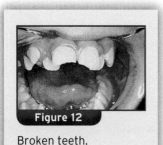

Figure 12

Broken teeth.

The front teeth are frequently broken by falls or direct blows **Figure 12**. Such damage is not unusual in the victims of violent acts or motor vehicle crashes. It is also common in children, especially those with an overbite.

Care for a Broken Tooth

1. Rinse the mouth with warm water to clean the area.
2. Apply an ice pack on the face in the area of the injured tooth to decrease swelling.
3. If you suspect a jaw fracture, stabilize the jaw by wrapping a bandage under the chin and over the top of the head.
4. Seek immediate dental care.

▶ Toothache

The most common reason for toothaches is dental decay. Victims frequently report pain limited to one area of the mouth, although it can be more widespread; pain can also affect the ear, eye, neck, or even the opposite side of the jaw. The tooth will be sensitive to heat and cold. Identify the diseased tooth by tapping the area with a spoon handle or similar object. A diseased tooth will hurt.

Care for a Toothache

1. Rinse the mouth with warm water to clean it out.
2. Use dental floss to remove any food that might be trapped between the teeth.
3. If you suspect a cavity, paint the tooth by using a small cotton swab soaked in oil of

CAUTION

DO NOT place pain medication (such as aspirin, acetaminophen, or ibuprofen) on the aching tooth or gum tissues or allow them to dissolve in the mouth. A serious acid burn can result.

DO NOT cover a cavity with cotton if there is any pus discharge or facial swelling. See a dentist immediately.

DO NOT stick anything into an exposed cavity or into a softened exposed root.

cloves (eugenol) (or Orajel) to help suppress the pain. Take care to keep the oil off the gums, lips, and inside surfaces of the cheeks. If applicable, follow the same procedures as for a broken tooth.
4. Give the victim acetaminophen or ibuprofen for pain.
5. Seek dental care.

Spinal Injuries

The *spine* is a column of vertebrae stacked on one another from the tailbone to the base of the skull. Each vertebra has a hollow center through which the spinal cord passes. The spinal cord consists of long tracts of nerves that join the brain with all other body organs and parts.

If a broken vertebra pinches spinal nerves, paralysis can result. All unresponsive victims should be treated as though they have a spinal injury. All responsive victims sustaining injuries from falls, diving accidents, or motor vehicle crashes should be carefully checked for a spinal injury before being moved **Figure 13**. Suspect a spinal injury in all head-injury victims.

A mistake in the handling of a spinal injury victim could mean a lifetime of paralysis for the victim. Suspect a spinal injury whenever a significant cause of injury occurs.

▶ Recognizing Spinal Injuries

Because the head may have been snapped suddenly in one or more directions, anytime there is a head injury, there may also be a spinal cord injury. About 15% to 20% of head-injury victims also have a spinal injury. Other signs and symptoms include the following:

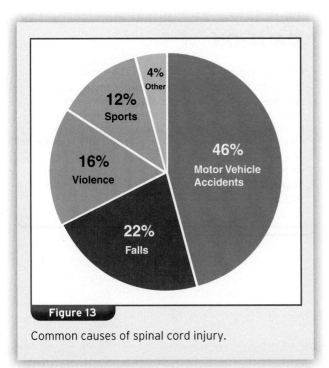

Figure 13

Common causes of spinal cord injury.

- Pain radiating into the arms or legs
- Neck or back pain
- Numbness, tingling, weakness, burning, or lessened sensation in the arms or legs
- Loss of bowel or bladder control
- Paralysis of the arms or legs
- Deformity (odd-looking angle of the victim's head and neck)

Ask a responsive victim these questions and follow these steps **Skill Drill 1**:

- Is there pain? Neck (cervical spine) injuries radiate pain to the arms; upper-back (thoracic spine) injuries radiate pain around the ribs; lower-back injuries usually radiate pain down the legs. Often, the victim will describe the pain as "electric."
- Can you wiggle your fingers? Moving the fingers is a sign that nerve pathways are intact (**Step ❶**).
- Can you feel this pressure on your finger? Pinch the tip of the victim's finger to check for spinal injury (**Step ❷**).
- Can you squeeze my hand? Ask the victim to grip your hand. A strong grip indicates that an upper spinal injury is unlikely (**Step ❸**).
- Can you wiggle your toes? Moving the toes is a sign that nerve pathways are intact (**Step ❹**).

- Squeeze the victim's toes (**Step ❺**).
- Can you push your foot against my hand? Ask the victim to press a foot against your hand (**Step ❻**). If the victim cannot perform this movement or if the movement is extremely weak against your hand, the victim may have a spinal injury.

If the victim is unresponsive, do the following:

- Look for cuts, bruises, and deformities.
- Test responses by pinching the victim's hand (the palm or back of the hand) and bare foot (the sole or the top of the foot). No reaction could mean spinal cord damage **Skill Drill 2**:

1. Pinch the victim's hand for a response (**Step ❶**).
2. Pinch the victim's foot for a response (**Step ❷**).
3. Test the spinal cord by using the Babinski test (**Step ❸**): Stroke the bottom of the foot firmly toward the big toe with a key or similar blunt object. The body's normal response is to move the big toe down (except in infants). If the spinal cord or brain is injured, the big toe in an adult and a child will flex upward.
4. Ask bystanders what happened. If you still are not sure about a possible spinal injury, assume the victim has one until it is proved otherwise.

▶ Care for a Spinal Injury

1. Monitor breathing. For an unresponsive victim, open the airway and check for breathing.
2. Stabilize the victim to prevent movement by using one of the following methods. Whichever method you use, tell the victim not to move.
   - Grasp the victim's head over the ears and hold the head and neck still until the EMS arrives **Figure 14**.
   - If you anticipate a long wait for EMS or you are tired from holding the victim's head in place, kneel with the victim's head between your knees or place objects on each side of the victim's head to prevent it from rolling from side to side.

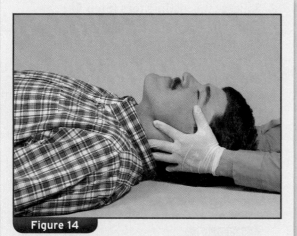

Figure 14

Steady and support the victim's head and neck as soon as possible. Have a bystander steady and support the feet. The head and feet should be continuously supported until medical help takes over. Stabilize by holding the head. Keep your arms steady by placing them on your thighs. To free yourself to help others, place heavy objects on each side of the head.

CAUTION

DO NOT move the victim, even if the victim is in water. (For a water-related rescue, manually stabilize the victim while floating on the water's surface.) Wait for EMS personnel to arrive; they have the proper training and equipment. Victims with suspected spinal injury require cervical collars and stabilization on a spine board. It is better to do nothing than to mishandle a victim with a spinal injury, unless the victim's location puts him or her in additional danger.

skill drill

1   Checking for Spinal Injuries in a Responsive Victim

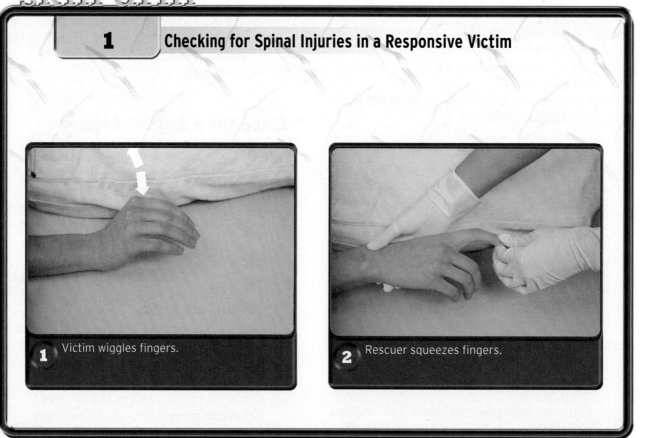

1   Victim wiggles fingers.

2   Rescuer squeezes fingers.

skill drill

1 | **Checking for Spinal Injuries in a Responsive Victim (*continued*)**

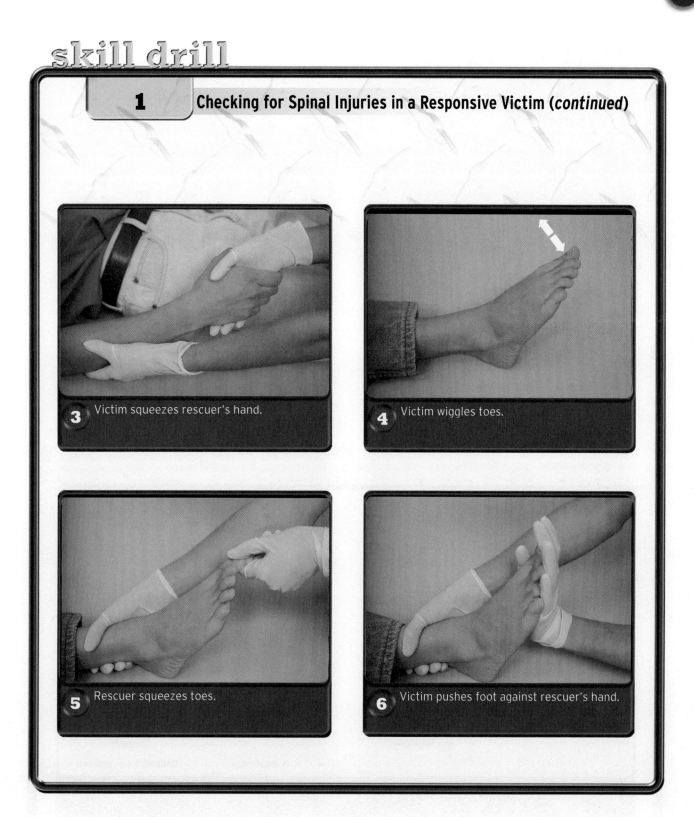

3 Victim squeezes rescuer's hand.

4 Victim wiggles toes.

5 Rescuer squeezes toes.

6 Victim pushes foot against rescuer's hand.

skill drill

2   Checking for Spinal Injuries in an Unresponsive Victim

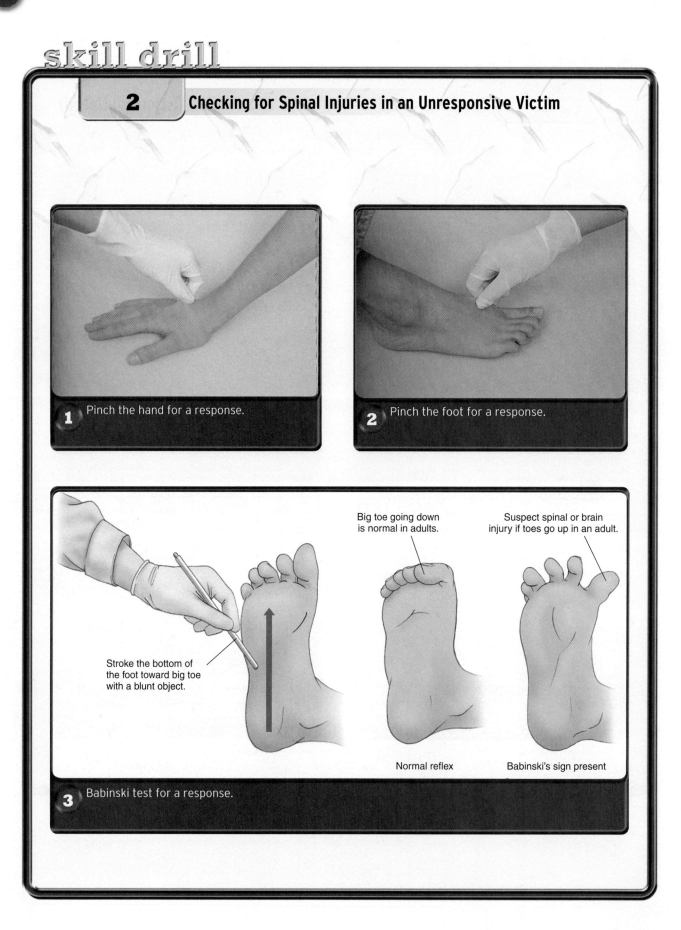

1   Pinch the hand for a response.

2   Pinch the foot for a response.

Stroke the bottom of the foot toward big toe with a blunt object.

Big toe going down is normal in adults.

Suspect spinal or brain injury if toes go up in an adult.

Normal reflex

Babinski's sign present

3   Babinski test for a response.

Spinal Injuries

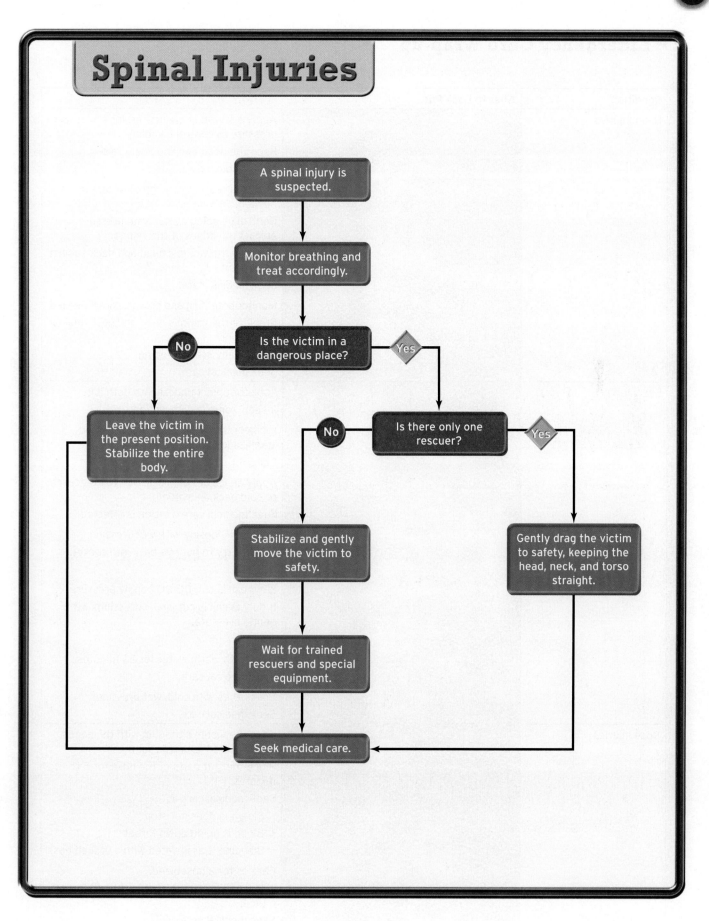

▶ Emergency Care Wrap-up

Condition	What to Look For	What to Do
Head Injuries	Scalp wound	Apply a sterile or clean dressing and direct pressure to control bleeding. Keep the head and shoulders raised. Seek medical care.
	Skull fracture	Monitor breathing and provide care if needed. Control bleeding by applying pressure around the edges of the wound. Stabilize the victim's head and neck against movement. Seek medical care.
	Brain injury (concussion)	Monitor breathing and provide care if needed. Stabilize the victim's head and neck against movement. Control any scalp bleeding. Seek medical care.
Eye Injuries	Loose object in eye	Look for object underneath both lids. If seen, remove with wet gauze.
	Penetrating eye injury	If object is still in eye, protect eye and stabilize long objects. Call 9-1-1.
	Blow to the eye area	Apply an ice or cold pack. DO NOT place ice or cold pack on eyeball. Seek medical care if vision is affected.
	Eye avulsion	Cover eye loosely with wet dressing. DO NOT try to put eye back into socket. Call 9-1-1.
	Cuts of eye or lid	If eyeball is cut, DO NOT apply pressure. If only eyelid is cut, apply dressings with gentle pressure. Call 9-1-1.
	Chemical in eye	Flush with warm water for 20 minutes. Seek medical care.
	Eye burns from light	Cover eyes with cold, wet dressings. Seek medical care.
Nose Injuries	Nosebleed	Keep the victim sitting up with the head level or tilted forward slightly. Pinch the soft parts of the nose for 5 to 10 minutes. Seek medical care if: • Bleeding does not stop • Blood is going down throat • Bleeding is associated with a broken nose
	Broken nose	Care as for a nosebleed. Apply an ice or cold pack for 15 minutes at a time. Seek medical care.

Condition	What to Look For	What to Do
Dental Injuries	Bitten lip or tongue	Apply direct pressure.
		Apply an ice or cold pack.
	Knocked-out tooth	Control bleeding (place rolled gauze in socket).
		Find tooth and preserve it in milk or the victim's saliva. Handle the tooth by the crown, not the root.
		Take the tooth with the victim to a dentist.
	Toothache	Rinse the mouth and use dental floss to remove trapped food.
		Give pain medication.
		Seek dental care.
Spinal Injuries	Spinal injury	Stabilize the head and neck against movement.
	Inability to move arms and/or legs or painful to move them	If unresponsive, open the victim's airway and check breathing.
	Numbness, tingling, weakness, or burning feeling in arms and/or legs	Call 9-1-1.
	Deformity (head and neck at an odd angle)	

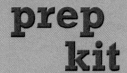

▶ Ready for Review

- Any head injury is potentially serious. If not properly treated, injuries that seem minor could become life threatening.
- Scalp wounds bleed profusely because the scalp has a rich supply of blood.
- A skull fracture is a break or crack in the cranium. Skull fractures may be open or closed.
- Injuries to the brain cause short- and long-term problems.
- An injured eye probably causes the most anxiety and concern in a victim.
- Penetrating eye injuries are severe injuries that result when a sharp object penetrates the eye.
- Blows to the eye can range in severity from minor to sight threatening.
- Cuts of the eye or lid require medical care.
- Chemicals in the eyes can threaten sight.
- A blow to the eye can knock it from its socket.
- Loose objects in the eye are the most frequent eye injury and can be very painful.
- Burns to the eye can result if a person looks at a source of ultraviolet light.
- Most ear injuries are not life threatening, but fast action may be needed to relieve pain or to prevent or reverse hearing loss.

- Most nosebleeds are self-limiting and seldom require medical attention.
- A foreign object in the nose is a problem mainly among small children who put small objects up their nostrils.
- Because dental emergencies generally cause considerable pain and anxiety, managing them promptly can provide great relief to the victim.
- Trauma can cause teeth to become loosened in their sockets.
- A knocked-out tooth is a dental emergency.
- The front teeth are frequently broken by falls or direct blows.
- The most common reason for toothaches is dental decay.
- A mistake in the handling of a spinal injury victim could mean a lifetime of paralysis for the victim.

▶ Vital Vocabulary

anterior nosebleed Bleeding from the front of the nose.

Battle's sign A contusion on the mastoid area of either ear; sign of a basilar skull fracture.

concussion A temporary disturbance of brain activity caused by a blow to the head.

contusion A bruise; an injury that causes a hemorrhage in or beneath the skin but does not break the skin.

posterior nosebleed Bleeding from the back of the nose, which may flow out of the nostrils and into the mouth or throat.

skull fracture A break of part of the skull (head bones).

▶ Assessment in Action

While working at a construction site, you witness a fellow worker fall to the ground after being struck by a piece of wood thrown by a table saw. He was not wearing his safety glasses and you see a cut to his eyeball and eyelid.

Directions: Circle Yes if you agree with the statement; circle No if you disagree.

Yes   No   **1.** Apply pressure immediately to the injured eyeball.

Yes   No   **2.** Tell the victim to keep both eyes closed. Both eyes can be covered with a cravat or roller bandage.

Yes   No   **3.** Position the victim with his head elevated.

Yes   No   **4.** Medical care is not necessary in this case.

▶ Check Your Knowledge

Directions: Circle Yes if you agree with the statement; circle No if you disagree.

Yes   No   **1.** Remove objects embedded in an eyeball.

Yes   No   **2.** Scalp wounds have very little bleeding.

Yes   No   **3.** Scrub and rinse the roots of a knocked-out tooth.

Yes   No   **4.** After a blow to the area around an eye, apply a cold pack.

Yes   No   **5.** Tears are sufficient to flush a chemical from the eye.

Yes   No   **6.** Use clean, damp gauze to remove an object from the eyelid's surface.

Yes   No   **7.** Preserve a knocked-out tooth in mouthwash.

Yes   No   **8.** Do not move a victim with a suspected spinal injury.

Yes   No   **9.** Inability to move the hands or feet, or both, may indicate a spinal injury.

Yes   No   **10.** To care for a nosebleed, have the injured person sit down and tilt his or her head back.

Chest, Abdominal, and Pelvic Injuries

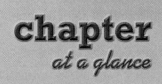

11

Chest Injuries

Chest injuries fall into two categories: open or closed. In open chest injuries, the chest wall is penetrated by some object (eg, knife, bullet). A closed chest injury is one in which the skin is not broken. The injury is caused by blunt trauma (eg, falling object, struck during a fight or assault).

All victims with chest injuries should have their breathing checked and rechecked. A responsive victim with a chest injury should usually sit up or, if the injury is on a side, be placed with the injured side down. This position prevents blood inside the chest cavity from seeping into the uninjured side and allows the uninjured side to expand.

▶ Closed Chest Injuries

In a **closed chest injury**, the skin is not broken. Closed chest injuries include rib fractures and flail chest.

Rib Fractures

The upper four ribs are rarely fractured because they are protected by the collarbone and the shoulder blades. The upper four ribs are so enmeshed with the muscles that they rarely need to be splinted or realigned like other broken bones. The lower two ribs are difficult to fracture because they are attached on only one end and have the freedom to move, which is why they are called *floating ribs*. Broken ribs usually occur along the side of the chest. The main symptom of a rib fracture is pain at the injured rib site when the victim breathes, coughs, or moves, or when the area is touched.

Recognizing Rib Fractures

The signs of rib fracture include:
- Sharp pain, especially when the victim takes a deep breath, coughs, or moves
- Victim holds the injured area, trying to reduce the pain
- Victim reports being hit where the pain is
- Area tender when pressed
- Shallow breathing

To assess for a rib fracture, gently press inward on both sides of the chest at the same time.

Care for Rib Fractures

1. Help the victim find a comfortable position. Stabilize the ribs by having the victim hold a pillow or other similar soft object against the injured area or use bandages to hold the pillow in place. You can also tie an arm over the injured area. Do not apply tight bandages around the chest because they will restrict breathing **Figure 1**.
2. Give pain medication.
3. Seek medical care.

Flail Chest

A **flail chest** is a serious injury that involves several ribs in the same area broken in more than one place. The area over the injury may move in a direction opposite to that of the rest of the chest wall during breathing (known as *paradoxical movement*). This injury is very painful and makes breathing difficult.

Recognizing Flail Chest

The signs and symptoms of a flail chest include:
- Paradoxical chest motion takes place. The area over the injury may move in a direction opposite to that of the rest of the chest wall during breathing.
- Breathing is very painful and difficult.
- Bruising of the skin over the injury may occur.

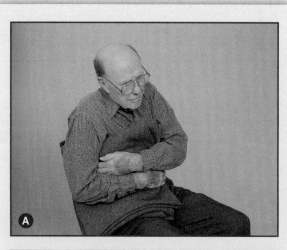

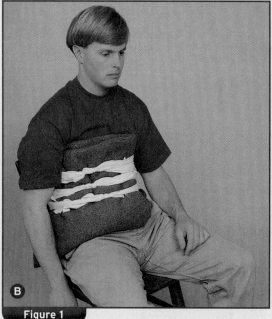

Figure 1

Stabilize the ribs with a soft object such as a pillow, coat, or blanket (hold or tie). Tell the victim to occasionally take a deep breath and to cough.

Care for Flail Chest

1. Support the chest by one of several methods:
   - Apply hand pressure. This is useful for a short time.
   - Place the victim on the injured side with a blanket or clothing underneath.
2. Monitor breathing.
3. Seek medical care.

Chest Injuries

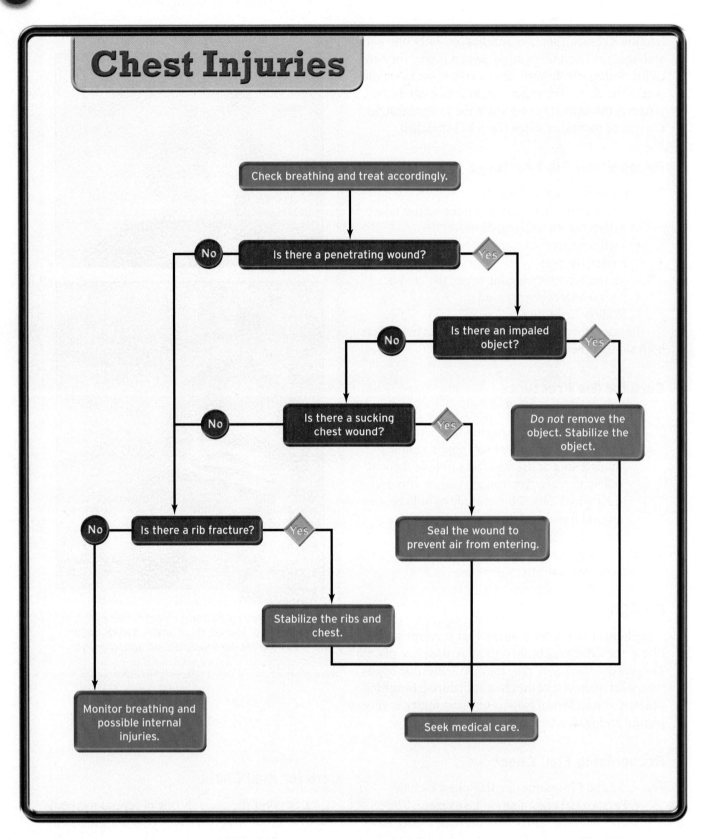

Check breathing and treat accordingly.

No ← Is there a penetrating wound? → Yes

Is there an impaled object? — No / Yes

Is there a sucking chest wound? — No / Yes

Do not remove the object. Stabilize the object.

Is there a rib fracture? — No / Yes

Seal the wound to prevent air from entering.

Stabilize the ribs and chest.

Monitor breathing and possible internal injuries.

Seek medical care.

▶ Open Chest Injuries

In an <u>open chest injury</u>, the skin has been broken and the chest wall is penetrated by an object such as a knife or bullet.

Impaled Object in the Chest

If an object penetrates the chest wall, air and blood escape into the space between the lungs and the chest wall. The air and blood cause the lung to collapse. Lung collapse can lead to shock and death.

Recognizing an Impaled Object in the Chest

An impaled object is usually easily recognized. However, in some cases the object may be below the skin surface and is difficult to see. Carefully look at wounds that could be hiding the object that caused the damage.

Care for an Impaled Object in the Chest

1. Stabilize the object in place with bulky dressings or clothes **Figure 2**. Do not try to remove an impaled object. Doing so can result in bleeding and air in the chest cavity.
2. Call 9-1-1.

Sucking Chest Wound

A <u>sucking chest wound</u> results when a chest wound allows air to pass into and out of the chest with each breath **Figure 3**. Bubbles may be seen at the wound

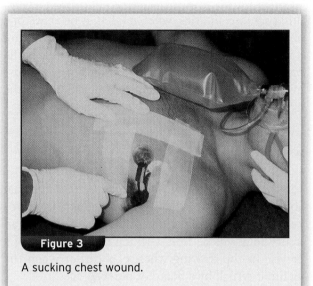

Figure 3

A sucking chest wound.

during exhalations and a sucking sound heard during inhalations.

Recognizing a Sucking Chest Wound

The signs of a sucking chest wound include:
- Blood bubbling out of a chest wound during exhalation
- Sucking sound heard during inhalations

Care for a Sucking Chest Wound

1. Seal the wound with anything available to stop air from entering the chest cavity. Plastic wrap or a plastic bag works well. Tape it in place, but leave one side untaped to create a flutter valve to prevent air from being trapped in the chest cavity. The open side of the dressing should be allowed to drain to gravity. If plastic wrap is not available, you can use your gloved hand.
2. Lean or lay the victim on the injured side.
3. If the victim has trouble breathing or seems to be getting worse, remove the plastic cover (or your hand) to let air escape, and then reapply.
4. Call 9-1-1.

Abdominal Injuries

Injuries to the abdomen are either open or closed and can involve hollow and/or solid organs. An internal abdominal injury is one of the most frequently

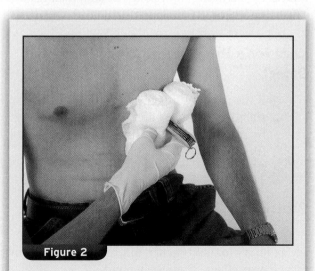

Figure 2

Stabilize a penetrating object with bulky padding. Secure the padding and object.

unrecognized injuries; when missed, it becomes one of the main causes of death. A hollow organ rupture (for example, of the stomach or intestines) spills the contents of the organ into the abdominal cavity, causing inflammation. Solid organ rupture (such as of the liver or spleen) results in severe internal bleeding.

▶ Closed Abdominal Injuries

Closed abdominal injuries occur when the internal abdominal tissues are damaged but the skin is unbroken. These are also known as blunt injuries. Such an injury might come from striking the handlebar of a bicycle or the steering wheel of a car, or when the victim is struck by a board or baseball bat.

A Blow to the Abdomen

Bruising and damage to internal organs can result from a severe blow to the abdomen.

Recognizing a Closed Abdominal Injury

Examine the abdomen by gently pressing all four quadrants of the abdomen with your fingertips **Figure 4**. A normal abdomen is soft and not tender when pressed. Signs of a closed abdominal injury include:

- Bruises or other marks
- Pain, tenderness, muscle tightness, or rigidity
- Distention (swelling)

Care for a Closed Abdominal Injury

1. If unresponsive, place the victim on the left side in a comfortable position with the legs bent and in a "fetal position."
2. If responsive, place the victim on one side in a comfortable position with the legs slightly bent. Roll onto side in case of vomiting.
3. Call 9-1-1.

▶ Open Abdominal Injuries

Open abdominal injuries are those in which the skin has been broken. These injuries are also known as *penetrating injuries*. Examples include stab wounds and

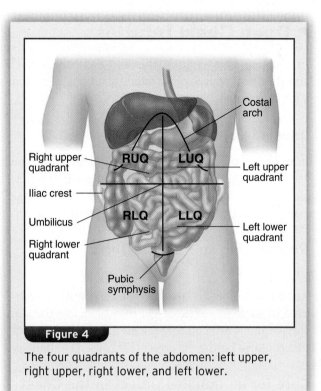

Figure 4

The four quadrants of the abdomen: left upper, right upper, right lower, and left lower.

gunshot wounds. It is difficult to know whether a penetrating injury involves more than just the abdominal wall. Always assume the worst—that internal organs have been damaged.

A Penetrating Wound/Impaled Object

Open abdominal wounds usually result from stabbing by a knife or other sharp object and are always serious injuries. Penetrating injuries to the abdomen usually cause internal organ damage.

Care for a Penetrating Wound/Impaled Object

1. If the penetrating object is still in place, stabilize the object and control the bleeding by placing bulky dressings around it. Do not try to remove the object.
2. Call 9-1-1.

Protruding Organs

A protruding organ injury (evisceration) refers to a severe injury to the abdomen in which internal organs escape or protrude from the wound.

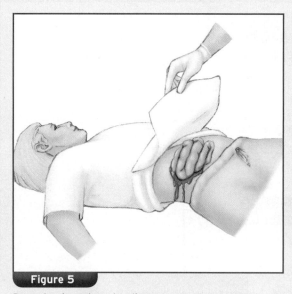

Figure 5

Do not reinsert protruding organs. Cover them with a moist, sterile dressing.

Care for Protruding Organs

1. Call 9-1-1.
2. Allow the victim to stay in a comfortable position with the legs pulled up toward the abdomen.
   Cover the protruding organs with a moist, sterile dressing or clean cloth, or a piece of plastic **Figure 5** .
3. Treat for shock.

CAUTION

DO NOT try to reinsert protruding organs into the abdomen. You could introduce infection or damage the intestines.

DO NOT cover the organs tightly.

DO NOT cover the organs with any material that clings or disintegrates when wet.

DO NOT give anything by mouth.

Pelvic Injuries

Pelvic fractures are usually caused by falling or a motor vehicle crash.

Recognizing Pelvic Injuries

The signs of a pelvic injury include:
- Pain in the hip, groin, or back that increases with movement
- Inability to stand or walk
- Signs of shock

Check the pelvis by gently pressing inward and downward on the tops of the hips. See Skill Drill 2, Steps 5a and 5b in the chapter entitled Finding Out What's Wrong.

Care for Pelvic Injuries

1. Treat the victim for shock.
2. Place padding between the victim's thighs, and then tie the victim's knees and ankles together. If the knees are bent, place padding under them for support.
3. Keep the victim on a firm surface.
4. Call 9-1-1.

CAUTION

DO NOT roll the victim–additional internal damage could result.

DO NOT move the victim. Whenever possible, wait for trained EMS personnel with their ambulance, backboard, and other specialized equipment.

Abdominal Injuries

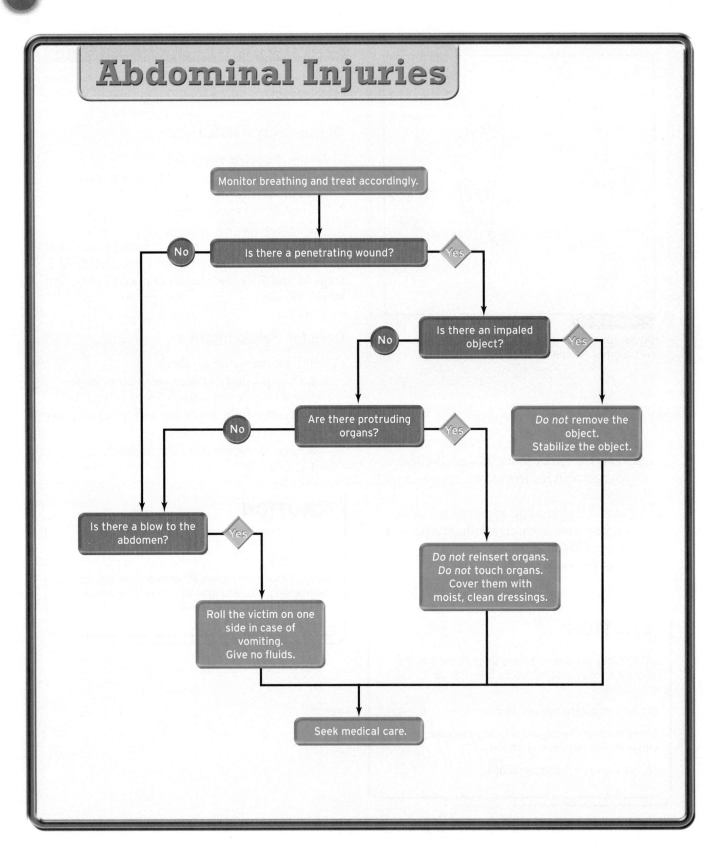

Monitor breathing and treat accordingly.

Is there a penetrating wound? — No / Yes

Is there an impaled object? — No / Yes

Do not remove the object.
Stabilize the object.

Are there protruding organs? — No / Yes

Do not reinsert organs.
Do not touch organs.
Cover them with moist, clean dressings.

Is there a blow to the abdomen? — Yes

Roll the victim on one side in case of vomiting.
Give no fluids.

Seek medical care.

▶ Emergency Care Wrap-up

Condition	What to Look For	What to Do
Chest Injuries	Rib fracture Sharp pain with deep breaths, coughing, or moving Shallow breathing Holding of injured area to reduce pain	Place victim in comfortable position. Support ribs with a pillow, blanket, or coat (either holding or tying with bandages). Seek medical care.
	Embedded (impaled) object Object remains in wound	DO NOT remove object from wound. Use bulky dressings or cloths to stabilize the object. Call 9-1-1.
	Sucking chest wound Blood bubbling out of wound Sound of air being sucked in and out of wound	Seal wound to stop air from entering chest; tape three sides of plastic or use gloved hand. Remove cover to let air escape if victim worsens or has trouble breathing. Call 9-1-1.
Abdominal Injuries	Blow to abdomen (closed) Bruise or other marks Muscle tightness and rigidity felt while gently pushing on abdomen	Place victim in comfortable position with legs pulled up toward the abdomen. Treat for shock. Seek medical care.
	Protruding organs (open) Internal organs escaping from abdominal wound	Place victim in a comfortable position with the legs pulled up toward the abdomen. DO NOT reinsert organs into the abdomen. Cover organs with a moist, sterile or clean dressing. Treat for shock. Call 9-1-1.
Pelvic Injuries	Pelvic fracture Pain in hip, groin, or back that increases with movement Inability to walk or stand Signs of shock	Keep victim still. Treat for shock. Call 9-1-1.

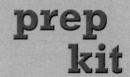

prep kit

▶ Ready for Review

- Chest injuries fall into two categories: open or closed.
- Closed chest injuries include rib fractures and flail chest.
- In an open chest injury, the skin has been broken and the chest wall is penetrated by an object such as a knife or bullet.
- Injuries to the abdomen are either open or closed and can involve hollow and/or solid organs.
- Closed abdominal injuries occur when the internal abdominal tissues are damaged but the skin is unbroken.
- Open abdominal injuries are those in which the skin has been broken and the abdominal wall penetrated.
- Pelvic fractures are usually caused by falling or a motor vehicle crash.

▶ Vital Vocabulary

<u>closed abdominal injuries</u> Injuries to the abdomen that occur as a result of a direct blow from a blunt object. There is no break in the skin.

<u>closed chest injury</u> An injury to the chest in which the skin is not broken; usually due to blunt trauma.

<u>flail chest</u> A condition that occurs when several ribs in the same area are broken in more than one place.

<u>open abdominal injuries</u> Injuries to the abdomen that include penetrating wounds and protruding organs.

<u>open chest injury</u> An injury to the chest in which the chest wall itself is penetrated by an external object such as a bullet or knife.

<u>protruding organ injury</u> A severe injury to the abdomen in which the internal organs escape or protrude from the wound; evisceration.

<u>sucking chest wound</u> A chest wound that allows air to pass into the chest cavity with each breath.

139

prep
kit

▶ Assessment in Action

You are on the first aid team at a local scout camp. The scout leaders are conducting a funny skit on a stage at the main lodge. One of the scouts in the skit jumps in the air and lands on his side. As he runs off the stage toward you, he is in obvious pain and is clutching his side. He lies down and a knife falls to the ground. You hear a sucking sound coming from the wound on his side whenever the victim inhales.

Directions: Circle Yes if you agree with the statement; circle No if you disagree.

Yes   No   **1.** You should check the victim's breathing and treat accordingly.

Yes   No   **2.** Blood bubbling out of the wound during breathing is a sign of a sucking chest wound.

Yes   No   **3.** This wound should be sealed on three sides to prevent air from being trapped in the chest cavity.

Yes   No   **4.** If the victim begins to have trouble breathing, do not remove the seal to reapply.

Yes   No   **5.** This is a medical emergency and 9-1-1 should be called immediately.

▶ Check Your Knowledge

Directions: Circle Yes if you agree with the statement; circle No if you disagree.

Yes   No   **1.** Stabilize a broken rib with a soft object, such as a pillow or blanket, tied to the chest.

Yes   No   **2.** Cover a sucking chest wound with a piece of plastic taped down on three sides.

Yes   No   **3.** Remove a penetrating or impaled object from the chest or the abdomen.

Yes   No   **4.** A flail chest refers to a single broken rib.

Yes   No   **5.** Keep the victim with a broken pelvis still.

Yes   No   **6.** Sharp pain while breathing can be a sign of a rib fracture.

Yes   No   **7.** Rib fractures should be treated by tightly taping the chest.

Yes   No   **8.** Most victims with abdominal injuries are more comfortable with their knees bent.

Yes   No   **9.** Leave a chest wound alone if you hear air being sucked in and out.

Yes   No   **10.** A broken pelvis can threaten life because of the large amount of blood lost.

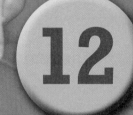

Bone, Joint, and Muscle Injuries

Bone Injuries

Bone, joint, and muscle injuries are among the most common reasons for seeking medical care. Although rarely fatal, they often result in short- or long-term disability.

▶ Fractures

The real problems are not the broken bones themselves but rather the potential injury to the vital organs next to them. People usually do not die of broken bones. They die of airway obstruction, blood loss, and brain injury. However, broken bones can be painful and debilitating and can cause lifelong aggravation, disability, and deformity.

The terms *fracture* and *broken bone* have the same meaning: a break or crack in a bone. There are two categories of fractures:

- **Closed fracture**. The skin is intact, and no wound exists anywhere near the fracture site **Figure 1A**.
- **Open fracture**. The skin over the fracture has been broken. The wound may result from the bone protruding through the skin or from a direct blow that cut the skin at the time of the fracture. The bone may not always be visible in the wound **Figure 1B**.

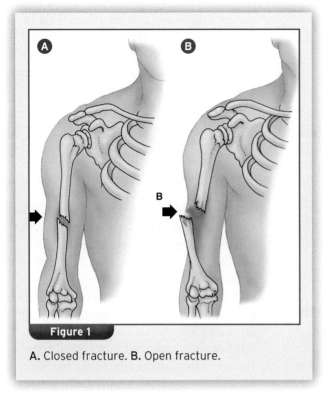

Figure 1

A. Closed fracture. B. Open fracture.

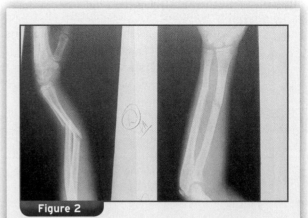

Figure 2

X-rays of a victim's forearm showing the fracture before and after setting.

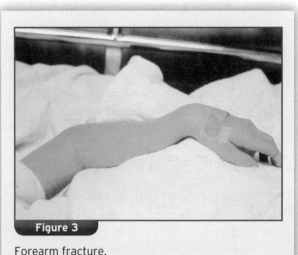

Figure 3

Forearm fracture.

Recognizing Fractures

It may be difficult to tell if a bone is broken **Figure 2**. When in doubt, treat the injury as a fracture. Use the mnemonic DOTS to assess for an injury—Deformity, Open wound, Tenderness, Swelling.

- *Deformity* might not be obvious. Compare the injured part with the uninjured part on the other side.
- *Open wound* may indicate an underlying fracture.
- *Tenderness* and pain are commonly found only at the injury site. The victim usually will be able to point to the site of the pain. A useful procedure for detecting a fracture is to feel along the bone gently; a victim's complaint about pain or tenderness serves as a reliable sign of a fracture.
- *Swelling* caused by bleeding happens rapidly after a fracture.

Additional signs and symptoms include the following:

- *Loss of use* may or may not occur.
- *Guarding* occurs when motion produces pain; the victim refuses to use the injured part. Sometimes, however, the victim is able to move a fractured limb with little or no pain.

- A *grating sensation*, called <u>crepitus</u>, can be felt and sometimes even heard when the ends of the broken bone rub together. Do not move the injured limb in an attempt to detect it **Figure 3**.
- The history of the injury can lead you to suspect a fracture whenever a serious accident has happened. The victim may have heard or felt the bone snap.

Care for Fractures

1. Perform a primary check for life-threatening conditions. A fracture, even an open fracture, seldom presents an immediate threat to life.

Treatment should be deferred until after you have handled any life-threatening conditions such as opening an airway or controlling massive bleeding. Only when all life-threatening conditions have been dealt with is it appropriate to identify and stabilize fractures. Determine what happened and the location of the injury.

2. Gently remove clothing covering the injured area. Cut clothing at the seams if necessary.

3. Examine the area by looking and feeling for DOTS.
   - Look at the injury site. Swelling and black-and-blue marks, which indicate escape of blood into the tissues, may come from the bone end or associated muscular and blood vessel damage. Shortening or severe deformity (angulation) between the joints or deformity around the joints, shortening of the extremity, and rotation of the extremity when compared with the opposite extremity indicate a bone injury. Lacerations or even small puncture wounds near the site of a bone fracture are considered open fractures.
   - Feel the injured area. If a fracture is not obvious, gently press, touch, or feel along the length of the bone for deformities, tenderness, and swelling.

4. Check blood flow and nerves. Use the mnemonic CSM (circulation, sensation, movement) as a way of remembering what to do **Skill Drill 1**:
   - *Circulation.* For an arm injury, feel for the radial pulse (located on the thumb side of the wrist); use the posterior tibial pulse (located between the inside ankle bone and the Achilles tendon) for a leg injury. A pulseless arm or leg is a significant emergency that requires immediate surgical care. If there is no pulse, gently realign the extremity to try to restore the blood flow. Some experts recommend the capillary refill test. (Press on a fingernail or toenail, then release it. If circulation is normal, the nail bed should return to its normal color within 2 seconds.) Performing the capillary refill test in the dark or the cold may limit its accuracy (**Steps ❶** and **❷**).
   - *Sensation.* This is the most useful early sign. Lightly touch or squeeze one of the victim's

toes or fingers and ask the victim what he or she feels (**Steps ❸** and **❹**). Loss of sensation is an early sign of nerve damage.
   - *Movement.* Inability to move develops later. Check for nerve damage by asking the victim to wiggle his or her toes or fingers (**Steps ❺** and **❻**). If the toes or fingers are injured, do not have the victim attempt to move them. A quick nerve and circulatory check is extremely important. The most serious complication of a fracture is inadequate blood flow in an extremity. The major blood vessels of an extremity tend to run close to the bones, which means that any time a bone is broken, the adjacent blood vessels are at risk of being torn by bone fragments or pinched off between the ends of the broken bone. The tissues of the arms and legs cannot survive for more than 3 hours without a continuing blood supply. If you note any disruption in the nerve or circulatory supply, seek immediate medical attention. Major nerve pathways also travel close to bone and may be torn or pinched off between the ends of the broken bone.

5. Stabilize the injured part to prevent movement.
   - If emergency medical services (EMS) will arrive soon, stabilize the injured part with your hands until they arrive.
   - If EMS will be delayed or if you are taking the victim to medical care, stabilize the injured part with a splint.

6. If the injury is an open fracture, do not push on any protruding bones **Figure 4**. Cover

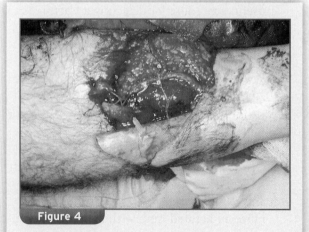

Figure 4

Open tibia, fibula fracture of the leg.

the wound and exposed bones with a dressing. Place rolls of gauze around the bone and bandage the injury without applying pressure on the bone.

7. Apply an ice pack, if possible, to help reduce swelling and pain.

8. Seek medical care. Call 9-1-1 for any open fractures or large bone fractures (such as the femur) or when transporting the victim would be difficult or would aggravate the injury.

skill drill

1   Checking CSM in an Extremity

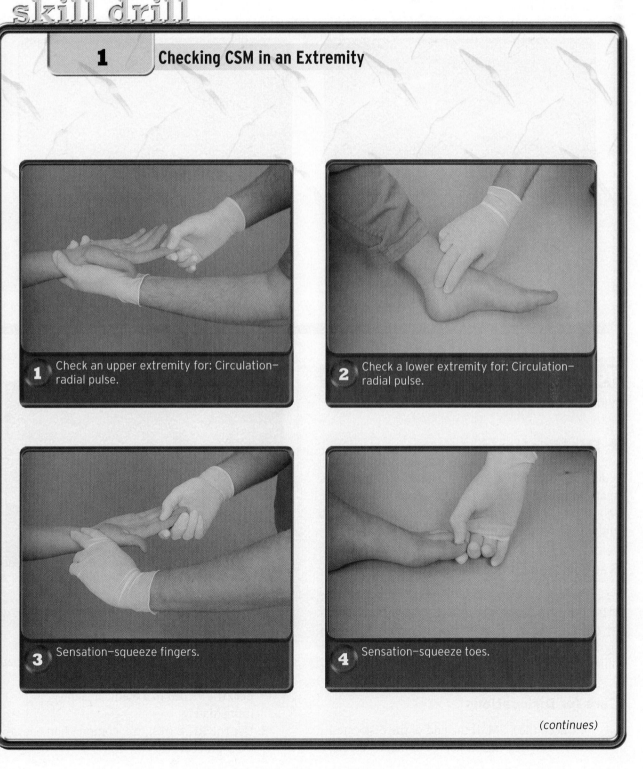

1 Check an upper extremity for: Circulation–radial pulse.

2 Check a lower extremity for: Circulation–radial pulse.

3 Sensation–squeeze fingers.

4 Sensation–squeeze toes.

(continues)

skill drill

1   **Checking CSM in an Extremity (*continued*)**

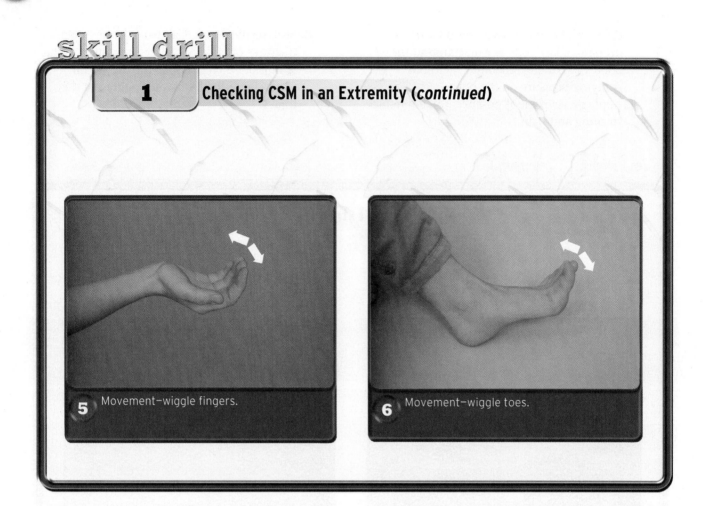

5 Movement–wiggle fingers.

6 Movement–wiggle toes.

Joint Injuries

A joint is where two or more bones come together.

▶ Dislocations

A *dislocation* occurs when a joint comes apart and stays apart with the bone ends no longer in contact. The shoulders, elbows, fingers, hips, kneecaps (patellas), and ankles are the joints most frequently affected.

Recognizing Dislocations

Dislocations cause signs and symptoms similar to those of fractures: deformity, severe pain, swelling, and inability of the victim to move the injured joint. The main sign of a dislocation is deformity. Its appearance will be different from that of an uninjured joint **Figure 5** .

Care for Dislocations

1. Check the CSM. If the end of the dislocated bone is pressing on nerves or blood vessels,

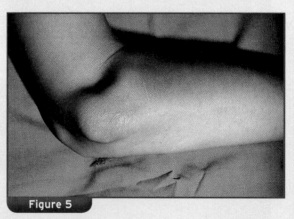

Figure 5

Dislocation

numbness or paralysis may exist below the dislocation. Always check the pulses. If there is no pulse in the injured extremity, transport the victim to a medical facility immediately.

2. Use the RICE (rest, ice, compression, elevation) procedures.

3. Use a splint to stabilize the joint in the position in which it was found.
4. Do not try to reduce the joint (put the displaced parts back into their normal positions) because nerve and blood vessel damage could result.
5. Seek medical care to reduce the dislocation. Call 9-1-1 for dislocations when transporting the victim would be difficult or would aggravate the injury.

▶ Sprains

A <u>sprain</u> occurs when a joint is twisted or stretched beyond its normal range of motion. Bones are held together at joints by tough bands of tissue called ligaments. When a joint is sprained, the ligaments are either partially or completely torn. There are different degrees of sprains, but it is difficult for a first aider to classify the degree of a sprain. Sprains most often occur in the knee and the ankle, but can occur in any joint.

Ankle sprains most often occur when the foot turns inward and stress is placed on the outside (lateral side) of the ankle. A severe lateral ankle sprain, if not correctly treated, can result in a chronically unstable ankle that is prone to sprains. Any ligament or bone injury on the inner side of the ankle usually represents a serious problem and requires medical care.

Recognizing Sprains

It is often difficult to distinguish between a severe sprain and a fracture because their signs and symptoms are similar.

- Severe pain
- Pain prevents the victim from moving or using the joint.
- Swelling
- Skin around the joint may be discolored because of bleeding from torn blood vessels.

Care for Sprains

1. Follow the RICE procedures. Apply an ice pack for 20 minutes; apply compression with an elastic bandage for 3 to 4 hours; repeat the cycles of an ice pack for 20 minutes and 3 hours of compression. Raise the injured part to reduce the flow of blood to the injury. For more information on the RICE procedure, see page 150.

2. Swelling in a joint can lead to stiffness in a matter of hours. It is important to keep a joint from swelling by using cold promptly; it is equally important to help the swelling recede as quickly as possible with compression and elevation.

Muscle Injuries

Although muscle injuries pose no real emergency, first aiders have ample opportunities to care for them.

▶ Strains

A *muscle strain*, also known as a *muscle pull*, occurs when a muscle is stretched beyond its normal range of motion and tears the muscle. There are different degrees of strains, but it is difficult for a first aider to classify the degree of a strain. When muscle fibers tear, fluid from nearby tissues leaks out and starts to build up near the injury. The area becomes inflamed, swollen, and tender. Inflammation begins immediately after an injury, but it can take 24 to 72 hours for enough tissue fluid to build up to cause pain and stiffness.

Recognizing Strains

Any of the following signs and symptoms may indicate a muscle strain:

- Sudden, sharp pain in the affected muscle
- Extreme tenderness when the area is touched
- Swelling
- Weakness and inability to use the injured part
- Stiffness and pain when the victim moves the muscle
- After a few days, the skin around the injury may be discolored because of bleeding from torn blood vessels.

Care for Strains

To care for strains, simply follow the RICE procedures.

▶ Cramps

A <u>cramp</u> occurs when a muscle goes into an uncontrolled spasm and contraction. Although scientific literature has yet to confirm the causes of muscle cramps, several factors are associated with them. For example, muscle cramping is associated with certain diseases such as diabetes and atherosclerosis. Muscle cramps are often associated with physical activity. Roughly, muscle cramps can be divided into two categories: *night cramps*, which include any cramp occurring at night or while an individual is at rest, and *heat cramps*, which are related to dehydration and electrolyte imbalance. (The electrolytes potassium and sodium carry an electric charge that helps trigger muscles to contract and relax.)

Recognizing Cramps

- Sudden, severe pain, usually in the legs
- A knotting of the muscle may be felt and sometimes seen.
- Restricted movement

Care for Cramps

Many treatments for cramps are available. Try one or more of the following:

1. Have the victim gently stretch the affected muscle. Because a muscle cramp is an uncontrolled muscle contraction or spasm, a gradual extension of the muscle may help lengthen the muscle fibers and relieve the cramp.
2. Relax the muscle by pressing and massaging it.
3. Apply an ice pack to help relieve the cramping pain (unless you are in a cold environment).

CAUTION

DO NOT give salt tablets to a person with muscle cramps. They can cause stomach irritation, nausea, and vomiting.

---

4. Pinch the upper lip hard (an acupressure technique) to reduce calf-muscle cramping.
5. Drink lightly salted cool water (dissolve ¼ teaspoon salt in a quart of water) or a commercial sports drink.

▶ Contusions

A muscle contusion or bruise results from a blow to the muscle.

Recognizing Contusions

- Swelling
- Pain and tenderness
- After a few days, the skin in the area may become discolored due to bleeding from torn blood vessels.

Care for Contusions

To care for muscle contusions, follow the RICE procedures.

▶ Emergency Care Wrap-up

Condition	What to Look For	What to Do
Bone Injuries	Fractures (broken bones) DOTS (deformity, open wound, tenderness, swelling) Inability to use injured part normally Grating or grinding sensation felt or heard Victim heard or felt bone snap	Expose and examine the injury site. Bandage any open wound. Splint the injured area. Apply ice or cold pack. Seek medical care: Depending on the severity, call 9-1-1 or transport to medical care.
Joint Injuries	Dislocation or sprain Deformity Pain Swelling Inability to use injured part normally	**Dislocation** Expose and examine the injury site. Splint the injured area. Apply ice or cold pack. Seek medical care. **Sprain** Use RICE procedures.
Muscle Injuries	**Strain** Sharp pain Extreme tenderness when area is touched Indentation or bump Weakness and loss of function of injured area Stiffness and pain when victim moves the muscle	Use RICE procedures.
	Contusion Pain and tenderness Swelling Bruise on injured area	Use RICE procedures.
	Cramp Uncontrolled spasm **Pain** Restriction or loss of movement	Stretch and/or apply direct pressure to the affected muscle.

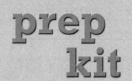

prep kit

▶ Ready for Review

- Broken bones can be painful and debilitating and can cause lifelong aggravation, disability, and deformity.
- A joint is where two or more bones come together. Joints can be dislocated or sprained.
- Muscles can be strained, bruised, or cramped.

▶ Vital Vocabulary

closed fracture A fracture in which there is no wound in the overlying skin.

cramp A painful spasm of a muscle.

crepitus A grating sound heard and the sensation felt when the fractured ends of a bone rub together.

fracture A break or rupture in a bone.

open fracture A fracture exposed to the exterior; an open wound lies over the fracture.

sprain A trauma to a joint that injures the ligaments.

▶ Assessment in Action

While walking through your neighborhood, you see two boys yelling for help on the sidewalk. One is on the ground in pain and clutching his arm. The other boy explains that the injured boy lost control while skateboarding and crashed. The victim said he heard a snap when he crashed and landed on his arm.

Directions: Circle Yes if you agree with the statement; circle No if you disagree.

Yes No 1. You should look and feel for DOTS.

Yes No 2. You notice a severe deformity on the victim's forearm but the skin is not broken. This is a closed fracture.

Yes No 3. You should check the injured arm for circulation, sensation, and movement.

Yes No 4. You should not splint the arm because of the deformity.

Yes No 5. Applying ice helps reduce swelling.

▶ Check Your Knowledge

Directions: Circle Yes if you agree with the statement; circle No if you disagree.

Yes No 1. Apply cold on a suspected sprain.

Yes No 2. The letters RICE stand for rest, ice, compression, and elevation.

Yes No 3. DOTS stands for deformity, open wound, tenderness, and swelling.

Yes No 4. Guarding occurs when motion produces pain.

Yes No 5. Crepitus cannot be heard, but it can be felt by the victim.

Yes No 6. A dislocation is cared for much differently than a fracture.

Yes No 7. Check a suspected fracture by having the victim move the extremity.

Yes No 8. Treat a muscle cramp by stretching the affected muscle.

Yes No 9. CSM stands for cold, swelling, and motion.

Yes No 10. Do not push on a protruding bone.

Extremity Injuries

13

Extremity Injuries

Injuries to the extremities are common because people are involved in active lifestyles that include sports and wilderness activities. This chapter focuses on bone, joint, and muscle injuries of the extremities; bleeding, wounds, and other soft-tissue injuries are covered elsewhere. Most of the conditions discussed result from sudden trauma, although some chronic injuries incurred over time, such as tennis elbow, are included.

▶ Assessment

Use these guidelines to assess injuries to the extremities:

- Look for signs and symptoms of fractures and dislocations.
- Examine the extremities, using the mnemonic DOTS (Deformity, Open wound, Tenderness, Swelling). Look at and gently feel the extremity, starting at the distal end (fingers or toes) and working upward.
- Compare one extremity with the other to determine size and shape differences.
- Use the "rule of thirds" for extremity injuries. Imagine each long bone as being divided into thirds. If deformity, tenderness, or swelling is located in the upper or lower third of a long bone, assume that the nearest joint is injured.

chapter
at a glance

- ▶ **Extremity Injuries**

- ▶ **RICE Procedure for Bone, Joint, and Muscle Injuries**

- ▶ **Splinting Extremities**

- Consider the cause of injury (COI) when evaluating the possibility of a fracture and its location. Forces that cause musculoskeletal injuries are direct forces (for example, a car bumper striking a pedestrian's leg), indirect forces along the long axis of bones (for example, a person falling onto an out-stretched hand and fracturing the collarbone), and twisting forces (for example, a person's foot fixed in one spot with the leg suddenly twisting).
- Use the mnemonic CSM as a reminder to check the extremity for circulation, sensation, and movement of fingers or toes.

▶ Types of Injuries

Types of injuries to the extremities range from a simple contusion to a complex open fracture:

- <u>Contusion</u>, or bruising of the tissue
- <u>Strain</u>, in which muscles are stretched or torn
- <u>Sprain</u>, which involves the tearing or stretching of the joints, causing mild to severe damage to the ligaments and joint capsules
- <u>Tendinitis</u>, which is inflammation of a tendon (cord that attaches muscle to bone) caused by overuse
- <u>Dislocation</u>, in which bones are displaced from their normal joint alignment, out of their sockets, or out of their normal positions
- <u>Fracture</u>, which is a break in a bone that may or may not be accompanied by an open wound

Care for Extremity Injuries

1. Use the RICE procedures for injuries described in this chapter (see Skill Drill 1, page 169).
2. Apply a splint to stabilize fractures and dislocations.

RICE Procedure for Bone, Joint, and Muscle Injuries

RICE is the acronym for rest, ice, compression, and elevation—the recommended immediate treatment for bone, joint, and muscle injuries. The steps during the first 48 to 72 hours after an injury can do a lot to relieve—even prevent—aches and pains. Treat all extremity bone, joint, and muscle injuries with the RICE procedure. In addition to RICE, fractures and dislocations should be splinted to stabilize the injured area.

▶ R = Rest

Injuries heal faster if rested. Rest means the victim does not use or move the injured part. Using any part of the body increases the blood circulation to that area, which can cause more swelling of an injured part. Crutches may be used to rest leg injuries.

▶ I = Ice

An ice pack should be applied to the injured area as soon as possible after the injury for 20 to 30 minutes as often as possible while awake, removing the ice pack for 5–10 minutes between each 20–30 minute period, during the first 24 to 48 hours. Never apply ice directly to the skin. Skin treated with cold passes through four stages: cold, burning, aching, and numbness. When the skin becomes numb, usually in 20 to 30 minutes, remove the ice pack. After removing the ice pack, compress the injured part with an elastic bandage and keep it elevated (the "C" and "E" of RICE).

CAUTION

DO NOT apply an ice pack for more than 20 to 30 minutes at a time. Frostbite or nerve damage can result.

DO NOT apply an ice pack on the back outside part of the knee. Nerve damage can occur.

DO NOT apply cold if the victim has a history of circulatory disease, Raynaud disease (spasms in the arteries of the extremities that reduce circulation), or abnormal sensitivity to cold, or if the injured part has been frostbitten previously.

DO NOT stop using an ice pack too soon. A common mistake is the early use of heat, which may result in swelling and pain. Use an ice pack three to four times a day for the first 24 hours, preferably up to 48 hours, before applying any heat. For severe injuries, using ice for up to 72 hours is recommended.

FYI

Heat and Cold: When to Use Which?

Many people use heat devices or ice packs to speed recovery from sports injuries—but when is the right time to use each technique? Cold usually should be applied immediately after an acute injury, such as an ankle sprain. Icing reduces pain, swelling, and muscle spasm immediately after injury, but its use should be discontinued after 2 or 3 days. Heat applications (heat packs, radiant heat, or whirlpool baths) can then be used to reduce muscle spasms and pain. In addition, heat increases blood flow and joint flexibility. Vigorous heat is used to treat chronic injuries, but mild heat can reduce muscle spasm. Heat is also effective for acute back pain, but ice massage is preferred if the back pain persists for 2 weeks or more.

Source: Kaul M P, Herring S A: Superficial heat and cold. *Physician and Sportsmedicine.* 22(12);65.

FYI

Homemade Ice Packs

- Ice bags kept in a freezer freeze solid and cannot be shaped to fit the injured area. One part isopropyl (rubbing) alcohol to three parts water prevents freezing, and the ice bag can be easily molded. Bags can be reused for months.
- An unopened bag of frozen vegetables is inexpensive; keeps its basic shape (unlike ice chips, which melt); molds to the shape of the injured area; is reusable; and is packaged in a fairly puncture-resistant, watertight bag.
- For cold therapy over a fairly large area, soak a face towel in cold water, wring it out, fold it, and place it in a large self-sealing plastic bag. Store the bag in the freezer. To use the cold pack, wrap it in a light cotton towel and apply for 20 minutes, after which it can be refrozen. A washcloth in a smaller bag can be used to treat a smaller area.
- Fill a plastic bag with snow.
- Fill a polystyrene plastic cup with water and freeze it. When you need an ice pack, peel the cup to below ice level; the remaining part of the cup forms a cold-resistant handle. Rub the ice over the injured area (movement is necessary to prevent skin damage). These ice "packs" are inexpensive and convenient and take up little space.
- To make a funnel for filling an ice bag, push out the bottom of a paper cup and fit it into the neck of the ice bag. The ice will slide through the cup and into the bag.

Cold constricts the blood vessels to and in the injured area, which helps reduce the swelling and inflammation, and it dulls the pain and relieves muscle spasms. Cold should be applied as soon as possible after the injury; healing time often is directly related to the amount of swelling that occurs. Heat has the opposite effect when applied to fresh injuries: It increases circulation to the area and increases the swelling and the pain.

Use either of the following methods to apply cold to an injury:

- Put crushed ice (or cubes) into a double plastic bag, hot water bottle, or wet towel. A layer of cloth should separate the ice from the skin. Secure it in place with an elastic bandage for 20 to 30 minutes. Ice bags can conform to the body's contours.
- Use a chemical "snap pack," a sealed pouch that contains two chemical envelopes. Squeezing the pack mixes the chemicals, producing a chemical reaction that has a cooling effect. Although they do not cool as well as other methods, they are convenient to use when ice is not readily available. They lose their cooling power quickly, however, and can be used only once. Also, they may be impractical because they are expensive.

▶ C = Compression

Compressing the injured area squeezes fluid out of the injury site. Compression limits the ability of the skin and other tissues to expand and reduces internal bleeding. Apply an elastic bandage to the injured area, especially the foot, ankle, knee, thigh, hand, or elbow. Fill the hollow areas with padding such as a sock or washcloth before applying the elastic bandage.

Elastic bandages come in various sizes for different body areas:

- 2″ width for the wrist, hand, and foot
- 3″ width for the elbow and arm
- 4″ width for the ankle, knee, and leg

Start the elastic bandage several inches below the injury and wrap in an upward, overlapping (about one half to three fourths of the bandage's width) spiral,

CAUTION

DO NOT apply an elastic bandage too tightly. If applied too tightly, elastic bandages will restrict circulation. Stretch a new elastic bandage to about one third its maximum length for adequate compression. Leave fingers and toes exposed so possible color change can be easily observed. Compare the toes or fingers of the injured extremity with those on the uninjured one. Pale skin, pain, numbness, and tingling are signs that the bandage is too tight. If any of these symptoms appears, immediately remove the elastic bandage. Leave the elastic bandage off until all the symptoms disappear, then rewrap the area less tightly. Always wrap from below the injury and move toward the heart.

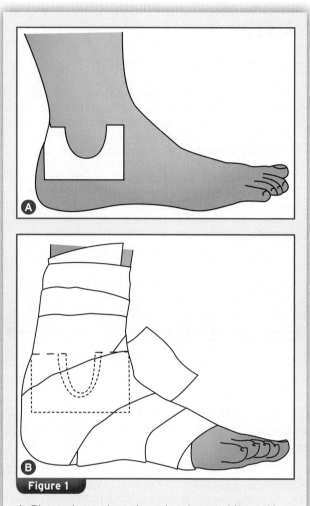

Figure 1

A. Place a horseshoe-shaped pad around the ankle knob. **B.** Secure the pad with an elastic bandage.

starting with even and somewhat tight pressure, then gradually wrapping more loosely above the injury. Stretch the elastic bandage no more than one third its ability to stretch.

Applying compression may be the most important step in preventing swelling. The victim should wear the elastic bandage continuously for the first 18 to 24 hours (except when cold is applied). At night, have the victim loosen but not remove the elastic bandage.

For an ankle injury, place a horseshoe-shaped pad around the ankle knob and secure it with the elastic bandage **Figure 1**. The pad can be made from various materials (eg, twisting a wash cloth, socks). The pad will compress the soft tissues and the bones. Wrap the bandage tightest nearest the toes and loosest above the ankle. It should be tight enough to decrease swelling but not tight enough to inhibit blood flow. For a contusion or a strain, place a pad between the injury and the elastic bandage.

▶ E = Elevation

Gravity slows the return of blood to the heart from the lower parts of the body. Once fluids get to the hands or feet, they have nowhere else to go, and those parts of the body swell. Elevating the injured area, in combination with ice and compression, limits circulation to that area, which in turn helps limit internal bleeding and minimize swelling.

It is simple to prop up an injured leg or arm to limit bleeding. Whenever possible, elevate the injured

part above the level of the heart for the first 24 hours after an injury. If a fracture is suspected, do not elevate an extremity until it has been stabilized with a splint. Along with the use of RICE procedures, fractures and dislocations should be splinted.

To perform the RICE procedure, follow the steps in **Skill Drill 1**:

1. R = Rest. Stop using the injured area.
2. I = Ice. Place an ice pack on the injured area. Use an elastic bandage to hold the ice pack in place for 20 to 30 minutes (**Step ❶**).
3. C = Compression. Remove the ice, apply a compression bandage, and leave in place for 3 to 4 hours (**Step ❷**).
4. E = Elevation. Raise the injured area higher than the heart, if possible (**Step ❸**).

skill drill

1 The RICE Procedure

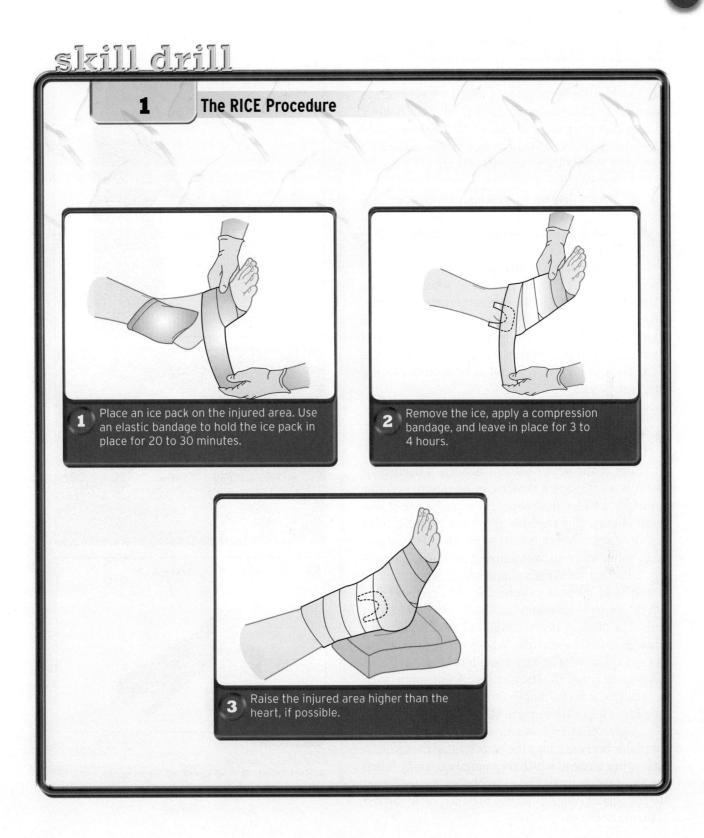

1 Place an ice pack on the injured area. Use an elastic bandage to hold the ice pack in place for 20 to 30 minutes.

2 Remove the ice, apply a compression bandage, and leave in place for 3 to 4 hours.

3 Raise the injured area higher than the heart, if possible.

Splinting Extremities

Injured extremities should be stabilized by splinting the extremity in the position in which it was found. To stabilize means to minimize further injury by holding a body part to prevent movement. All fractures should be stabilized before a victim is moved. The reasons for splinting to stabilize an injured area are to:

- Reduce pain.
- Prevent damage to muscles, nerves, and blood vessels.
- Prevent a closed fracture from becoming an open fracture.
- Reduce bleeding and swelling.

All fractures are complicated to some degree by damage to the soft tissue and structures surrounding the bone. The major cause of tissue damage at a fracture site is movement by the end of the broken bone. The end of a broken bone is sharp, and it is important to prevent a fractured bone from moving into soft tissues.

▶ Types of Splints

A **splint** is any device used to stabilize a fracture or a dislocation. Such a device can be improvised (for example, a folded newspaper), or it can be one of several commercially available splints (for example, SAM splint). Lack of a commercial splint should never prevent you from properly stabilizing an injured extremity. Splinting sometimes requires improvisation.

A rigid splint is an inflexible device attached to an extremity to maintain stability. It can be a padded board, a piece of heavy cardboard, or a SAM splint molded to fit the extremity. Whatever its construction, a rigid splint must be long enough to be secured well above and below the fracture site. A soft splint, such as a pillow, is useful mainly for stabilizing fractures of the lower leg or the forearm **Figure 2** .

A self-splint, or anatomic splint, is almost always available because it uses the body itself as the splint. A self-splint is one in which the injured extremity is tied to an uninjured part (for example, an injured finger to the adjacent finger, the legs together, or an injured arm to the chest).

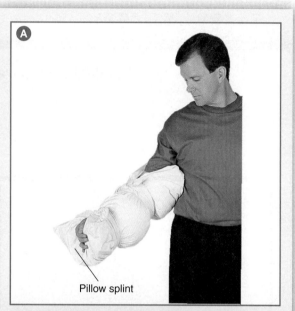

Pillow splint

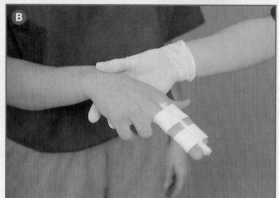

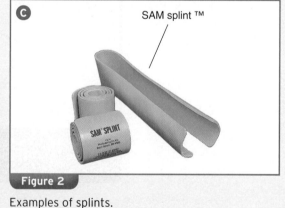

SAM splint ™

Figure 2

Examples of splints.
A. Soft splint. **B.** Self-splint. **C.** Rigid splint.

▶ Splinting Guidelines

All fractures and dislocations should be stabilized before the victim is moved. When in doubt, apply a splint. To apply a splint:

1. Cover any open wounds with a sterile dressing before applying a splint.

2. Check the CSM in the extremity. If pulses are absent and medical help is hours away, gently line up a fracture or a dislocation to restore blood flow. Support the limb and move gently to line up the parts. Joints may be left in a position of comfort. Line up the limb above and below the joint, do not force anything into position. Any movement of a fracture is expected to cause pain; you should be aware of this and warn the victim. You do not have to align the limb perfectly, just align it enough to allow the return of circulation.

3. Determine what to splint by using the rule of thirds. Imagine each long bone as being divided into thirds. If the injury is located in the upper or lower third of a bone, assume that the nearest joint is injured. Therefore, the splint should extend to stabilize the bones above and below the unstable joint. For example, for a fracture of the upper third of the tibia (shinbone), the splint must extend above the knee to include the upper leg, as well as the lower leg, because the knee is unstable. For a fracture of the middle third of a bone, stabilize the joints above and below the fracture (for example, the wrist and elbow for a fractured radius or ulna; the shoulder and elbow for a fractured humerus; the knee and ankle for a fractured tibia or fibula). In addition to splinting an upper extremity fracture, place the injured arm in an arm sling and a swathe (binder).

4. If two first aiders are present, one should support the injury site and minimize movement of the extremity until splinting is completed.

5. When possible, place splint materials on both sides of the injured part, especially when two bones are involved, such as the radius and ulna in the lower arm or the tibia and fibula in the lower leg. This sandwich splint prevents the injured extremity from rotating and keeps the two bones from touching. With rigid splints, use extra padding in natural body hollows and around any deformities.

6. Apply splints firmly but not so tightly that blood flow into an extremity is affected. Check the CSM before and periodically after the splint is applied. If the pulse disappears, loosen the splint enough so you can feel the pulse. Leave the fingers or toes exposed so the CSM can be checked easily.

7. Use RICE (rest, ice, compression, and elevation) on the injured part. When practical, elevate the injured extremity after it is stabilized to promote drainage and reduce swelling. Do not, however, apply ice packs if a pulse is absent.

If the victim has a possible spinal injury and an extremity injury, the spinal injury takes precedence. Splinting the spine is always a problem. Tell the victim not to move. Then stabilize the spine with rolled blankets or similar objects placed on each side of the neck and torso. In most cases, it is best to wait until EMS personnel arrive with proper equipment to handle spinal injuries.

Most fractures do not require rapid transportation. An exception is an arm or a leg without a pulse, which means there is insufficient blood flow to the injured extremity. In that case, immediate medical care is necessary.

CAUTION

DO NOT straighten dislocations or fractures of the spine, elbow, wrist, hip, or knee because of the proximity of major nerves and arteries. Instead, if the CSM assessment findings are normal, splint joint injuries in the position in which you find them.

DO NOT apply traction on open fractures. Instead, cover the wound with a sterile dressing and apply a splint.

Seek medical care for the following injuries or situations:

- Any open fracture
- Any dislocation (injury that causes joint deformity)
- Any joint injury with moderate to severe swelling
- Any injury in which there is deformity, tenderness, or swelling over the bone
- If the victim is unable to walk or bear weight after a lower extremity injury
- If a snap, crackle, or pop was heard at the time of injury
- If the injured area, especially a joint, becomes hot, tender, swollen, or painful
- If you are unsure whether a bone was broken
- If the injury does not improve rapidly, especially over the first few days

▶ Slings

An open triangular bandage can be used as a **sling**. A folded triangular bandage known as a cravat can be used as a **swathe** (binder) in conjunction with a sling. A cravat may also be applied using the same procedures as an open triangular sling but placed around the wrist when long splints on an upper arm or forearm may be in the way. To apply an arm sling to the upper arm, forearm, or hand/wrist injuries, follow the steps below:

1. Hold the victim's arm slightly away from the chest, with the wrist and hand slightly higher (about 40″) than the tip of the elbow. Place a triangular bandage between the forearm and chest with the point of the triangular bandage toward the elbow and stretch the bandage well beyond the elbow. Pull the upper end of the bandage over the uninjured shoulder.
2. Bring the lower end of the bandage over the forearm.

▶ Ready for Review

- Injuries to the extremities are common.
- There are many types of injuries to the extremities, ranging from simple contusions to complex open fractures.
- RICE is the acronym for Rest, Ice, Compression, and Elevation.

▶ Vital Vocabulary

contusion A bruise; an injury that causes a hemorrhage in or beneath the skin but does not break the skin.

dislocation Bone is displaced from its normal joint alignment, out of its socket, or out of its normal position.

fracture A break or crack in the bone.

sling A triangular bandage applied around the neck to support an injured upper extremity; any material long enough to suspend an upper extremity by passing the material around the neck; used to support and protect an injury of the arm, shoulder, or clavicle.

splint Any support used to immobilize a fracture or to restrict movement of a part.

sprain A trauma to the joint that injures the ligaments.

strain An injury to a muscle caused by a violent contraction or an excessive, forcible stretching.

swathe A cravat tied around the body to decrease movement of a part.

tendinitis Inflammation of a tendon caused by overuse.

▶ Assessment in Action

During a flag football game at a neighborhood park, your teammate is going back for a sure interception. He jumps for the ball, catches it, and comes down, twisting his ankle in a small hole on the field. Your teammate is in pain and is feeling nauseous.

Directions: Circle Yes if you agree with the statement; circle No if you disagree.

Yes No **1.** It is difficult to distinguish between a severely sprained ankle and a fractured ankle.

Yes No **2.** If the victim cannot walk at least four steps and reports tenderness when you press on the ankle knob bone (malleous), suspect a fractured ankle.

Yes No **3.** Heat should be applied immediately to a sprained ankle to increase blood flow and decrease pain.

Yes No **4.** Swelling on both sides of the ankle usually indicates a sprained ankle.

prep kit

▶ Check Your Knowledge

Directions: Circle Yes if you agree with the statement; circle No if you disagree.

Yes   No   **1.** Injuries heal faster if rested.

Yes   No   **2.** Compression increases internal bleeding, helping the injury to heal faster.

Yes   No   **3.** A strain is actually a tear in the muscle.

Yes   No   **4.** The three bones in the fingers are very strong and do not break easily.

Yes   No   **5.** The hip joint is easily dislocated.

Yes   No   **6.** Considerable force is required to break the femur.

Yes   No   **7.** A strain is actually a tear in the muscle.

Yes   No   **8.** Knee injuries are not serious.

Yes   No   **9.** Shin splints are a pain that runs down the back of the leg.

Yes   No   **10.** Most ankle injuries are not fractures.

Sudden Illnesses

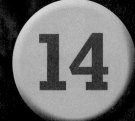

14

▶ Unexplained Change in Responsiveness

Victims can be fully alert (responsive), completely unresponsive, or can range anywhere between these two. Not all responsive victims are fully alert and they may respond to different levels of stimulation (eg, respond to your voice or squeezing of shoulder muscle). The level of responsiveness and mental status indicate how well the brain is functioning.

The main causes for a decrease in a person's alertness and responsiveness are brain injury and lack of either oxygen or glucose reaching the brain. The mnemonic STOP offers clues to the cause(s) of changes in responsiveness **Table 1**.

▶ Heart Attack

Heart muscle needs oxygen to survive. A coronary attack (heart attack) occurs when the blood flow that brings oxygen to the heart muscle is severely reduced or cut off completely. This happens when coronary arteries that supply the heart with blood slowly become thicker and harder from a buildup of plaque (ie, fat, cholesterol, and other substances). This slow process is known as atherosclerosis **Figure 1A**. When plaque in a heart artery breaks free, a blood clot forms around the plaque, this blood clot can block the artery and shut off blood flow to the heart muscle. When the heart muscle is starved for oxygen and nutrients, it is called ischemia. When damage or death of part of

Table 1 STOP Mnemonic

S	Sugar	Blood glucose too low (insulin reaction) or too high (diabetic coma)
	Seizures	
	Stroke	
	Shock	
T	Temperature	Too high (heatstroke) or too low (hypothermia)
O	Oxygen	Inadequate oxygen
P	Poisoning	Drug/alcohol overdose
		Carbon monoxide poisoning
	Pressure on brain	Head injury

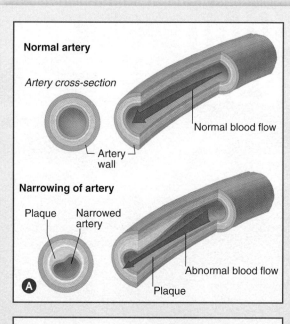

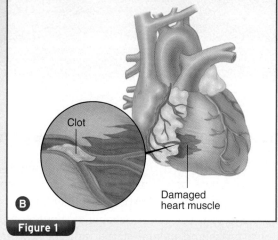

Figure 1

A. A normal artery with normal blood flow and an artery with plaque buildup. B. A heart attack occurs when a clot prevents blood flow to a part of the heart.

the heart muscle occurs as a result of ischemia, it is called a **heart attack** or myocardial infarction (MI) Figure 1B .

Heart and blood vessel disease is America's number one killer. About half of the deaths from heart and blood vessel disease are from coronary heart disease, which includes heart attack. About 325,000 people a year die of coronary attack before they get to a hospital emergency department.

Difference Between Heart Attack and Cardiac Arrest

The conditions *heart attack* and *cardiac arrest* confuse many people. The two are very different, and so is the first aid and emergency care for them.

- **Heart attack.** When one or more of the arteries delivering blood to the heart becomes blocked, a heart attack results. Oxygen-rich blood cannot reach the heart muscle, and the heart muscle becomes damaged. This damage to the heart muscle can lead to disturbances of the heart's electrical system and can lead to a cardiac arrest.
- **Cardiac arrest.** Cardiac arrest occurs when either the heart stops beating (asystole) or when the heart's lower chambers (ventricles) suddenly develop a rapid irregular rhythm (ventricular fibrillation), causing the ventricles to quiver rather than contract. The quivering motion of the ventricles renders the heart an ineffective pump that can no longer

supply the body and brain with oxygen-rich blood. Within seconds, the victim becomes unresponsive and has no pulse. Only immediate action such as cardiopulmonary resuscitation (CPR) and external defibrillation can offer hope of survival.

Recognizing a Heart Attack

Some heart attacks are sudden and intense, leaving no doubt about what is happening. Most heart attacks, however, start slowly, with mild pain or discomfort.

Heart attack victims are often not sure what is wrong and wait too long before getting help.

The National Heart, Lung and Blood Institute offer these signs of a possible heart attack:

- **Chest discomfort**. Most heart attacks involve discomfort in the center of the chest that lasts more than a few minutes or that goes away and comes back. It can feel like uncomfortable pressure, squeezing, fullness, or pain.
- **Discomfort in other areas of the upper body**. Symptoms can include pain or discomfort in one or both arms, the back, neck, jaw, or stomach.
- **Shortness of breath** with or without chest discomfort.
- **Other signs** may include breaking out in a cold sweat, nausea, or lightheadedness.

The most common heart attack symptom for both men and women is chest pain or discomfort. However, women are somewhat more likely than men to experience some of the other symptoms, especially shortness of breath, nausea/vomiting, and back or jaw pain.

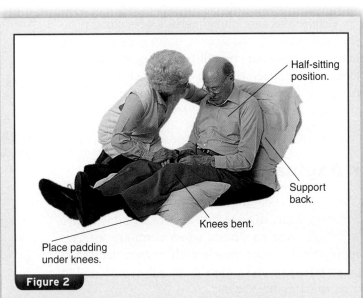

Figure 2

Help the victim into a relaxed position to ease strain on the heart.

Half-sitting position.

Support back.

Knees bent.

Place padding under knees.

No Chest Pain in One Third of Heart Attacks

A study of hundreds of thousands of heart attack victims found that as many as one third had no chest pain and that they were less likely to seek help and twice as likely to die.

The study found that women, people of color, people older than 75 years, and people with previous heart failure, stroke, or diabetes were most likely to have painless heart attacks. Although doctors have long known about painless heart attacks, many said they did not realize the number was so high.

Patients with chest pain were more than twice as likely to be diagnosed at admission and to receive clot-busting drugs or undergo angioplasty to open clogged arteries.

Source: Canto JG, Shlipak MG, Rogers WJ, et al. Prevalence, clinical characteristics, and mortality among patients with myocardial infarction presenting without chest pain. *JAMA.* 2000. 283:3223-3229.

Care for Heart Attack

Treat a suspected heart attack in the following manner:

1. Immediately call 9-1-1 if a heart attack is suspected or if the chest pain does not go away in a victim taking nitroglycerin. Medications to dissolve a clot must be given early. Do not drive yourself or anyone else to the hospital.
2. Monitor breathing. If the victim becomes unresponsive and stops breathing, begin CPR.
3. Help the victim to the most comfortable resting position, usually sitting **Figure 2**. Loosen clothing around the neck and waist. Be calm and reassuring.
4. If the victim is alert, able to swallow, and not allergic to aspirin, help the victim take one adult aspirin (325 mg) or two chewable children's aspirin (81 mg each). Pulverize them or have the victim crunch them with his or her teeth before swallowing.

Find out if the victim is using nitroglycerin. Nitroglycerin tablets, spray, or ointment can relieve chest pain from angina but not always from a heart attack. Nitroglycerin dilates the coronary arteries, which increases blood flow to the heart muscle. It also lowers blood pressure and dilates the veins, thus decreasing the work of the heart and the heart muscle's need for oxygen.

Caution: Because nitroglycerin lowers blood pressure, the victim should sit or lie down once it is taken. Let the victim take one pill or one spray under the tongue. If necessary, help him or her take it. If the chest pain or discomfort does not improve within 5 minutes after the one dose, call 9-1-1. Previously, victims were told to take up to three doses, 5 minutes apart.

▶ Angina

Chest pain called **angina pectoris** can result from coronary heart disease just as a heart attack does Table 2. Angina occurs when coronary arteries supplying the heart muscle with oxygen-rich blood become narrow and cannot carry sufficient blood to meet the demands during:

- Physical exertion
- Excitement
- Emotional upset
- Eating of a heavy meal
- Extreme hot or cold temperature exposure
- Cigarette smoking

Recognizing Angina

It can be difficult to differentiate a heart attack from angina, even for physicians. Chest pain from a heart attack is as likely to happen at rest as during activity, the pain lasts longer than 10 minutes, and it is not relieved by nitroglycerin. Differentiate angina from a heart attack by these signs and symptoms:

- Chest pain is described as crushing, squeezing, or like somebody standing on the victim's chest.
- Pain can spread to the jaw, the arms (frequently the left arm), and the mid-back.
- Pain usually lasts from 3 to 10 minutes, but rarely longer than 10 minutes.
- The pain is almost always relieved by the victim's prescribed nitroglycerin.
- Pain can be associated with shortness of breath, nausea, or sweating.
- Victim feels anxious.

Table 2 Chest Pain

Cause of Pain	Characteristics	Care
Muscle or rib pain from exercise or injury	Reproduced by movement Tender spot when pressed	Rest Aspirin or ibuprofen
Respiratory infection (eg, pneumonia, bronchitis, pleuritis)	Cough Fever Sore throat Production of sputum	Antibiotics
Indigestion	Belching Heartburn Nausea Sour taste	Antacids
Angina pectoris	Lasts less than 10 minutes (but pain is similar to that of a heart attack)	Rest Victim's nitroglycerin
Heart attack (myocardial infarction)	Lasts more than 10 minutes Pressure, squeezing, or pain near center of the chest Pain spreads to shoulders, neck, or arms Lightheadedness, fainting, sweating, nausea, shortness of breath	Call 9-1-1 Check breathing Resting position Victim's nitroglycerin

Other Causes of Chest Pain

Not all causes of chest pain relate to the heart, including:

- Muscle or rib pain due to exercise, excessive coughing, or injury. The victim can reproduce the pain by movement, and often the area of complaint is tender when pressed. Rest and aspirin or ibuprofen relieves the pain.
- Respiratory infections such as pneumonia, bronchitis, pleuritis, or lung injury. Chest pain due to these conditions usually worsens when the victim coughs or breaths deeply. Fever and colored sputum might be present. The victim needs medical care and may require prescribed medications.
- Indigestion, usually accompanied by belching, heartburn, nausea, and a sour taste in the mouth. This type of pain is relieved by antacids.

Why Don't They Call?

A study asked heart attack victims who waited for more than 20 minutes before getting help why they delayed. Their answers included the following:

- They thought the symptoms would go away.
- The symptoms were not severe enough.
- They thought it was a different illness.
- They were worried about medical costs.
- They were afraid of hospitals.
- They feared being embarrassed.
- They wanted to wait for a better time.
- They did not want to find out what was wrong.

The average time that elapsed between symptom onset and hospital arrival was 2 hours; 28% waited at least 1 hour, 33% waited 1 to 3 hours, 15% waited 3 to 6 hours, and 23% waited more than 6 hours. Most victims reported they were not sure their symptoms were severe enough to merit action as drastic as calling 9-1-1.

The same study concluded that one way to shorten out-of-hospital delay is to encourage victims with heart-related symptoms to use EMS rather than slower transportation methods.

Source: Meischke H, Eisenberg MS, Schaeffer SM, Larsen MP. 1995. Reasons patients with chest pain delay or do not call 911. *Ann Emerg Med.* 25(2):193-197.

Care for Angina

Angina can be treated with drugs that affect the blood supply to the heart muscle, the heart's demand for oxygen, or both. Drugs that affect the blood supply are coronary vasodilators; they cause blood vessels to relax. When this happens, the opening inside the vessels (the lumen) gets bigger. Then blood flow improves, letting more oxygen and nutrients reach the heart muscle.

Nitroglycerin mainly relaxes the veins and relaxes the coronary arteries a little. By relaxing the veins, it reduces the amount of blood that returns to the heart and eases the heart's workload. By relaxing the coronary arteries, it increases the heart's blood supply. Physicians often prescribe nitroglycerin for those with angina.

1. Have the victim stop what he or she is doing and sit down. Keep bystanders away. Provide calm reassurance to help reduce the victim's anxiety.
2. If the victim has medically prescribed nitroglycerin, either tablets or a spray, let the victim use it. This is one pill or one spray under the tongue. Follow the prescription label's directions. If necessary, help him or her use it.
3. If the chest pain or discomfort does not improve within 5 minutes after taking one

dose of nitroglycerin, call 9-1-1. Previously, victims were told to take up to three nitroglycerin tablets, 5 minutes apart, when they had chest pain or discomfort. This procedure has been changed so that if there is no improvement within 5 minutes after taking one dose, 9-1-1 should be called.

▶ Stroke (Brain Attack)

A **stroke**, also called a brain attack, occurs when there is a sudden interruption of blood flow to the brain. This occurs when arteries in the brain rupture or become blocked so part of the brain does not receive the blood flow it needs **Figure 3** . Deprived of oxygen-rich blood, nerve cells in the affected area of the brain cannot function and die within minutes. Because dead brain cells are not replaced, the devastating effects of strokes often are permanent. When nerve cells do

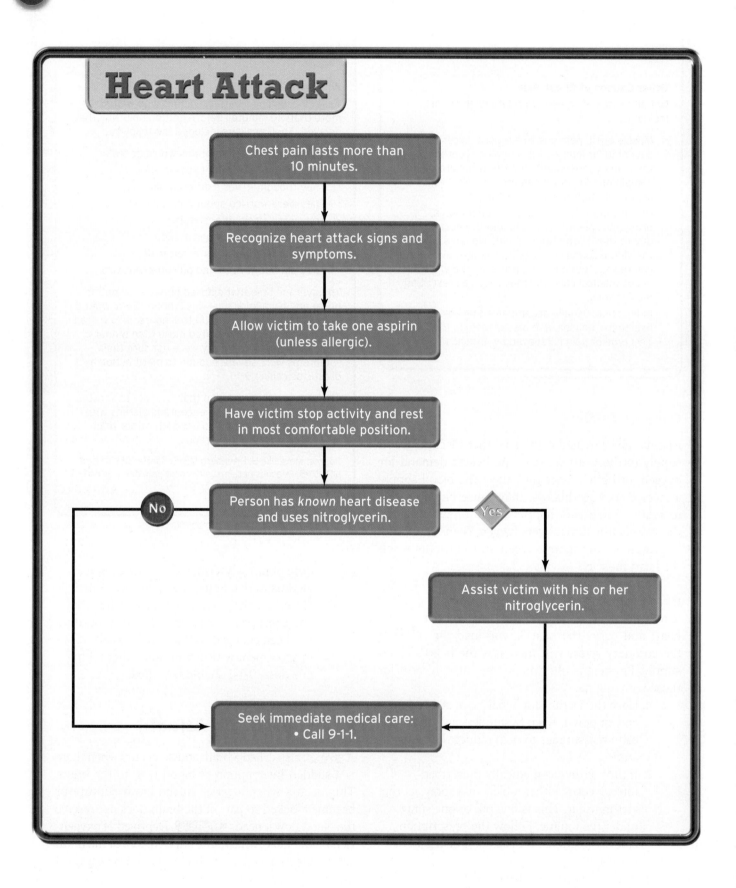

Heart Attack

Chest pain lasts more than 10 minutes.

↓

Recognize heart attack signs and symptoms.

↓

Allow victim to take one aspirin (unless allergic).

↓

Have victim stop activity and rest in most comfortable position.

↓

No ← Person has *known* heart disease and uses nitroglycerin. → **Yes**

Assist victim with his or her nitroglycerin.

Seek immediate medical care:
• Call 9-1-1.

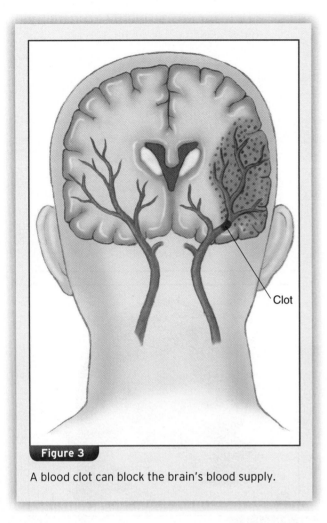

Figure 3

A blood clot can block the brain's blood supply.

Give Me 5 for Stroke

The American Academy of Neurology, the American College of Emergency Physicians, and the American Heart Association/American Stroke Association formed a joint campaign known as "Give Me 5" for Stroke. Women especially need to know the warning signs, because they account for over 60% of the deaths from stroke. They are also often the health information keepers for their families. Give Me 5 for Stroke uses easy-to-remember words to help identify the five signs of stroke. The key words are:

- Walk: Is their balance off?
- Talk: Is their speech slurred or face droopy?
- Reach: Is one side weak or numb?
- See: Is their vision all or partly lost?
- Feel: Is their headache severe?

not function, the part of the body they control cannot function either. Each year, about 800,000 Americans suffer a new or recurrent stroke, and about one fourth of these victims die, making it the third leading cause of death.

Strokes are classified as ischemic or hemorrhagic:

- **Ischemic stroke**. This type of stroke occurs when blood vessels to the brain become narrowed or clogged with fatty deposits called plaque, cutting off blood flow to brain cells. High blood pressure is the most important risk factor for ischemic stroke and can be controlled. Ischemic strokes are the most common type of stroke and account for about 85% of all strokes. Ischemic strokes usually occur at night or first thing in the morning.

Because tissue plasminogen activators (tPA) and other clot-busting drugs must be given as soon as possible after stroke onset (within 3 hours), it is important to recognize a stroke and to seek immediate medical care.

- **Hemorrhagic stroke**. About 15% of all strokes happen when a blood vessel ruptures in or near the brain. This kind of stroke is often associated with a very severe headache, nausea, and vomiting. Usually the symptoms appear suddenly.

Immediately seek medical care if there is a possibility of stroke. Any or all of the following procedures might be needed:

- Medication to control high blood pressure
- Medication to reduce brain swelling
- Surgery to repair an aneurysm or remove a blood clot

Recognizing Stroke

Symptoms of stroke include the following:

- Weakness, numbness, or paralysis of the face, an arm, or a leg on only one side of the body
- Blurred or decreased vision, especially in one eye
- Problems speaking or understanding
- Dizziness or loss of balance
- Sudden, severe, and unexplained headache
- Deviation of the eyes from PEARL (pupils equal and reactive to light), which might mean the brain is being affected by lack of oxygen

Table 3 Cincinnati Prehospital Stroke Scale

Test	Normal	Abnormal
Facial droop **Figure 4** (Ask victim to show teeth or smile.)	Both sides of face move equally well.	One side of the face does not move as well as the other.
Arm drift **Figure 5** (Ask victim to close eyes and hold out both arms with palms up.)	Both arms move the same, or both arms do not move.	One arm does not move, or one arm drifts down compared with the other side.
Speech (Ask victim to say, "The sky is blue in Cincinnati.")	Victim uses correct words with no slurring.	Victim slurs words, uses inappropriate words, or is unable to speak.

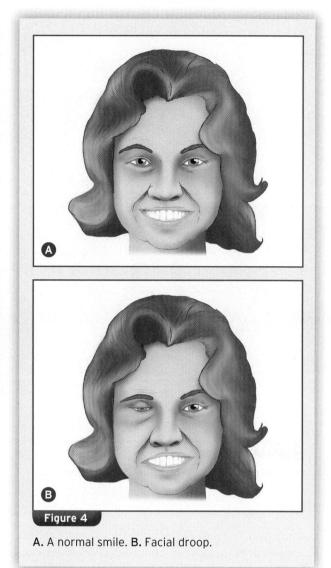

Figure 4

A. A normal smile. B. Facial droop.

CAUTION

DO NOT give a stroke victim anything to drink or eat. The throat can be paralyzed, which restricts swallowing.

The Cincinnati Stroke Scale is a proven method for quickly identifying stroke victims. When you suspect a stroke, apply these three simple tests **Table 3**:

- Facial droop
- Arm drift
- Speech

Care for a Stroke Victim

First aid for a stroke victim is limited to supportive care:

1. Call 9-1-1 immediately. Minimize brain damage by getting the victim to medical care.
2. Check the time at which the first signs appeared. A physician can use the information to determine whether a clot-busting drug can be given.
3. Monitor breathing. If the victim becomes unresponsive and stops breathing, begin CPR.
4. If the victim is unresponsive and breathing, place the victim in the recovery position to keep the airway open and to permit possible secretions and vomit to drain from the mouth.
5. If the victim is responsive, get the victim into a comfortable position with the head elevated. Be sure that the victim does not exert himself or herself.
6. Do not give the victim anything to drink or eat.
7. Reassure and keep the victim warm until EMS arrives.

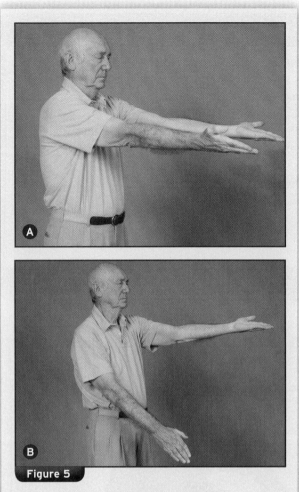

Figure 5

A. Normal arm position. **B.** Arm droop.

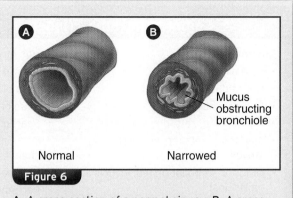

Figure 6

A. A cross-section of a normal airway. **B.** A cross-section of an airway during asthma symptoms, with the airway narrowed and inflamed, a thickened airway wall, and mucus.

▶ Asthma

<u>Asthma</u> is a chronic (long-term) lung disease that inflames and narrows the airways. Asthma causes recurring periods of wheezing (a whistling sound when a person breathes), chest tightness, shortness of breath, and coughing. The coughing often occurs at night or early in the morning.

Asthma affects people of all ages, but it most often starts in childhood and has the highest prevalence rate in those ages 5 to 17 years. In the United States, about 23 million people are known to have asthma.

The airways are tubes that carry air into and out of the lungs. People who have asthma have inflamed airways. This makes the airways swollen and very sensitive. They tend to react strongly to certain substances that are breathed in.

When the airways react, the muscles around them tighten. This causes the airways to narrow, allowing less air to flow to the lungs. Swelling makes the airways even narrower. Cells in the airways may make more mucus than normal **Figure 6**. Mucus is a sticky, thick liquid that can further narrow a person's airways.

This chain reaction can result in asthma symptoms. Symptoms can happen each time the airways are irritated. Sometimes symptoms are mild and go away on their own or after minimal treatment with an asthma medicine. At other times, symptoms continue to get worse. An asthma attack is when symptoms get more intense and/or additional symptoms appear.

It is important to treat symptoms when they are first noticed. This helps prevent the symptoms from worsening and causing a severe asthma attack. Severe asthma attacks may require medical care, and they can cause death.

Some of the known triggers of asthma are listed in **Table 4**.

Recognizing an Asthma Attack

Asthma varies a great deal from one person to another. Symptoms can range from mild to moderate to severe and can be life-threatening. The episodes can come occasionally or often. Between episodes, the person has no breathing difficulties.

The common asthma signs and symptoms include:

- **Excessive coughing**. Coughing from asthma is often worse at night or early in the morning.
- **Wheezing**. Wheezing is a whistling or squeaky sound that occurs when the victim breathes.

Table 4 Common Asthma Triggers

Environmental	Drugs or Chemicals	Conditions or Events
• Cold air	• Aspirin	• Gastroesophageal reflux
• House dust mites	• Beta blocker medicine	• Allergic rhinitis
• Cockroaches	• Food or drug preservatives	• Panic attacks
• Animals (eg, cats, dogs, rodents)	• Seafood, shellfish	• Menstruation, pregnancy
• Indoor irritants (eg, wood-burning stoves)	• Occupational exposure to chemicals	• Viral respiratory infections
• Outdoor air pollution (eg, vehicle emissions)	• Household cleaning agents	• Emotional stress, excitement
• Indoor or outdoor molds and fungi	• Perfumes	• Exercise
• Tobacco smoke		
• Pollen (eg, grass, trees)		

- **Chest tightness**. This may feel like something is squeezing or sitting on the chest.
- **Shortness of breath**. Some people who have asthma say they cannot catch their breath or they feel out of breath.
- **Sitting in the tripod position**. This position involves leaning forward with hands on knees or other support, trying to breathe.
- **Inability to speak in complete sentences** without pausing for breath.
- **Nostrils flaring** with each breath.

Not all people who have asthma have these symptoms. Likewise, having these symptoms does not always mean that the person has asthma.

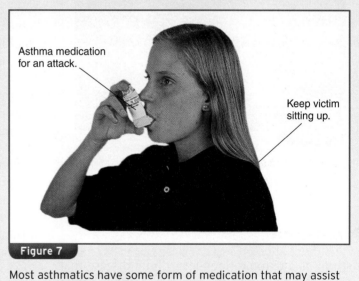

Asthma medication for an attack.

Keep victim sitting up.

Figure 7

Most asthmatics have some form of medication that may assist them during an asthma attack.

Care for an Asthma Attack

1. Place the victim in a comfortable, upright position, leaning slightly forward (tripod position).
2. Ask the victim about any asthma medication he or she uses. Most asthmatics have some form of medication, usually administered through physician-prescribed, handheld inhalers or a device (nebulizer) that turns liquid medicine into a mist for inhalation **Figure 7** .

Asthma is treated with two types of medicines: long-term control and quick-relief medicines. Quick-relief, or "rescue," medicines relieve asthma symptoms that may flare up; a first aider should know about these medications.

All people who have asthma need a quick-relief medicine to help relieve asthma symptoms that may flare up. Inhaled short-acting beta-agonists are the first choice for quick relief. These inhaled medicines act quickly to relax tight muscles around the airways during a flare-up, allowing the airways to open up so

FYI

Using a Physician-Prescribed Quick-Relief Inhaler (Metered-Dose Inhaler)

Check the inhaler's expiration date.

The inhaler should be at room temperature.

If there is a spacer/holding chamber, attach the inhaler to it.

Shake the inhaler several times.

The victim should blow out the air in the lungs.

The victim's lips should be placed around the inhaler and the victim should begin to inhale deeply.

The victim depresses the handheld inhaler to release the medicine as he or she breathes in slowly until the lungs are full.

If using a spacer/holding chamber, the victim should press down on the inhaler and then wait 5 seconds before breathing in.

The victim should hold his or her breath for at least 10 seconds, allowing the medication to be absorbed into the lungs.

Wait for several breaths before taking a second dose.

air can flow through them. Asthma symptoms should respond to inhaled medicine quickly (within 1 hour).

The quick-relief medicine should be taken when the first asthma symptoms are noticed. The quick-relief inhaler should be with the person at all times. Most people who have asthma can safely manage their symptoms using their medications.

3. If asthma signs and symptoms (eg, coughing, wheezing, tight chest) begin, the victim can take two puffs of the quick-relief medicine. If the victim's condition does not improve but symptoms are mild, call the victim's physician for advice and administer up to four more puffs over 30 minutes.

4. If the medicine is not helping, breathing is hard and fast, the nose opens wide during breathing, or the victim cannot walk or talk well, call 9-1-1 or take the victim to the nearest emergency department if that would be faster. The victim can take four more puffs of the quick-relief medicine (two puffs at a time, waiting 15 minutes between each set of two puffs) while awaiting EMS or traveling to the hospital.

▶ Hyperventilation

Fast, deep breathing, called hyperventilation, is common during emotional stress. The victim might be hysterical or quite calm. Other factors that can cause rapid breathing include untreated diabetes, severe shock, certain poisons, and brain swelling due to injury or high altitude.

Recognizing Hyperventilation

Signs of hyperventilation include:

- Shortness of breath
- Fast breathing (more than 40 breaths per minute)
- Tingling or numbness of the hands, feet, and around the mouth
- Dizziness or lightheadedness

Care for Hyperventilation

If you encounter someone who is hyperventilating, these steps can help:

1. Calm and reassure the victim.
2. Take the victim to a quiet place or ask bystanders to leave. Have the victim sit down.
3. Encourage the person to breathe slowly, using the abdominal muscles: inhale through the nose, hold the full inhalation for 1 to 2 seconds, then exhale slowly through pursed lips.

FYI

Breathing Into a Paper Bag

A popular remedy for anxiety-related hyperventilation is to breathe into a paper bag. Do not do this. Tests on healthy people show that bag rebreathing rarely restores blood-gas balance but often causes dangerous stress to the heart and respiratory system, especially in people with a chronic respiratory disease.

Source: Callaham M. Hypoxic hazards of traditional paper bag rebreathing in hyperventilating patients. *Ann Emerg Med.* 18(6):622-628.

▶ Chronic Obstructive Pulmonary Disease

Chronic obstructive pulmonary disease (COPD) is a broad term applied to emphysema, chronic bronchitis, and related lung diseases. The incidence of COPD is very high in North America, and the most common causative factor is cigarette smoking.

Chronic obstructive pulmonary disease describes a disease that makes it hard for a person to breathe because the normal flow of air into and out of the person's lungs is partially obstructed.

Because COPD takes many years to develop before a person notices difficulty breathing, COPD is usually considered a disease of older adults and is most commonly diagnosed in people older than 60 years.

Chronic bronchitis is caused by chronic infection, which can be brought on by irritations such as tobacco smoke. The bronchi become thick, unable to stretch, and partially blocked. Early symptoms include a cigarette cough or a cough due to a cold. Later, more severe symptoms include difficulty breathing, increased sputum, and severe coughing.

Emphysema often occurs with chronic bronchitis. The alveoli of the lungs are partially destroyed, and the lungs have lost their elasticity, making it difficult for the victim to exhale. Common symptoms include coughing, wheezing, and shortness of breath. Breathing is extremely difficult for people with emphysema.

Recognizing Chronic Obstructive Pulmonary Disease

The signs and symptoms of COPD are similar to those of asthma. Most victims will wheeze; coughing and shortness of breath might be more prominent in people with COPD than in asthma. Many people with COPD depend on a constant low level of artificially supplied oxygen to maintain breathing.

Care for Chronic Obstructive Pulmonary Disease

Use the following guidelines when caring for someone with COPD:
1. Persons with COPD usually will have their own physician-prescribed medications. Assist the victim to take any prescribed medications.
2. Place the victim in the sitting position that provides the greatest comfort.
3. Encourage the victim to cough up any secretions.
4. For acute breathing distress, obtain immediate medical assistance. The victim might need oxygen, which is available from EMS and at hospital emergency departments.

▶ Fainting

A sudden, brief loss of responsiveness not associated with a head injury is known as **syncope** (fainting) or **psychogenic shock**.

Simple fainting is common and benign and can have physical or emotional causes. Fainting can happen suddenly when blood flow to the brain is interrupted. The nervous system dilates blood vessels to three to four times their normal size and allows blood to pool in the legs and lower body.

Syncope, or simple fainting, can be precipitated by unpleasant emotional stimuli such as the sight of blood or strong fear. It usually occurs when the victim is in the upright position.

Most fainting episodes are associated with decreased blood flow causing deficient oxygen or glucose in the brain. The decreased blood flow can be caused by a slow heart rate (vagal reaction, in which the vagus nerve, which slows the heart rate, is overstimulated by fright, anxiety, drugs, or fatigue), heart-rhythm disturbances, dehydration, heat exhaustion, anemia (low hemoglobin), or bleeding. Decreased glucose (**hypoglycemia**) can be caused by diabetes, medications used to treat diabetes, or infections.

Sitting or standing for a long time without moving, especially in a hot environment, can cause blood to pool in dilated vessels, which results in a loss of effective circulating blood volume, causing the blood pressure to drop. As the blood flow to the brain decreases, the person loses consciousness and collapses.

Recognizing Fainting

A person who is about to faint usually will have one or more of the following signs and symptoms:
- Dizziness
- Weakness
- Seeing spots
- Visual blurring
- Nausea
- Pale skin
- Sweating

Care for Fainting

If a person appears about to faint:
1. Prevent the person from falling.
2. Help the person lie down.
3. Loosen tight clothing at the neck and waist.
4. Stay with the victim until he or she recovers.

Fainting

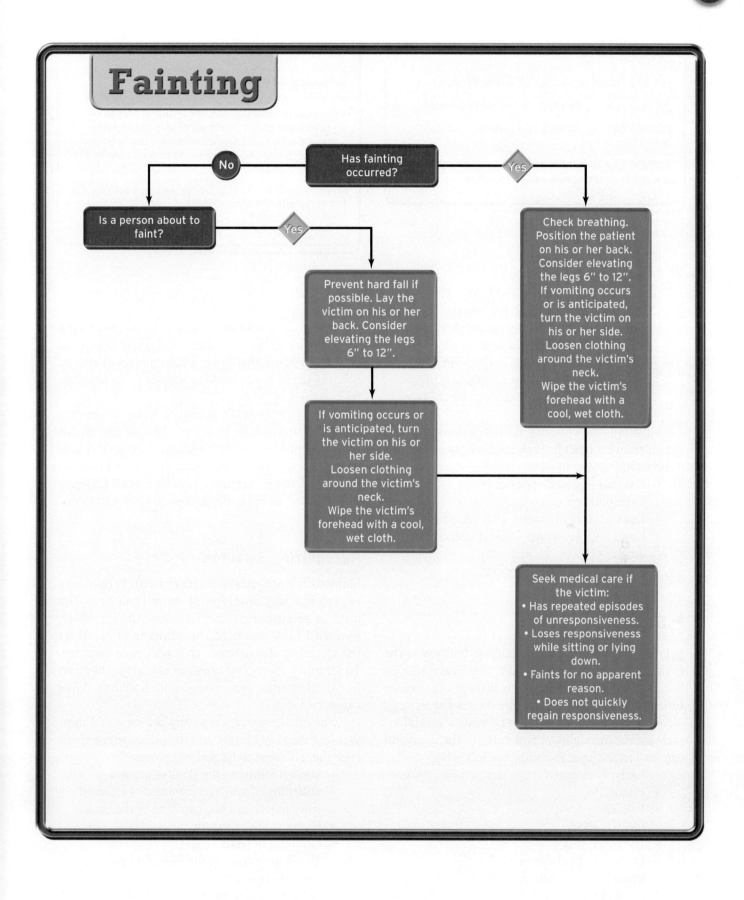

Has fainting occurred?

No → Is a person about to faint?

Yes →

Is a person about to faint? — **Yes** → Prevent hard fall if possible. Lay the victim on his or her back. Consider elevating the legs 6" to 12".

↓

If vomiting occurs or is anticipated, turn the victim on his or her side. Loosen clothing around the victim's neck. Wipe the victim's forehead with a cool, wet cloth.

Has fainting occurred? — Yes → Check breathing. Position the patient on his or her back. Consider elevating the legs 6" to 12". If vomiting occurs or is anticipated, turn the victim on his or her side. Loosen clothing around the victim's neck. Wipe the victim's forehead with a cool, wet cloth.

↓

Seek medical care if the victim:
• Has repeated episodes of unresponsiveness.
• Loses responsiveness while sitting or lying down.
• Faints for no apparent reason.
• Does not quickly regain responsiveness.

CAUTION

DO NOT splash or pour water on the victim's face.

DO NOT use smelling salts or ammonia inhalants.

DO NOT slap the victim's face in an attempt to revive him or her.

DO NOT give the victim anything to drink until he or she has fully recovered and can swallow.

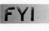

FYI

Knowledge of Epilepsy

A survey found that about half of all persons have witnessed an epileptic seizure either in person or on television; about one third of all persons know someone with epilepsy, but relatively few are familiar with epilepsy, how to respond to a seizure, or the Epilepsy Foundation.

Source: Kobau R, Price P. 2003. Knowledge of epilepsy and familiarity with this disorder in the U.S. population. *Epilepsia.* 44(11):1449-1454.

If fainting has happened:
1. Monitor breathing.
2. Loosen tight clothing and belts.
3. If the victim fell, check for injuries.
4. After recovery, have the victim sit for a while, and when he or she is able to swallow, give cool, sweetened liquids to drink and help the victim slowly regain an upright posture.
5. Fresh air and a cold, wet cloth for the face usually aid recovery.

Most fainting episodes are not serious, and the victim recovers quickly. Seek medical care, however, if the victim:

- Has had repeated episodes of unresponsiveness
- Does not quickly regain responsiveness
- Loses responsiveness while sitting or lying down
- Faints for no apparent reason

▶ Seizure

Seizures are a symptom of epilepsy. Epilepsy is the underlying tendency of the brain to produce sudden bursts of electrical energy that disrupt other brain functions. Having a single seizure does not necessarily mean a person has epilepsy. Several medical conditions increase the instability or irritability of the brain and can lead to seizures, including the following:

- Lack of oxygen
- Heatstroke
- Poisoning
- Electric shock
- Hypoglycemia
- High fever in children
- Brain injury, tumor, or stroke
- Alcohol withdrawal, drug abuse, or overdose

Epilepsy, on the other hand, is an underlying condition (or permanent brain injury) that affects the delicate systems that govern how electrical energy behaves in the brain, making it susceptible to recurring seizures.

Most people with seizures have idiopathic epilepsy; that is, the cause of the seizures is not known. Epilepsy is not a mental illness, and it is not a sign of low intelligence. It also is not contagious. Between seizures, a person with epilepsy can function as normally as a person who does not have epilepsy.

Recognizing Seizures

Many different types of seizures exist. People may experience just one type or more than one. The kind of seizure a person has depends on which part and how much of the brain is affected by the electrical disturbance that produces seizures. To simplify the many types of seizures, they can be divided into convulsive and nonconvulsive categories.

Convulsive seizures typically last for 1 to 2 minutes (but may last longer), and the person may experience the following signs and symptoms:

- Sudden falling to the floor or ground
- Stiffening of arm and leg muscles followed by jerky movement with arching of the back
- Foaming at the mouth
- Grinding of teeth
- Bluish-gray color of the face and lips
- Eyes roll upward
- Loss of bladder and bowel control

Nonconvulsive seizures last only a few seconds, and the person may experience the following signs and symptoms:

- Staring, confused, or inattentive
- Frequent eye blinking
- Involuntary movements (eg, lip smacking, picking at clothes, fumbling)

Nonconvulsive seizures are so brief that they often escape detection.

Status Epilepticus

Most seizures end after a few seconds or a few minutes. If they are prolonged, or occur in a series, it is called **status epilepticus**. This is an emergency situation and requires immediate medical care. Repeated, uncontrolled seizures can lead to brain damage, fractures, severe dehydration, and aspiration. In adults, the most common cause of status epilepticus is failure to take prescribed medicines for epilepsy.

Caring for a Seizure

The following information is adapted from the Epilepsy Foundation and can be used for seizure victims with a known seizure disorder.

First Aid for a Convulsive Seizure

- Do not restrain or hold the person down or try to stop his or her movements.
- Clear the area around the person of anything hard or sharp. Remove glasses.
- Loosen ties, scarves, or anything around the neck that could interfere with breathing.
- Place something flat and soft, like a folded jacket, under the head.

CAUTION

DO NOT restrain the victim.

DO NOT put anything between the victim's teeth during the seizure.

DO NOT splash or pour water or any other liquid on the victim's face.

DO NOT move the victim to another place (unless it is the only way to protect the victim from injury).

DO NOT leave a victim until he or she is fully alert and recovered.

- Turn him or her gently onto one side to help keep the airway open.
- Do not try to force the mouth open with any hard implement or with fingers. Efforts to hold the tongue down can injure the teeth or jaw. A person having a seizure cannot swallow his or her tongue.
- Stay with the person until the seizure ends naturally. Do not leave him or her alone until the person is fully conscious, alert, and able to speak normally.
- Ask if there is anyone who should be called to help him or her get home.
- Look for a medical ID (although its absence does not rule out a seizure).

This may not be a medical emergency, even though it looks like one. It stops naturally after a few minutes. The average person with a known seizure disorder who has a typical seizure should rest and then continue about his or her activities. The person will need limited assistance, if any, unless he or she needs to be driven home. People who have just seized should not be permitted to drive. If this is a person's first seizure or if it represents a change in a person's seizure disorder (eg, more frequent, different kind), call 9-1-1.

First Aid for a Nonconvulsive Seizure

- Watch the person carefully and explain to others what is happening. They may think that the dazed person is drunk or on drugs.
- Guide the person gently away from any danger (eg, steps, highway, hot stove). Do not grab and hold them because they may struggle or lash out.
- Stay with the victim until he or she has fully recovered.

When to Call 9-1-1

- A seizure lasts more than 5 minutes.
- A second seizure starts soon after the first has ended.
- Alertness does not start to return after shaking has stopped.
- The seizure happened in water.
- The victim is injured (eg, bleeding from the head, unequal pupils, vomiting), diabetic, or pregnant.
- No medical identification tag is found, and there is no way of knowing whether the seizure is caused by epilepsy.
- The victim has never had a seizure before.

Seizures

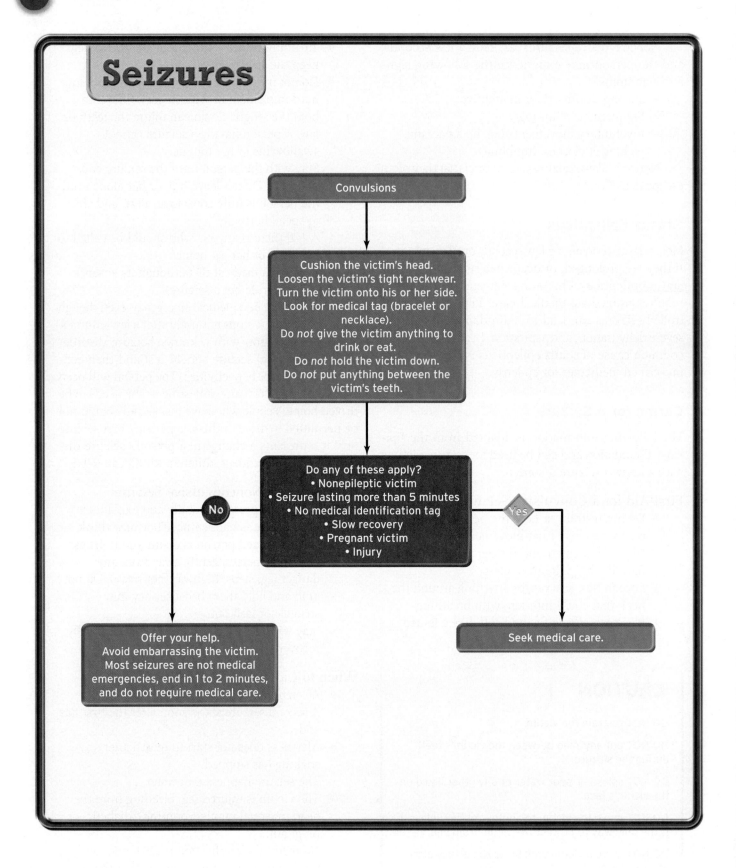

Convulsions

Cushion the victim's head.
Loosen the victim's tight neckwear.
Turn the victim onto his or her side.
Look for medical tag (bracelet or necklace).
Do *not* give the victim anything to drink or eat.
Do *not* hold the victim down.
Do *not* put anything between the victim's teeth.

Do any of these apply?
• Nonepileptic victim
• Seizure lasting more than 5 minutes
• No medical identification tag
• Slow recovery
• Pregnant victim
• Injury

No → Offer your help.
Avoid embarrassing the victim.
Most seizures are not medical emergencies, end in 1 to 2 minutes, and do not require medical care.

Yes → Seek medical care.

▶ Diabetic Emergencies

Insulin is a hormone produced by the pancreas that assists the body in using energy from food **Figure 8**. Insulin takes glucose from the blood and then carries it into the cells where it is used. When excess glucose remains in the blood and is not transferred to the cells, they must rely on fat for fuel. Because blood glucose is a major source of fuel used by the body, when it cannot be used it will build up in the blood. The blood glucose then overflows into the urine, passing through the body unused and discarded. When this occurs, a condition called <u>diabetes</u> develops **Table 5**. Insulin is either ineffective or lacking in the body. Diabetes is not contagious and in most cases special diet and/or medication can control it.

The body is continuously balancing glucose and insulin. Too much insulin and not enough glucose leads to low blood glucose and possibly insulin reaction. Insulin reaction results from severe low blood glucose, causing unconsciousness and possibly death. Too much glucose and not enough insulin leads to high blood glucose, the production of ketones, and possibly diabetic coma. Ketones cause a sweet or fruity odor on the breath.

Types of Diabetes

Type 1 Diabetes

Type 1 diabetes (formerly called juvenile-onset or insulin-dependent diabetes) is most commonly diagnosed in childhood, but it may present at any age in life. About 2 million of the individuals with diabetes have type 1 diabetes. This type of diabetes requires external insulin (not made by the body), which enables the glucose to enter the cells. External insulin is necessary because the body is unable to produce the insulin the cells require. When a person with type 1 diabetes is deprived of external insulin, he or she will become very ill. Type 1 diabetics will usually be thin or not overweight.

Type 2 Diabetes

Type 2 diabetes used to be known as non-insulin-dependent or adult-onset diabetes. The incidence of type 2 diabetes is reaching epidemic proportions in the United States. More than 21 million people currently have type 2 diabetes. Excess body weight and a sedentary lifestyle are widely recognized risk factors, especially because type 2 diabetes is being diagnosed in a growing number of children and adolescents. Other risk factors include a family history of type 2 diabetes and age older than 45 years. The age of onset is usually over the age of 40 years, but it can occur at any age. This type of diabetes may require insulin replacement and other medication.

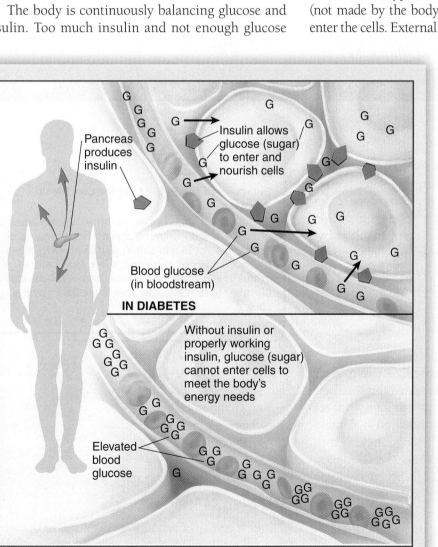

Figure 8

Normal metabolism (top) and diabetes (bottom).

Table 5 Diabetic Emergencies

	Diabetic Coma (high blood glucose)	Insulin Shock (low blood glucose)
Cause	Not enough insulin; too much glucose	Too much insulin; not enough glucose
Insulin level	Insufficient	Excessive
Onset of symptoms	Gradual	Sudden
Skin	Flushed, dry, warm	Pale, clammy
Breath	Fruity odor	Normal
Thirst	Severe	Normal
Urination	Frequent	Normal
Behavior	Normal to disorientation, drowsiness, and change in mood	Appearance of intoxication: combativeness, bad temper, anger, confusion, disorientation
Other symptoms	Drowsiness, vomiting, heavy breathing, eventual stupor or unconsciousness	Sudden hunger, eventual stupor, or unresponsiveness
First aid	If in doubt, give sugar. Give fluids to fight dehydration. Take victim to hospital.	Give sugar. Seek medical care.

Gestational Diabetes

Gestational diabetes occurs in some pregnancies. It usually ends after a baby is born, but when women who had gestational diabetes get older, type 2 diabetes can develop. Gestational diabetes results from the body's resistance to the action of insulin. This resistance is caused by hormones produced during pregnancy. Gestational diabetes is usually treated with diet, but some women need insulin.

Recognizing Low Blood Glucose (Hypoglycemia)

The condition of low blood glucose, called hypoglycemia, is sometimes referred to as an insulin reaction.

This condition occurs in a diabetic for several reasons: too much insulin, too little or delayed food intake, exercise, alcohol, or any combination of these factors.

The American Diabetes Association lists the following signs and symptoms in insulin reaction and hypoglycemia as diabetic emergencies requiring first aid:

- Sudden onset
- Staggering, poor coordination, clumsiness
- Anger, bad temper
- Pale face color
- Confusion, disorientation
- Sudden hunger

FYI

Summary of the Rule of 15s for Low Blood Glucose

The diabetic should check his or her blood glucose level. If it is not within the appropriate range, he or she should eat 15 g of sugar, wait 15 minutes, check the blood glucose again and, if low, eat 15 more grams of sugar, wait 15 minutes and check the blood glucose again. If still low, seek immediate medical care.

- Excessive sweating
- Trembling, shakiness
- Seizure
- Eventual unconsciousness

Care for Low Blood Glucose (Hypoglycemia)

The best course of action is giving sugar to the victim using the rule of 15s.

1. The diabetic should check his or her blood glucose. If it is not within a proper range, he or she should eat 15 g of sugar. If the diabetic

Table 6 Fast-Acting Sugar (10 to 15 grams)

- Two to five glucose tablets
- One tube of glucose gel
- 4 oz of regular soda (not diet)
- 4 oz of orange or apple juice
- 2 Tbsp of raisins
- Five to seven Lifesavers candy
- 6 to 8 oz of skim or 1% milk
- Two tsp of honey or corn syrup

is not able to test his or her blood glucose, and you strongly suspect that the victim has low blood glucose, give the victim 10 to 15 g of fast-acting sugar if all the following conditions are present (Table 6):

- The victim is a known diabetic.
- The victim's mental status is not altered.
- The victim is alert enough to swallow.

2. Wait 15 minutes for the sugar to get into the blood.
3. If the diabetic is able, check the blood glucose level again. If it is still low, he or she should consume 15 more grams of sugar. If testing is not available, and there is no

improvement in 15 minutes, give the victim 15 more grams of sugar.

4. If there is no improvement, seek immediate medical care.

If the victim is or becomes unresponsive, call 9-1-1 immediately. In all cases, seek medical care following a diabetic episode and advise the victim's physician of the incident. Hypoglycemia can be a life-threatening emergency.

Another emergency procedure uses an injected medication called glucagon, available by a physician's prescription, to raise blood glucose quickly. Glucagon works the opposite of insulin. It mobilizes glucose stored in the muscles and liver as glycogen. Be aware that many people vomit after receiving glucagon. A family member or friend should learn when and how to inject glucagon in an emergency.

Recognizing High Blood Glucose (Diabetic Coma, Hyperglycemia)

The opposite reaction of hypoglycemia is called diabetic coma or **hyperglycemia**. This condition occurs when a diabetic has too much glucose in their blood. There are several scenarios that can cause this medical condition, such as insufficient insulin, overeating, illness, inactivity, stress, or a combination of these factors.

The American Diabetes Association lists the following signs and symptoms as warranting first aid in the case of a diabetic emergency involving hyperglycemia and diabetic coma:

- Gradual onset
- Drowsiness
- Extreme thirst
- Very frequent urination
- Flushed skin
- Vomiting
- Fruity breath odor
- Heavy breathing
- Eventual unconsciousness

Care for High Blood Glucose (Diabetic Coma, Hyperglycemia)

If you are uncertain whether the victim has a high or low blood glucose level and the victim is responsive and able to drink, give him or her a beverage or food containing sugar. If there is no improvement in the victim's condition within 15 minutes, seek medical care immediately.

Q&A

How can you tell the difference between hypoglycemia (insulin reaction) and hyperglycemia (diabetic coma)?

It is difficult to determine whether a person has hypoglycemia or hyperglycemia. Sugar helps the person with hypoglycemia, but not the person with hyperglycemia. However, do not debate whether to give sugar; sugar will cause no harm in either condition.

Ask the diabetic two questions: "Have you eaten today?" and "Have you taken your insulin today?" If the diabetic has taken his or her insulin but has not eaten, suspect hypoglycemia. If the diabetic has eaten but has not taken insulin, suspect hyperglycemia. If you are unsure which condition exists, give sugar.

Diabetic Emergencies

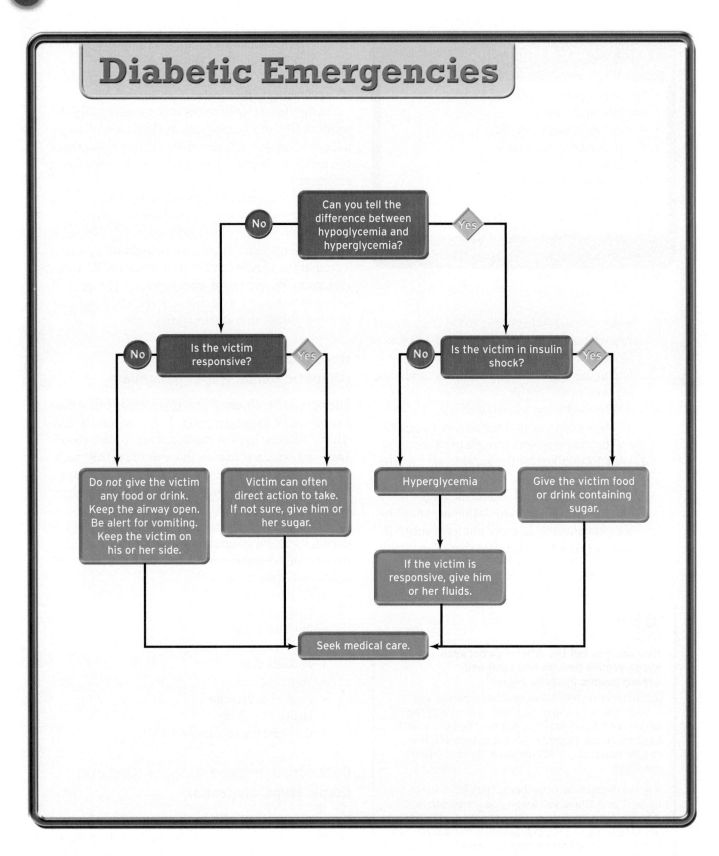

Can you tell the difference between hypoglycemia and hyperglycemia?

No → Is the victim responsive?

- **No** → Do *not* give the victim any food or drink. Keep the airway open. Be alert for vomiting. Keep the victim on his or her side.
- **Yes** → Victim can often direct action to take. If not sure, give him or her sugar.

Yes → Is the victim in insulin shock?

- **No** → Hyperglycemia → If the victim is responsive, give him or her fluids.
- **Yes** → Give the victim food or drink containing sugar.

Seek medical care.

▶ Emergencies During Pregnancy

Most pregnancies are normal and occur without complications. However, sometimes problems do arise and medical care is required. It is essential that you remain calm, focused, and considerate of the mother during this unforeseen and stressful situation.

Recognizing Emergencies During Pregnancy

Immediately notify a doctor to report the following signs and symptoms in a pregnant woman:

- Vaginal bleeding
- Cramps in lower abdomen
- Swelling of the face or fingers
- Severe continuous headache
- Dizziness or fainting
- Blurring of vision or seeing spots
- Uncontrollable vomiting

Care for Pregnancy Emergencies

If the victim is experiencing vaginal bleeding or abdominal pain:

1. Keep the woman quiet, warm, and on her left side.
2. Have victim or another woman place a sanitary napkin or any sterile or clean pad over the opening of the vagina.
3. Have victim or another woman replace, but save, any blood-soaked pads and all tissues that are passed. Send this with the woman to medical help for examination by the physician.
4. Seek medical care immediately.

If the victim has injuries to her lower abdomen:

1. Keep the woman quiet, warm, and on her left side.
2. Monitor breathing.
3. Seek medical care.

▶ Emergency Care Wrap-up

Condition	What to Look For	What to Do
Heart Attack	Chest pressure, squeezing, or pain Pain spreading to shoulders, neck, jaw, or arms Dizziness, sweating, nausea Shortness of breath	Help victim take his or her prescribed medication. Call 9-1-1. Help victim into a comfortable position. Give one adult or two children's aspirin. Monitor breathing.
Angina	Chest pain similar to a heart attack Pain seldom lasts longer than 10 minutes	Have victim rest. If victim has his or her own nitroglycerin, help the victim use it. If pain continues beyond 10 minutes, suspect a heart attack and call 9-1-1.
Stroke	Sudden weakness or numbness of the face, an arm, or a leg on one side of the body Blurred or decreased vision Problems speaking Dizziness or loss of balance Sudden, severe headache	Call 9-1-1. If responsive, help victim into a comfortable position with head and shoulders slightly raised. If unresponsive, move onto his or her side.

Condition	What to Look For	What to Do
Breathing Difficulty	Abnormally fast or slow breathing Abnormally deep or shallow breathing Noisy breathing Bluish lips Need to pause while speaking to catch breath	**Unknown Reason** Help victim into a comfortable position. Call 9-1-1. **Asthma Attack** Help victim into a comfortable position. Help victim use inhaler. Call 9-1-1 if victim does not improve. **Hyperventilation** Encourage victim to inhale, hold breath a few seconds, then exhale. Call 9-1-1 if condition does not improve.
Hyperventilation	Fast breathing (> 40 breaths per minute)	Calm and reassure victim. Inhale slowly through nose, hold for 1-2 seconds, exhale slowly through pursed lips.
COPD	Similar to asthma—wheeze, cough, short of breath	Help in taking prescribed medicine. Place in comfortable sitting position. Drink clear fluids. Might need medical care for oxygen.
Fainting	Sudden, brief unresponsiveness Pale skin Sweating	Check breathing. Check for injuries if victim fell. Consider raising feet 6 to 12 inches. Call 9-1-1 if needed.
Seizures	Sudden falling Unresponsiveness Rigid body and arching of back Jerky muscle movement	Prevent injury. Loosen any tight clothing. Roll victim onto his or her side. Call 9-1-1 if needed.
Diabetic Emergencies	**Low blood glucose** Develops very quickly Anger, bad temper Hunger Pale, sweaty skin **High blood glucose** Develops gradually Thirst Frequent urination Fruity, sweet breath odor Warm and dry skin	If uncertain about high or low blood glucose level, give sugar. Repeat in 15 minutes if no improvement. Call 9-1-1 if victim does not improve.
Pregnancy Emergencies	Vaginal bleeding Cramps in lower abdomen Swelling of face or fingers Severe continuous headache Dizziness or fainting Blurring of vision or seeing spots Uncontrollable vomiting	Keep the woman warm. For vaginal bleeding, place sanitary napkin or sterile or clean pad over opening of vagina. Send blood-soaked pad and tissues with the woman to medical care. Seek medical care.

prep kit

▶ Ready for Review

- A heart attack occurs when the heart muscle tissue dies because its blood supply is reduced or stopped.
- Angina pectoris can result from coronary heart disease just as a heart attack does.
- A stroke occurs when part of the blood flow to the brain is suddenly cut off.
- Asthma is chronic, inflammatory lung disease characterized by repeated breathing problems. Hyperventilation is fast, deep breathing and is common during emotional stress.
- Chronic obstructive pulmonary disease (COPD) is a broad term applied to emphysema, chronic bronchitis, and related lung diseases.
- Fainting is a sudden brief loss of responsiveness not associated with head injury.
- A seizure results from an abnormal stimulation of the brain's cells causing uncontrollable muscle movements.
- Diabetes is a condition in which insulin is lacking or ineffective.
- Hypoglycemia is very low blood glucose and can be caused by too much insulin, too little or delayed food intake, exercise, alcohol, or a combination of these factors.
- Hyperglycemia occurs when the body has too much glucose in the blood and can be caused by insufficient insulin, overeating, inactivity, illness, stress, or a combination of these factors.

▶ Vital Vocabulary

__angina pectoris__ A spasmodic pain in the chest, characterized by a sensation of severe constriction or pressure on the anterior chest; associated with insufficient blood supply to the heart, aggravated by exercise or tension, and relieved by rest or medication.

__asthma__ A condition marked by recurrent attacks of breathing difficulty, often with wheezing, due to spasmodic constriction of the air passages, often as a response to allergens or to mucus plugs in the bronchioles.

__diabetes__ A condition that develops when glucose builds up in the blood, overflows into the urine, and passes through the body unused.

__heart attack__ Lay term for a condition resulting from blockage of a coronary artery and subsequent death of part of the heart muscle; an acute myocardial infarction; sometimes called simply a coronary.

__hyperglycemia__ An abnormally increased concentration of glucose in the blood.

__hypoglycemia__ An abnormally diminished concentration of glucose in the blood.

__psychogenic shock__ A shock-like state due to severe emotional distress; may result in a fainting spell resulting from a transient decrease in blood flow to the brain.

__seizure__ Generalized, uncoordinated muscular activity associated with a loss of responsiveness; a convulsion; an attack of epilepsy.

__status epilepticus__ The occurrence of two or more seizures without a period of complete consciousness between them.

__stroke__ A brain injury due to bleeding in the brain tissue or to a blockage of blood flow, causing permanent damage.

__syncope__ Fainting; a brief period of unresponsiveness.

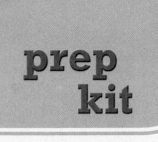

prep kit

▶ Assessment in Action

You are on a 5-day backpack trip in the mountains with your friends. On day three, and after several tough miles into the hike, your friend seems to be disoriented and is stumbling over rocks and tree roots on the trail. He falls to the ground and is responsive. You know that this friend has type 1 diabetes and did take his insulin in the morning.

Directions: Circle Yes if you agree with the statement; circle No if you disagree.

Yes   No   **1.** This person is very likely suffering from hyperglycemia.

Yes   No   **2.** Low blood glucose levels can be caused by too much insulin, too little or delayed food intake, exercise, and alcohol.

Yes   No   **3.** To give sugar in this scenario, the victim must be a known diabetic, have an altered mental status, and must be awake enough to swallow.

Yes   No   **4.** You should follow the rule of 15s when giving sugar to the victim in this scenario.

▶ Check Your Knowledge

Directions: Circle Yes if you agree with the statement; circle No if you disagree.

Yes   No   **1.** Heart attack victims can experience chest pain.

Yes   No   **2.** You can help the victim of chest pain take his or her nitroglycerin.

Yes   No   **3.** A responsive stroke victim should lie down with his or her head slightly raised.

Yes   No   **4.** Asthma victims may have a prescribed inhaler.

Yes   No   **5.** A victim who is breathing fast (hyperventilation) should be encouraged to breathe slowly by holding inhaled air for several seconds and then exhaling slowly.

Yes   No   **6.** Immobilize the spine of a victim having a seizure.

Yes   No   **7.** Some seizure victims display a rigid arching of the back.

Yes   No   **8.** A person having seizures always requires medical attention.

Yes   No   **9.** If in doubt about the type of diabetic emergency a victim is experiencing, give sugar to a responsive victim who can swallow.

Yes   No   **10.** Nitroglycerin can relieve chest pain associated with angina.

Poisoning

Poison

▶ What Is a Poison?

The American Association of Poison Control Centers defines a **poison** (also known as a toxin) as anything that can harm someone if it is: (1) used in the wrong way, (2) used by the wrong person, or (3) used in the wrong amount.

Poisons can be classified by how they enter the body:

- Ingested (swallowed)—through the mouth
- Inhaled (breathed)—through the lungs
- Injected—through needlelike device (eg, snake's fangs, bee's stinger)
- Absorbed (direct contact)—through the skin or eyes

Poisons come in four forms: solids (such as pain medicine pills or tablets), liquids (such as household cleaners, including bleach), sprays (such as spray cleaners), and gases (such as carbon monoxide [CO]).

Most consumer products are safe if label directions are followed, but some can be poisonous if used incorrectly. The most common poisons are not necessarily the most dangerous ones. Some of the more dangerous poisons that could be found in a home include the following:

- Antifreeze and windshield washer products
- Some medicines
- Corrosive cleaners such as drain openers, oven cleaners, toilet bowl cleaners, and rust removers
- Fuels such as kerosene, lamp oil, gasoline
- Pesticides

▶ Ingested (Swallowed) Poisons

<u>Ingested poisoning</u> occurs when the victim swallows a toxic substance. Fortunately, most poisons have little toxic effect or are ingested in such small amounts that severe poisoning rarely occurs. However, the potential for severe or fatal poisoning is always present. About 80% of all poisonings happen by ingesting a toxic substance **Figure 1**.

Recognizing Ingested Poisoning

The following are signs of ingested poisoning:
- Abdominal pain and cramping
- Nausea or vomiting
- Diarrhea

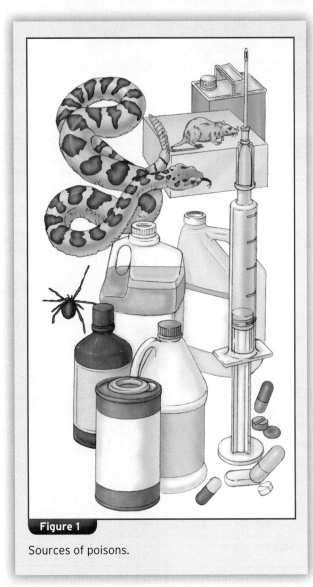

Figure 1

Sources of poisons.

- Burns, odor, or stains around and in the mouth
- Drowsiness or unconsciousness
- Seizure
- Poison container nearby

Care for Ingested Poisoning Victims

If you think someone has been poisoned:
1. Check the condition of the victim. Call 9-1-1 immediately if the person:
   - Has collapsed (is unresponsive)
   - Is having trouble breathing; monitor for breathing and, if absent, begin CPR
   - Has severe pain in the chest
   - Shows other life-threatening signs
2. Call <u>Poison Help</u> (1-800-222-1222) even if there are no signs of poisoning. Try to identify what poison is involved. If possible, bring its container to the phone.

CAUTION

DO NOT give water or milk to dilute poisons other than caustic or corrosive substances (acids and alkalis) unless told to do so by staff at a poison center. Fluids can dissolve a dry poison such as tablets or capsules more rapidly and fill up the stomach, forcing the stomach contents (the poison) into the small intestine, where it will be absorbed faster. Vomiting and aspiration could occur.

CAUTION

DO NOT gag or tickle the back of the victim's throat with a finger or a spoon handle. This method is usually ineffective in causing vomiting, and any vomiting produced is not very forceful.

DO NOT give dish soap, raw eggs, or mustard powder. They are not effective.

DO NOT use syrup of ipecac.

3. A nurse, pharmacist, or other poison expert will answer your call. Be ready to tell the person:
   - The name of the product (found on the container's label)
   - The amount of product involved (eg, half the bottle, a dozen tablets)
   - How long ago the poison contacted the victim
   - The age and weight of the victim
   - What signs of poisoning you notice
4. A poison expert will decide whether the person is in danger. The poison expert will give you the advice you need and may stay on the phone with you while you get help or call you later to follow up.
5. Most calls (about 70%) can be handled outside of a hospital. If you need a physician or an ambulance, the poison expert will tell you right away.

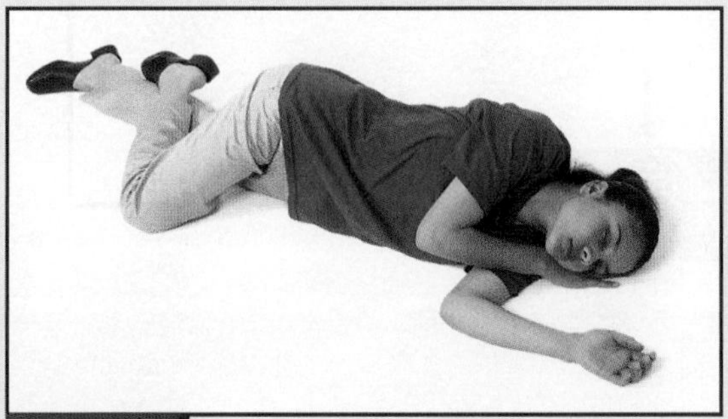

Figure 2

The left-side position delays the advance of the poison into the small intestine.

6. Place the victim on his or her left side (recovery position) **Figure 2**. For ingested poisoning, the left side is best because it positions the end of the stomach where it enters the small intestine (pylorus) straight up. Gravity will delay (by as much as 2 hours) the advance of the poison into the small intestine, where absorption into the victim's circulatory system is faster. The side position also helps prevent aspiration (inhalation) into the lungs if vomiting begins.
7. Save poison containers, plants, and the victim's vomitus to help medical personnel identify the poison.

Alcohol Emergencies

▶ Alcohol Intoxication

Alcohol is a depressant, not a stimulant. It affects a person's judgment, vision, reaction time, and coordination. In very large amounts, it can cause death by paralyzing the respiratory center of the brain.

Alcohol is the most commonly used and abused drug in the United States, possibly even the world. It is also one of the most lethal because it is implicated as a cofactor in up to 40% of drownings, over 40% of

CAUTION

DO NOT follow the first aid procedures or recommendations on a container label without first getting confirmation from a medical source. Many labels are incorrect or out of date.

DO NOT try to neutralize a poison. Giving weak acids, such as lemon juice or vinegar, is not safe, contrary to the advice given on many drain cleaner and lye product labels. Chemical neutralization releases large quantities of heat that can burn sensitive tissues.

DO NOT think that a specific antidote exists for most poisons. An antidote is a substance that counteracts a poison's effects. Few poisons have specific antidotes that will effectively block their toxic effects.

DO NOT think that there is a universal antidote. No product is effective in treating most or all poisons.

Poisoning (Ingested)

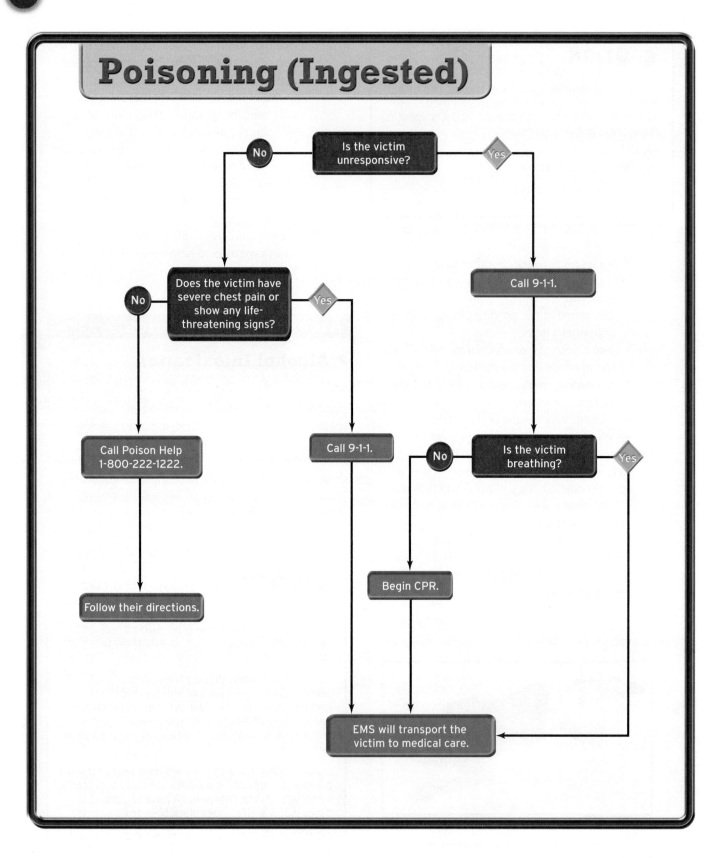

Is the victim unresponsive?
- No →
- Yes →

No → Does the victim have severe chest pain or show any life-threatening signs?
- **Yes** → Call 9-1-1.

Yes (unresponsive) → Call 9-1-1.

No (no chest pain) → Call Poison Help 1-800-222-1222. → Follow their directions.

Is the victim breathing?
- **No** → Begin CPR.
- **Yes** →

EMS will transport the victim to medical care.

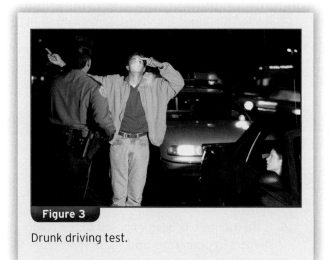

Figure 3

Drunk driving test.

traffic deaths **Figure 3**, 67% of homicides, and 33% of suicides. It directly affects more than 12 million people annually (10% of all males and 3% of all females) and causes more than 200,000 deaths. Alcohol abuse is a major national health problem, ranking with heart disease and cancer. Lack of data makes it difficult to assess the actual number of alcohol-related injuries. It is estimated, however, that about 25% of the patients treated in hospital emergency departments were for intoxication alone. Nearly 50% of patients in trauma centers were injured while under the influence of alcohol.

Helping an intoxicated person is often difficult because the person could be belligerent and combative. However, it is important that people who abuse alcohol be helped and not labeled as drunks. Their condition can be quite serious, even life-threatening.

Occasionally, a person will have consumed so much alcohol that there are signs of central nervous system depression. In such cases, complete respiratory support might be necessary. Death can result from the excessive consumption of alcohol.

The consumption of alcohol is deeply embedded in our society. Because of the widespread use of alcohol, people whose lives are affected directly or indirectly by alcohol abuse should be educated so they can recognize problems and know what to do in an emergency.

Recognizing Intoxication

Although the following signs indicate alcohol intoxication, some might also mean illness or injury other than alcohol abuse, such as diabetes or heat injury:

- The odor of alcohol on a person's breath or clothing

- Unsteady, staggering walking
- Slurred speech and the inability to carry on a conversation
- Nausea and vomiting
- Flushed face

Seizures can result from alcohol ingestion or alcohol withdrawal. Any seizures related to alcohol require medical evaluation. Diabetic coma can mimic alcohol intoxication, as can poisoning and neurologic problems.

Care for Intoxicated Individuals

First aid for an intoxicated person includes these steps:

1. Look for any injuries. Alcohol can mask pain.
2. Monitor breathing and treat accordingly.
3. If the intoxicated person is lying down, place him or her in the recovery (left-side) position to reduce the likelihood of vomiting and aspiration of vomit and to delay the absorption of alcohol into the bloodstream. Be sure to check that the victim is breathing and does not have a spinal injury before you move him or her. The recovery position can be used for responsive and unresponsive persons.
4. Call the poison center for advice or the local emergency number for help. It might be best to let EMS personnel decide whether the police should be alerted.
5. If the victim becomes violent, leave the scene and find a safe place until police arrive.
6. Provide emotional support.
7. Assume that an injured or unresponsive victim has a spinal injury and needs to be stabilized against movement. Because of decreased pain perception, an intoxicated victim cannot be assessed reliably. If you suspect a spinal injury, wait for EMS personnel to arrive. They have

the proper equipment and training to stabilize and move a victim.

8. Because many intoxicated people have been exposed to the cold, suspect hypothermia (dangerously low body temperature) and move the person to a warm place whenever possible. Remove wet clothing and cover the person with warm blankets. Handle a hypothermic victim gently because rough handling could induce a deadly heart rhythm.

Drug Emergencies

Drugs are classified according to their effects on the user:

- Uppers are stimulants of the central nervous system. They include amphetamines, cocaine, and caffeine.
- Downers (sedative-hypnotic) are depressants of the central nervous system. They include barbiturates, tranquilizers, marijuana, and narcotics.
- Hallucinogens alter and often enhance the sensory and emotional information in the brain centers. They include LSD (lysergic acid diethylamide), mescaline, peyote, and PCP (phencyclidine hydrochloride, or angel dust). Marijuana also has some hallucinogenic properties.
- Volatile chemicals usually are inhaled and can cause serious damage to many body organs. They include plastic model glue and cement, paint solvent, gasoline, spray paint, and nail polish remover.

Recognizing Drug Overdose

The condition of a person suffering from drug overdose may be quite serious, even life-threatening. The signs of drug overdose include the following:

- Drowsiness, anxiety, or agitation
- Dilated (large) or constricted (small) pupils
- Confusion
- Hallucinations

Care for a Drug Overdose

Care for a drug overdose is the same as that for alcohol intoxication:

1. Look for injuries. Drugs can mask pain.
2. Monitor breathing.

3. If the victim is lying down, place him or her in the recovery position. Rolling the victim onto the left side not only reduces the likelihood of vomiting and aspiration of vomit, but also delays absorption of drugs into the bloodstream.
4. Call the poison control center (1-800-222-1222) for advice or 9-1-1 for help.
5. Provide emotional support, but if the victim becomes violent, leave the scene, call 9-1-1, and find a safe place until police arrive.
6. If the victim has been exposed to the cold, suspect hypothermia and move the person to a warm environment whenever possible. Remove wet clothing and cover the individual with warm blankets. Handle a hypothermic victim gently because rough handling could induce a cardiac arrest.

Carbon Monoxide Poisoning

Carbon monoxide (CO), because of its common presence in our environment, along with its insidious nature, is the leading cause of poisoning death in the United States each year. Carbon monoxide is an odorless, colorless, nonirritating gas produced by the incomplete combustion of carbon-based fuels.

Recognizing Carbon Monoxide Poisoning

It is difficult to determine whether a person is a victim of CO poisoning. Sometimes, a complaint of having the flu is really a symptom of CO poisoning. Although many symptoms of CO poisoning resemble those of the flu, there are differences. For example, CO poisoning does not cause low-grade fever or generalized aching or involve the lymph nodes.

The signs and symptoms of CO poisoning are as follows:

- Headache
- Ringing in the ears (tinnitus)
- Chest pain (angina)
- Muscle weakness
- Nausea and vomiting
- Dizziness and visual changes (blurred or double vision)
- Unresponsiveness
- Respiratory and cardiac arrest

The traditionally cited sign of CO poisoning is cherry-red skin and lips. This sign is uncommon, however, and occurs only at death; therefore, it is a poor initial indicator of CO poisoning. The following are earmarks of possible CO poisoning:

- The symptoms come and go.
- The symptoms worsen or improve in certain places or at certain times of the day.
- People around the victim have similar symptoms.
- Pets seem ill.

Care for Carbon Monoxide Poisoning Victims

1. Get the victim out of the toxic environment and into fresh air immediately.
2. Call 9-1-1, who will send EMS personnel who will be able to give the victim 100% oxygen, improving oxygenation and disassociating the linkage between the CO and the hemoglobin. For a responsive victim, it takes 4 to 5 hours with ordinary air (21% oxygen) or 30 to 40 minutes with 100% oxygen to reverse the effects of CO poisoning.
3. Monitor breathing.
4. Place an unresponsive breathing victim in the recovery position.
5. Seek medical care. All suspected victims of CO poisoning should obtain a blood test to determine the level of CO.

Plant-Induced Dermatitis: Poison Ivy, Poison Oak, and Poison Sumac

About 85% of the population is sensitive to poison ivy, poison oak, and poison sumac. If a person reaches adulthood without experiencing a reaction, the risk falls from 85% to 50%. With more people venturing into the outdoors, episodes of dermatitis caused by exposure to poison ivy, poison oak, and poison sumac are increasing **Figure 4**, **Figure 5**, **Figure 6**. (Actually, more than 60 plants can cause allergic reactions, but these three are by far the most common offenders.) Of those who do react, 15–25% will have incapacitating swelling and blistering eruptions that require medical care **Figure 7**. There is no routine test to determine an individual's degree of sensitivity—a history of dermatitis is the most reliable indicator.

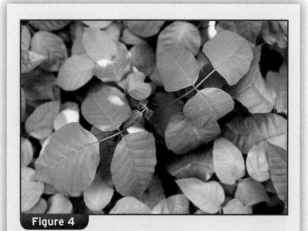

Figure 4

Poison ivy, found in all 48 contiguous states in the United States.

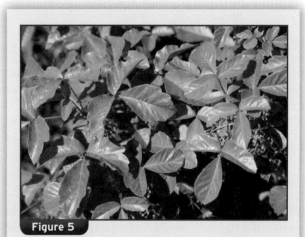

Figure 5

Poison oak.

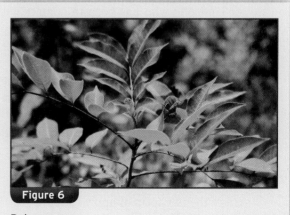

Figure 6

Poison sumac.

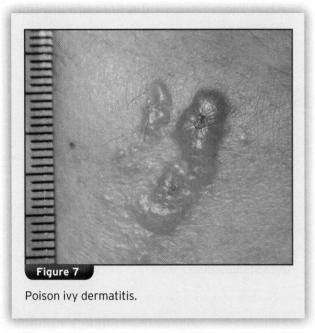

Figure 7

Poison ivy dermatitis.

Recognizing Plant-Induced Dermatitis

Most people do not realize they have come in contact with a poisonous plant until the rash erupts. Reactions can range from mild to severe.

- Mild: itching
- Mild to moderate: itching and redness
- Moderate: itching, redness, and swelling
- Severe: itching, redness, swelling, and blisters

Severity is important, but so is the amount of skin affected. The greater the amount of skin affected, the greater the need for medical care. A day or two is the usual time between contact and the onset of signs and symptoms.

Care for Plant-Induced Dermatitis

To care for someone who has been in contact with poisonous plants:

1. People who know they have been in contact with a poisonous plant should wash the skin with soap and water as soon as possible (within 5 minutes for sensitive people and within 1 hour for moderately sensitive people). Unfortunately, most victims do not know about their contact until several hours or days later, when the itching and rash begin. Use soap and water to cleanse the skin of the oily resin or apply rubbing (isopropyl) alcohol liberally (not in swab-type dabs). If too little isopropyl alcohol is used, the oil will be spread to another site and enlarge the injury. Other solvents, such as paint thinner, can be used, but they can irritate or damage the skin. Rinse with water to remove the solubilized material. Water removes urushiol from the skin, oxidizes and inactivates it, and does not penetrate the skin (as solvents do).

2. For a mild reaction, have the victim soak in a lukewarm bath sprinkled with 1 to 2 cups of colloidal oatmeal. Colloidal oatmeal makes a tub slick, so take appropriate precautions. Or, apply one of the following:
   - Wet compresses soaked with aluminum acetate for 20 to 30 minutes three or four times a day
   - Calamine lotion (calamine ointment if the skin becomes dry and cracked) or zinc oxide
   - Baking soda paste: 1 teaspoon of water mixed with 3 teaspoons of baking soda

3. For a mild to moderate reaction, care for the skin as you would for a mild reaction and use a physician-prescribed corticosteroid ointment.

4. For a severe reaction, care for the skin as you would for mild and moderate reactions and use a physician-prescribed oral corticosteroid such as prednisone. Apply a physician-prescribed topical corticosteroid ointment or cream, cover the area with a transparent plastic wrap, and lightly bind the area with an elastic or self-adhering bandage. A physician-prescribed antihistamine can be used for itching.

Poison Ivy, Oak, and Sumac

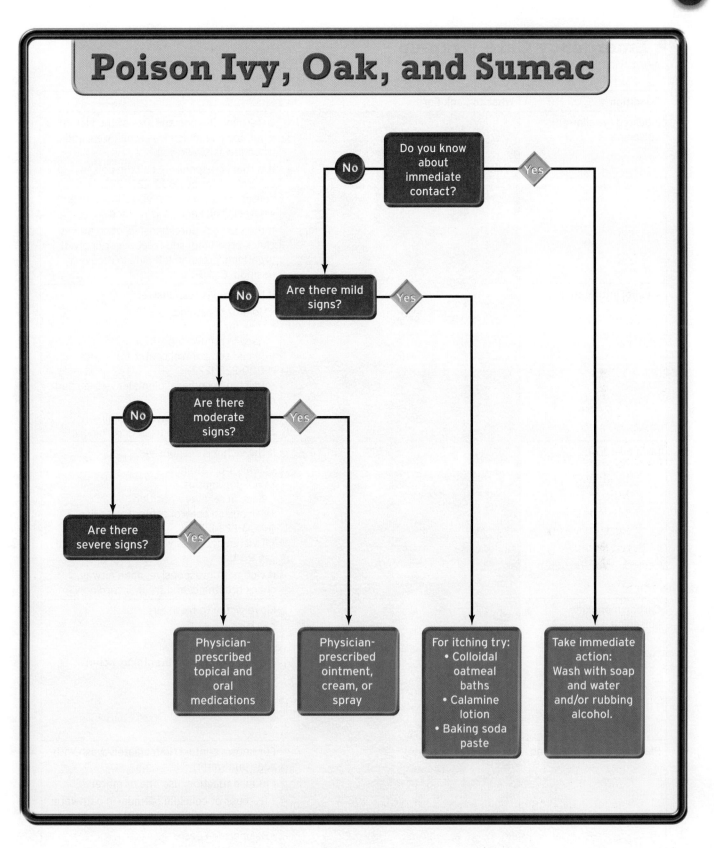

▶ Emergency Care Wrap-up

Condition	What to Look For	What to Do
Ingested (swallowed) poisoning	Abdominal pain and cramping Nausea or vomiting Diarrhea Burns, odor, or stains around and in mouth Drowsiness or unresponsiveness Poison container nearby	Determine the age and size of the victim, what and how much was swallowed, and when it was swallowed. If victim is responsive, call the poison control center at 1-800-222-1222. The center will advise what you should do and whether medical care is needed. If the victim is unresponsive, open airway, check breathing, and treat accordingly. If breathing, place on left side in recovery position. Call 9-1-1.
Alcohol intoxication	Alcohol odor on breath or clothing Unsteadiness, staggering Confusion Slurred speech Nausea and vomiting Flushed face	If the victim is responsive: • Monitor breathing. • Look for injuries. • Place in recovery position. • Call poison control center for advice (1-800-222-1222). • If victim becomes violent, leave area and call 9-1-1. If victim is unresponsive, open airway, check breathing, and treat accordingly.
Drug overdose	Drowsiness, agitation, anxiety, hyperactivity Change in pupil size Confusion Hallucinations	If the victim is responsive: • Monitor breathing. • Look for injuries. • Place in recovery position. • Call poison control center for advice (1-800-222-1222). • If victim becomes violent, leave area and call 9-1-1. If victim is unresponsive, open airway, check breathing, and treat accordingly.
Carbon monoxide poisoning	Headache Ringing in ears Chest pain Muscle weakness Nausea and vomiting Dizziness and vision difficulties Unresponsiveness Breathing and heart stopped	Move victim to fresh air. Call 9-1-1. Monitor breathing. Place unresponsive breathing victim in recovery position.
Plant (contact) poisoning	Rash Itching Redness Blisters Swelling	For known contact, immediately wash with soap and water. For mild reaction, use one or more: • 1–2 cups of colloidal oatmeal in bathwater • Calamine lotion • Baking soda paste For severe reactions, perform step 2 and seek medical care.

▶ Ready for Review

- A poison is any substance that impairs health or causes death by its chemical action when it enters the body or comes in contact with the skin.
- Poisons are classified by how they enter the body. They can be ingested, inhaled, absorbed, and injected.
- Ingested poisoning occurs when the victim swallows a toxic substance.
- Alcohol is a depressant that affects a person's judgment, vision, reaction time, and coordination.
- Drugs are classified according to their effects on the user:
- Uppers (stimulants)
- Downers (depressants)
- Hallucinogens
- Volatile chemicals
- Carbon monoxide is the leading cause of poisoning death in the United States each year.
- About 85% of the population is sensitive to poison ivy, poison oak, and poison sumac.

▶ Vital Vocabulary

carbon monoxide A colorless, odorless, poisonous gas formed by incomplete combustion, such as in fire.

ingested poisoning Poisoning caused by swallowing a toxic substance.

poison Any substance that impairs health or causes death by its chemical action when it enters the body or comes in contact with the skin; also known as a toxin.

Poison Help Medical facility providing immediate, free, expert advice any time; can be reached by calling 1-800-222-1222.

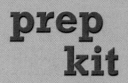

prep kit

▶ Assessment in Action

You have been helping your sister paint three rooms in her home. While taking a break, your 2-year-old niece enters the room with a small cup of paint used for touch up. There is paint around and inside her mouth.

Directions: Circle Yes if you agree with the statement; circle No if you disagree.

Yes   No   **1.** Immediately give your niece water or milk to dilute the ingested paint.

Yes   No   **2.** Use syrup of ipecac to induce vomiting.

Yes   No   **3.** Determine how much of the paint was swallowed, when it was swallowed, and the age and size of the victim.

Yes   No   **4.** Call the poison control center for advice (1-800-222-1222).

▶ Check Your Knowledge

Directions: Circle Yes if you agree with the statement; circle No if you disagree.

Yes   No   **1.** Swallowing a poison can produce nausea.

Yes   No   **2.** Milk should be given to all victims of ingested poison.

Yes   No   **3.** A victim of alcohol intoxication does not require medical care.

Yes   No   **4.** Carbon monoxide has a unique smell.

Yes   No   **5.** Everyone who touches a poison ivy, poison oak, or poison sumac plant will have some type of skin reaction.

Yes   No   **6.** Causing a poisoned victim to vomit is a recommended first aid practice.

Yes   No   **7.** Some cases of poison ivy, poison oak, or poison sumac require medical care.

Yes   No   **8.** Calamine lotion can help relieve itching caused by poison ivy, poison oak, or poison sumac.

Yes   No   **9.** If an intoxicated or drugged person becomes violent, leave the area.

Yes   No   **10.** Move a victim of carbon monoxide poisoning to fresh air.

16

Bites and Stings

▶ Animal Bites

It is estimated that one of every two Americans will be bitten at some time by an animal or by another person. Dogs are responsible for about 80% of all animal bite injuries **Figure 1**. Of the nearly 5 million dog bites that occur yearly, 80% are trivial or minor, and medical care is not required or sought, which demonstrates the importance of knowing first aid. The remainder account for about 1% of all emergency department and physician office visits. Each year, about 19 bite-related deaths occur in the United States **Table 1**.

Animal bites represent a major, largely unrecognized public health problem. Two concerns result from an animal bite: immediate tissue damage and later infection from microorganisms. A dog's mouth can carry more than 60 species of bacteria, some of which are dangerous to humans. Two examples of infection—tetanus and rabies—have been almost eradicated by medical advances, but they still pose a potential problem.

Although cat bites are less mutilating than dog bites, cat bites have a much higher rate of infection than dog bites. Cats have very sharp teeth, which can create deep puncture wounds and involve muscle, tendon, and bone.

Besides children, elderly people and people unable to help themselves are especially prone to animal bites because they are sometimes unable to detect or prevent a dangerous situation. Many animal-related deaths occur when the victim is left alone with the offending pet. Contrary to popular belief, wild or stray dogs seldom are involved in fatal attacks.

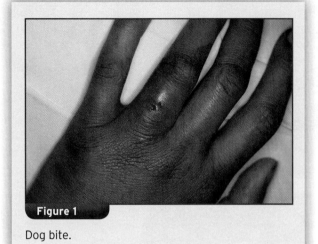

Figure 1

Dog bite.

Table 1 Animal-Related Human Deaths in the United States (1991-2001)

Animal	Average number of deaths each year
Venomous animals	
Snake	5.2
Spider	6
Scorpion	0.45
Hornet, bee, wasp	48.5
Centipede	0.45
Other specified venomous arthropod	6
Venomous marine animal	0.18
Other specified venomous animal	2.1
Total venomous	68.88
Nonvenomous animals	
Dog	18.9
Rat	0.27
Nonvenomous snake	0
Other animals except arthropod	4
Other specified animal*	76.9
Unspecified animal	4
Total nonvenomous	104.07
Overall total	172.95

*Note that this category includes bitten or struck by other mammals, contact with marine animal, bitten or stung by nonvenomous insect or other nonvenomous arthropods, bitten or struck by crocodile or alligator, bitten or confronted by other reptiles.

Source: Adapted from Langley RL. 2005. Animal-related fatalities in the United States: An update. *Wilderness Environ Med* 16(2):67-74.

Damage mostly occurs on the hands, arms, legs, and face. A damaged face presents several problems because the proximity of blood vessels to the skin surface makes it susceptible to copious bleeding. Facial disfigurement and scarring can result in emotional trauma. Complete or partial loss of an eye also is possible.

Wild animal attacks occur most often in rural or wilderness locations. Not all injuries are bites. Severe injuries result from victims being thrown in the air, gored by an antler, butted, or trampled on the ground.

Rabies

Rabies is one of the most ancient and feared of diseases. Although human rabies rarely occurs in the United States or in other industrialized nations, it remains a scourge in developing countries. A virus found in warm-blooded animals causes rabies, which spreads from one animal to another in the saliva, usually through a bite or by licking. Bites from cold-blooded animals such as reptiles do not carry the danger of rabies.

A bite or a scratch is considered a significant rabies exposure if it penetrates the skin. Unprovoked attacks are more likely to have been inflicted by a rabid animal than are provoked attacks. Nonbite exposure consists of contamination of wounds, including scratches, abrasions, and weeping skin rashes.

Consider an animal as possibly rabid if any of the following applies:

- The animal made an unprovoked attack.
- The animal acted strangely, that is, out of character (for example, a usually friendly dog

is aggressive, or a wild fox seems docile and friendly).
- The animal was a high-risk species (skunk, raccoon, or bat).

Report animal bites to the police or animal control officers; they should be the ones to capture the animal for observation. If a healthy domestic dog or cat up to date with its rabies vaccination bit the victim, the animal should be confined and observed for 10 days for any illness. If a wild animal bit the victim, it should be considered a possible rabies exposure and medical care should be sought immediately.

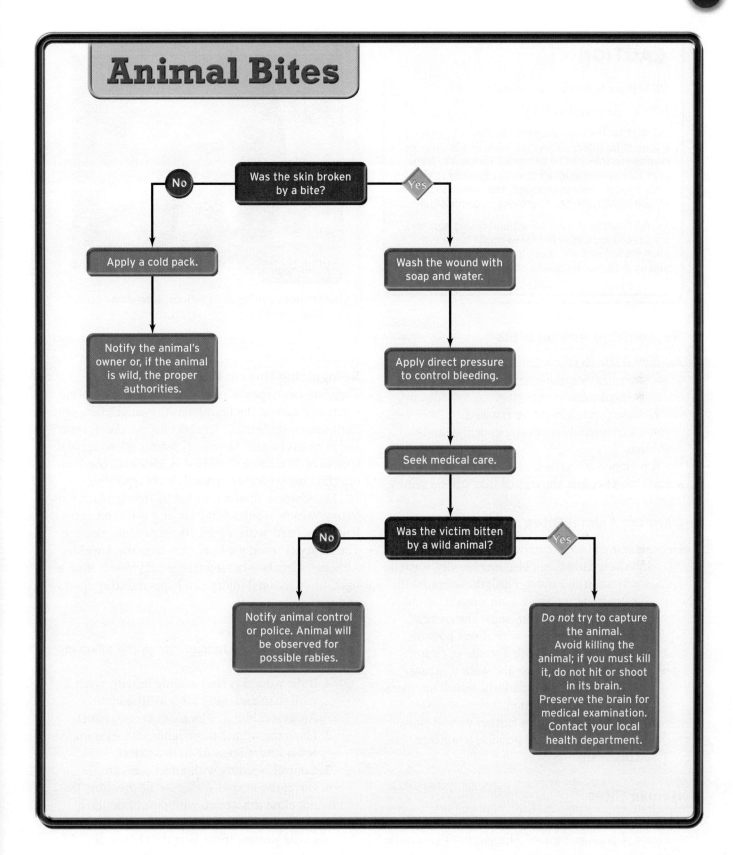

CAUTION

DO NOT try to capture the animal yourself.

DO NOT get near the animal.

DO NOT kill the animal unless absolutely necessary. If it must be killed, protect the head and brain from damage so they can be examined for rabies. Transport a dead animal intact to limit exposure to potentially infected tissues or saliva. The animal's remains should be refrigerated to prevent decomposition.

DO NOT handle the animal without taking appropriate precautions. Infected saliva might be on the animal's fur, so wear heavy gloves or use a shovel if you have to move a dead animal.

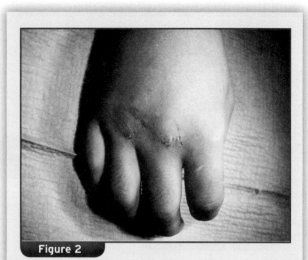

Figure 2

Human bites can result in serious, spreading infection.

Recognizing Animal Bites

An animal bite has the following characteristics:
- Puncture wound from animal's sharp, pointed teeth
- Tissue and skin can be crushed
- Open wound on fingers, knuckles, and/or hand

It is important to be cautious when dealing with animal bites because the animal may still be nearby.

Care for Animal Bites

Help an animal bite victim by doing the following:
1. If the wound is not bleeding heavily, wash it with soap and water. Flush the wound with water under pressure from a faucet. Avoid scrubbing, which can bruise the tissues.
2. Control the bleeding with direct pressure.
3. Cover the wound with a sterile or clean dressing. Do not close the wound because doing so could trap bacteria, which increases the chances of infection.
4. Seek medical care for further wound cleaning and closure, and possible tetanus or rabies care.

Human Bites

After dogs and cats, the animal most likely to bite humans is another human. Human bites can cause severe injury, often more so than other animal bites. The human mouth contains a wide range of bacteria and viruses, so the chance of infection is great from a human bite, especially on the hand **Figure 2**.

Recognizing Human Bites

There are two types of human bites. True bites occur when any part of the body's flesh is caught between teeth, usually deliberately. True bites happen during fights and in cases of abuse. Mandatory reporting laws apply if spousal or child abuse is involved. A schoolyard bite, with one child biting another, generally is not reportable.

Much worse than a true bite is the clenched-fist injury, which results from cutting a fist on teeth. It is associated with a high likelihood of infection. The injury is usually a laceration over the knuckles. Although clenched-fist injuries usually result from a fight, unintentional injury can happen during sports and play.

Care for Human Bites

Help someone with a human bite in the following manner:
1. If the wound is not bleeding heavily, wash it with soap and water for 5 to 10 minutes. Avoid scrubbing, which can bruise tissues.
2. Flush the wound thoroughly with running water under pressure from a faucet.
3. Control bleeding with direct pressure.
4. Cover the wound with a sterile dressing. Do not close the wound with tape or butterfly bandages. Closing the wound traps bacteria in the wound, increasing the chance of infection.
5. Seek medical care for possible further wound cleaning, a possible tetanus shot, and sutures to close the wound, if needed.

▶ Snake Bites

Throughout the world, about 50,000 people die of snake bites each year. Each year in the United States, 40,000 to 50,000 people are bitten by snakes, 7,000 to 8,000 of them by venomous snakes **Figure 3**.

Victims who die of snake bites in the United States usually do so during the first 48 hours after the bite. Only four snake species in the United States are venomous: rattlesnakes (which account for about 65% of all venomous snake bites and nearly all the snake bite deaths in the United States), copperheads, water moccasins (also known as cottonmouths), and coral snakes **Figure 4**, **Figure 5**, **Figure 6**, and **Figure 7**. Although uncommon, snake bites can be painful, costly, and potentially deadly. Other than death, disabilities such as partial or complete loss of an extremity or finger or loss of movement in a joint can occur. Most victims fully recover.

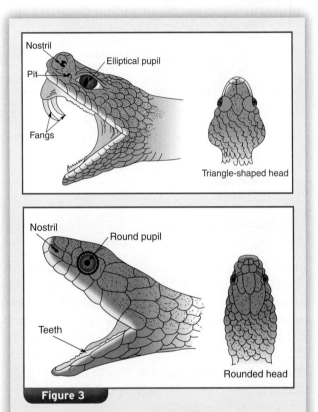

Figure 3

Characteristic features of venomous snakes (pit vipers) and of harmless snakes.

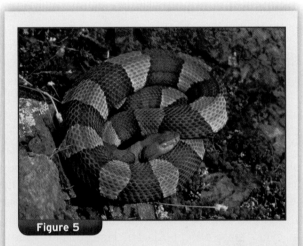

Figure 5

Copperhead snake.

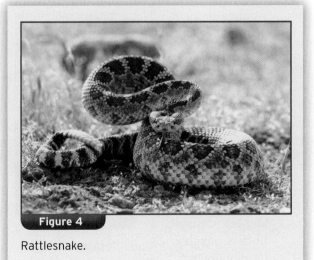

Figure 4

Rattlesnake.

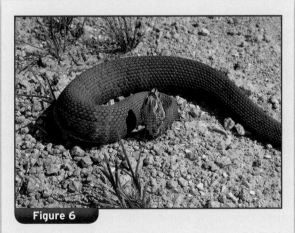

Figure 6

Water moccasin (cottonmouth).

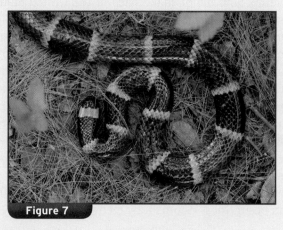

Figure 7

Coral snake; the United States' most venomous snake.

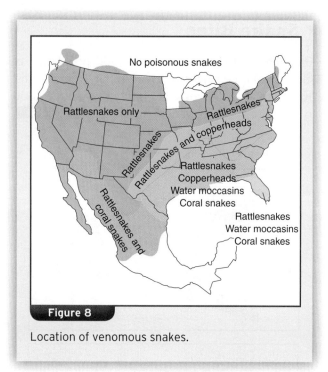

Figure 8

Location of venomous snakes.

The first three are pit vipers, which have three characteristics in common:

- Triangular, flat heads wider than their necks
- Elliptical pupils (cat-like eyes)
- A heat-sensitive pit between the eye and the nostril on each side of the head

The coral snake is small and colorful, with a series of bright red, yellow, and black bands around its body (every other band is yellow). Coral snakes are found in Arizona, the southeastern United States, and Texas.

At least one species of venomous snakes is found in every state except Alaska, Hawaii, and Maine **Figure 8** . Exotic snakes, whether imported legally or smuggled into the United States, can be found in zoos, schools, snake farms, and amateur and professional collections, and account for at least 15 bites a year. Some of the exotic snakes can be poisonous.

Pit Vipers

Pit vipers are found in every state but Alaska, Maine, and Hawaii. Rattlesnakes are the most widespread of the pit vipers. Copperheads are found in the central southeastern United States and westward into the Big Bend of Texas. Cottonmouth water moccasins are found in the southeast from Virginia to Florida and into Texas. Snakes benefit us by keeping the rodent population from exploding out of control. They consume hundreds of thousands of mice and rats every year. Few snakes act aggressively toward a human unless provoked. The vast majority of bites are not deadly and can be effectively treated.

Ninety-eight percent of snake bites are on the extremities. Alcohol intoxication of the victim is a factor in many bites. The majority of bites in the United States occur in the southwestern part of the country—partly due to the near-extinction of pit vipers in the eastern United States. The eastern and western diamondback rattlesnakes account for almost 95% of the deaths. These deaths occur most often in children, in the elderly, and in victims to whom **antivenom** is not given or is inappropriately given.

Recognizing Pit Viper Bites

Signs of a pit viper bite include:

- Severe burning pain at the bite site.
- Two small puncture wounds about ½″ apart (some cases have only one fang mark) **Figure 9** .
- Swelling (occurs within 10 to 15 minutes and can involve an entire extremity).
- Discoloration after 2–3 hours and blood-filled blisters possibly developing in 6 to 10 hours.

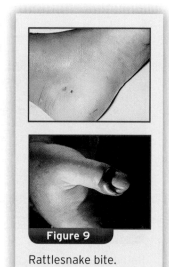

Figure 9

Rattlesnake bite.

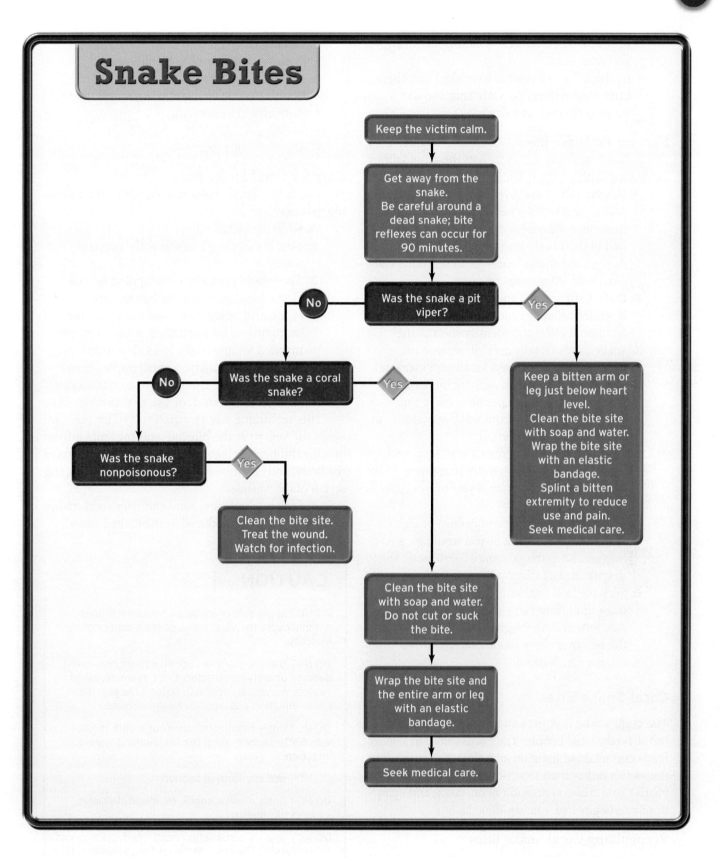

Snake Bites

Keep the victim calm.

Get away from the snake.
Be careful around a dead snake; bite reflexes can occur for 90 minutes.

Was the snake a pit viper?

No → Was the snake a coral snake?

Yes → Keep a bitten arm or leg just below heart level.
Clean the bite site with soap and water.
Wrap the bite site with an elastic bandage.
Splint a bitten extremity to reduce use and pain.
Seek medical care.

Was the snake a coral snake?

No → Was the snake nonpoisonous?

Yes → Clean the bite site with soap and water.
Do not cut or suck the bite.

Was the snake nonpoisonous?

Yes → Clean the bite site.
Treat the wound.
Watch for infection.

Clean the bite site with soap and water.
Do not cut or suck the bite.

Wrap the bite site and the entire arm or leg with an elastic bandage.

Seek medical care.

- In severe cases, nausea, vomiting, sweating, and weakness.
- In about 25% of venomous snake bites, there is no venom injection, only fang and tooth wounds (known as a dry bite).

Care for Pit Viper Bites

The Wilderness Medical Society lists these guidelines for dealing with pit viper bites:

1. Get the victim and bystanders away from the snake. Snakes have been known to bite more than once. Pit vipers can strike about one half of their body length. Be careful around a decapitated snake head—head reactions can persist for 90 minutes or more.
2. Do not attempt to capture or kill the snake. It wastes valuable time, there is a risk of additional bites, and identification of the snake is not usually needed because the same antivenom is used for all pit viper bites.
3. Keep the victim quiet. Activity increases venom absorption. If possible, carry the victim or have the victim walk very slowly to help to minimize exertion.
4. Gently wash the bitten area with soap and water. Any ring(s) or jewelry that might reduce blood circulation if swelling occurs should be removed.
5. Stabilize the bitten extremity (arm or leg) with a sling or a splint as you would for a fracture. Keep the extremity below heart level despite the fact that swelling might occur.
6. Seek medical care immediately. This is the most important thing to do for the victim. Antivenom must be given within 4 hours of the bite (not every venomous snake bite requires antivenom).

Coral Snake Bites

The coral snake is America's most venomous snake, but it rarely bites people. The coral snake has short fangs and tends to hang on and chew its venom into the victim rather than to strike and release, like a pit viper. Coral snake venom is a neurotoxin, and symptoms can begin 1 to 5 hours after the bite.

Recognizing Coral Snake Bites

Someone who has been bitten by a coral snake might exhibit the following symptoms:

- Minimal pain
- Sagging or drooping of upper eyelids

- Weakness
- Pricking, tingling of skin (often numb at bite site)
- Double vision (seeing two of a single object)
- Difficulty in swallowing
- Sweating
- Abnormal flow of saliva

Care for Coral Snake Bites

You can help a coral snake bite victim in the following manner:

1. Keep the victim calm.
2. Gently clean the bite site with soap and water.
3. Apply mild pressure by wrapping several elastic bandages over the bite site and the entire arm or leg. Applying mild pressure (as tightly as for a sprained ankle) is recommended for any snake bites. The technique originated in Australia, where it has been very successful. Do not cut the victim's skin, suck on the wound, or use a suction device.

This technique has two parts: (1) The pressure holds the venom at the bite site and prevents it from moving through the lymphatic system to other parts of the body, and (2) immobilization limits the pumping action of the muscles.

4. Seek medical care. Antivenom for coral snakes is no longer produced in the United States.

CAUTION

DO NOT apply cold or ice to a snake bite. It does not inactivate the venom and poses a danger of frostbite.

DO NOT use the cut-and-suck procedure—you could damage underlying structures (for example, blood vessels, nerves, or tendons). Cutting the skin may cause infection and a poorly healing wound.

DO NOT apply mouth suction. Your mouth is filled with bacteria, increasing the likelihood of wound infection.

DO NOT use any form of suction.

DO NOT apply electric shock. No medical studies support this method.

DO NOT apply a constriction band—their use remains controversial. They may increase tissue damage. If applied too tightly or if swelling occurs, they can act as a tourniquet.

Dead Snakes Can Still Bite
Data collected at the Good Samaritan Regional Medical Center in Phoenix show that fatal injuries do not prevent rattlesnakes from biting humans. Of the 34 patients admitted to the Phoenix Center for Rattlesnake Bites in a recent 11-month period, five were bitten by snakes that had been fatally injured and were presumed dead. One patient was bitten on the index finger after picking up a snake he had bludgeoned in the head and assumed was dead. Another was bitten after picking up a snake he had shot, then decapitated.

Source: Suchard JR, LoVecchio F. 1999. Envenomations by rattlesnakes thought to be dead. *N Engl J Med* 340(24):1930.

Nonpoisonous Snake Bites

Nonvenomous snakes inflict the most snake bites. If you are not positive about a snake, assume it was venomous. Some so-called nonpoisonous North American snakes such as the hognose and garter snakes have venom that can cause painful local reactions but no systemic (whole-body) symptoms.

Recognizing Nonpoisonous Snake Bites
A nonpoisonous snake bite results in the following:
- Feeling of a mild to moderate pinch
- Curved lines (horseshoe shaped) of tiny pinpricks on the skin that correspond with the rows of sharp, pointy teeth
- Bleeding
- Mild itching

Care for Nonpoisonous Snake Bites
A victim of a nonpoisonous snake bite should be treated as follows:
1. Gently clean the bite site with soap and water.
2. Care for the bite as you would a minor wound.
3. Seek medical care.

▶ Insect Stings

Generally, venomous flying insects are aggressive only when threatened or when their hives or nests are disrupted. Under such conditions, they sting, sometimes in swarms. Honeybees and some yellow jackets have barbed stingers that become embedded in the victim's skin during the sting **Figure 10**. After injecting its venom, the bee flies away, tearing and leaving behind the embedded stinger and venom sac, which causes it to die. Honeybees and bumblebees do not release all their venom during the initial injection; some remains in the stinger embedded in the victim's skin. If the stinger and venom sac are not removed properly, additional venom can be released and worsen the victim's reaction.

In contrast, the stingers of wasps, yellow jackets, hornets, and fire ants are not barbed and do not become embedded in the victim. Thus, these insects can sting multiple times, and most species (with a few exceptions, such as some yellow jacket species) do not die as a result of the stinging.

Recognizing Insect Stings

A rule of thumb is that the sooner symptoms develop after a sting, the more serious the reaction will be.
- Usual reactions are instant pain, redness around the sting site, and itching.
- Worrisome reactions include hives, swelling of lips or tongue, a tickle in the throat, and wheezing.
- Life-threatening reactions are bluish or grayish skin color, seizures, unresponsiveness, and an inability to breathe because of swelling and spasm of the airway.

About 60% to 80% of anaphylactic deaths are caused by the victim not being able to breathe because swollen airway passages obstruct airflow to the lungs. The second most common cause of death is shock, caused by collapse of blood circulation through the body.

Care for Insect Stings

The following outlines how to assist someone who has been bitten or stung by an insect.
1. Most people who have been stung can be treated on site, and everyone should know what to do if a life-threatening allergic reaction (anaphylaxis) occurs. In particular, people who have had a severe reaction to an insect sting should be instructed about what they can do to protect themselves. They also should be advised to wear a medical-alert identification tag identifying them as allergic to insect stings.

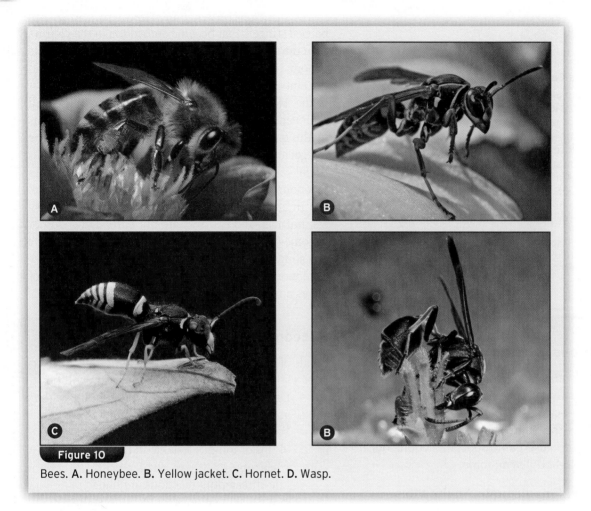

Figure 10

Bees. **A.** Honeybee. **B.** Yellow jacket. **C.** Hornet. **D.** Wasp.

2. Look at the sting site for a stinger and venom sac embedded in the skin. Bees are the only stinging insects that leave their stingers and venom sac behind. If the stinger is embedded, remove it or it will continue to inject poison for 2 or 3 minutes. Remove the stinger and venom sac as soon as possible by any method.

3. Wash the sting site with soap and water to prevent infection.

4. Apply an ice pack over the sting site to slow absorption of the venom and relieve pain. Use a commercial sting stick containing a topical anesthetic such as Xylocaine (unless the victim is known to be allergic to the drug). Because bee venom is acidic, a paste made of baking soda and water can help. Sodium bicarbonate is an alkalinizing agent that draws out fluid and reduces itching and swelling. Wasp venom, on the other hand, is alkaline, so apply vinegar or lemon juice. A paste made of unseasoned meat tenderizer

can help a bee sting victim if the paste comes in direct contact with the venom. That generally is not possible, however, because the bee will have injected the venom through too small a hole and too deeply into the victim's skin.

5. To further relieve pain and itching, use aspirin (adults only), acetaminophen, or ibuprofen. A topical steroid cream, such as hydrocortisone, can help combat local swelling and itching. An antihistamine can prevent some local symptoms if given early, but it works too slowly to counteract a life-threatening allergic reaction.

6. Observe the victim for at least 30 minutes for signs of an allergic reaction. For a person having a severe allergic reaction, a dose of epinephrine is the only effective treatment. A person with a known allergy to insect stings should have a physician-prescribed emergency kit that includes a prefilled, spring-loaded device that automatically injects

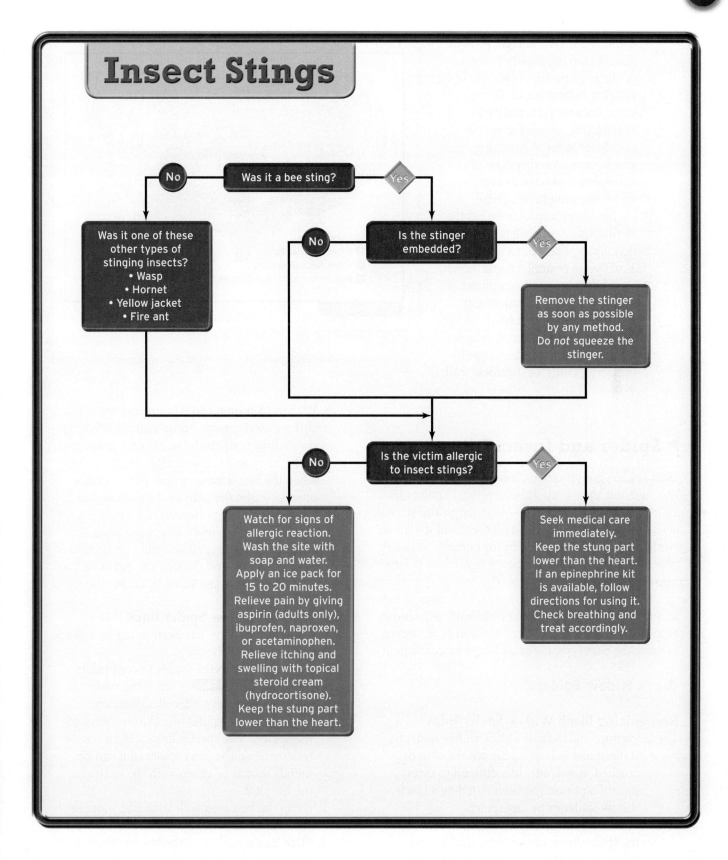

Insect Stings

Was it a bee sting?

No → Was it one of these other types of stinging insects?
- Wasp
- Hornet
- Yellow jacket
- Fire ant

Yes → Is the stinger embedded?

No

Yes → Remove the stinger as soon as possible by any method. Do *not* squeeze the stinger.

Is the victim allergic to insect stings?

No → Watch for signs of allergic reaction. Wash the site with soap and water. Apply an ice pack for 15 to 20 minutes. Relieve pain by giving aspirin (adults only), ibuprofen, naproxen, or acetaminophen. Relieve itching and swelling with topical steroid cream (hydrocortisone). Keep the stung part lower than the heart.

Yes → Seek medical care immediately. Keep the stung part lower than the heart. If an epinephrine kit is available, follow directions for using it. Check breathing and treat accordingly.

epinephrine. The allergic person should take the kit whenever he or she is going someplace where stinging insects are known to exist. Because epinephrine is short-acting, watch the victim closely for signs of returning anaphylaxis. Another dose of epinephrine as often as every 15 minutes might be needed.

7. Do not use epinephrine unless the victim has a severe allergic reaction. Epinephrine has a shelf life of 1 to 3 years or until it turns brown.

8. Watch for signs and symptoms of a delayed allergic reaction, especially during the first 6 to 24 hours. If the victim develops difficulty breathing, facial swelling, fever, chills, or dizziness, call 9-1-1.

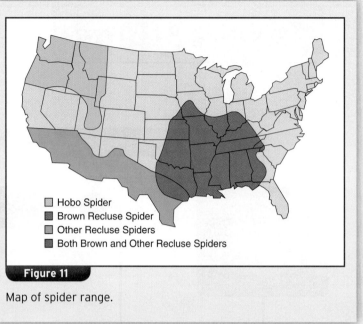

- ☐ Hobo Spider
- ■ Brown Recluse Spider
- ☐ Other Recluse Spiders
- ■ Both Brown and Other Recluse Spiders

Figure 11

Map of spider range.

▶ Spider and Insect Bites
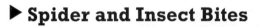

Most spiders are venomous, which is how they paralyze and kill their prey. However, most spiders lack an effective delivery system—long fangs and strong jaws—to bite a human. About 60 species of spiders in North America are capable of biting humans, although only a few species have produced significant poisonings **Figure 11**.

The number of deaths from spider bites is not accurately known. A spider bite is difficult to diagnose, especially when the spider was not seen or recovered, because the bites typically cause little immediate pain.

Black Widow Spiders

Recognizing Black Widow Spider Bites
The following could indicate a black widow spider bite:
- If the spider is trapped against the skin or crushed, it will bite. It is difficult to determine if a person has been bitten by a black widow spider or by any spider.
- The victim might feel a sharp pinprick when the spider bites, but some victims are not aware of the bite. Within 15 minutes, a dull, numbing pain develops in the bite area.
- Two small fang marks might be seen as tiny red spots.

- Within 15 minutes to 4 hours, muscle stiffness and cramps occur, usually affecting the abdomen when the bite is on a lower part of the body and the shoulders, back, or chest when the bite is on an upper part. Victims often describe the pain as the most severe they have ever experienced.
- Headache, chills, fever, heavy sweating, dizziness, nausea, and vomiting occur next. Severe pain around the bite site peaks in 2 to 3 hours and can last 12 to 48 hours.

Care for Black Widow Spider Bites
To care for someone who has been bitten by a black widow spider, do the following:
1. If possible, catch the spider to confirm its identity **Figure 12**. Even if the body has been crushed, save it for identification (although most spider bite victims never see the spider). The species helps determine the treatment, so the dead spider (if it can be found) should be taken with the victim to the hospital.
2. Clean the bite area with soap and water or rubbing alcohol.
3. Place an ice pack over the bite to relieve pain and delay the effects of the venom.
4. Give aspirin (adults only), ibuprofen, or acetaminophen.
5. Monitor breathing.

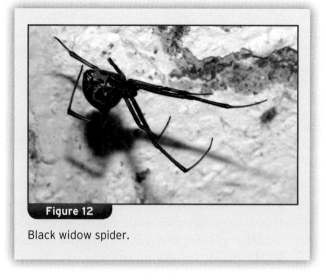

Figure 12

Black widow spider.

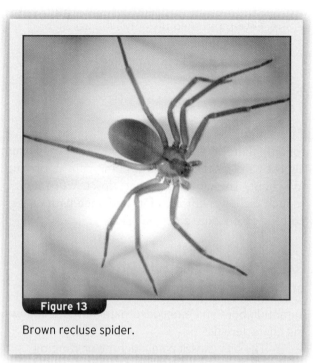

Figure 13

Brown recluse spider.

6. Seek medical care immediately. For black widow spider bites, an antivenom exists. It is usually reserved for children younger than 6 years, people older than 60 years and with high blood pressure, pregnant women, and victims with severe reactions. The antivenom will give relief within 1 to 3 hours.

Brown Recluse Spiders

Brown recluse spiders are also known in North America as fiddle-back and violin spiders **Figure 13**. They have a violin-shaped figure on their backs (several other spider species have a similar configuration on their backs). Color varies from fawn to dark brown, with darker legs. Male and female spiders are venomous. Brown recluse spiders are found primarily in the southern and midwestern states, with other less toxic but related spiders throughout the rest of the country. They are absent from the Pacific Northwest.

Recognizing Brown Recluse Spider Bites

If you suspect a brown recluse spider bite, remember the following:

- The brown recluse spider bites only when it is trapped against the skin.
- A local reaction usually occurs within 2 to 8 hours with mild to severe pain at the bite site and the development of redness, swelling, and local itching.
- In 48 to 72 hours, a blister develops at the bite site, becomes red, and bursts. During the early stages, the affected area often takes on a bull's-eye appearance, with a central white area surrounded by a reddened area, ringed by a whitish or blue border. A small, red crater remains, over which a scab forms. When the scab falls away in a few days, a larger crater remains. That too scabs over and falls off, leaving a larger crater. The craters are known as volcano lesions. This process of slow tissue destruction can continue for weeks or months. The ulcer sometimes requires skin grafting.
- Fever, weakness, vomiting, joint pain, and a rash could occur.
- Stomach cramps, nausea, and vomiting might occur. Death is rare.

Care for Brown Recluse Spider Bites

This is how you can care for someone who has been bitten by a brown recluse spider:

1. If possible, catch the spider to confirm its identity. Even if the body has been crushed, save it for identification (although most spider bite victims never see the spider). The species helps determine the treatment, so the dead spider (if it can be found) should be taken with the victim to the hospital.
2. Clean the bite area with soap and water or rubbing alcohol.
3. Place an ice pack over the bite to relieve pain and delay the effects of the venom.

4. Give aspirin (adults only), ibuprofen, or acetaminophen.
5. Seek medical care immediately.

Tarantulas

Tarantulas bite only when vigorously provoked or roughly handled **Figure 14**. The bite varies from almost painless to a deep throbbing pain lasting up to 1 hour. The tarantula, when upset, will roughly scratch the lower surface of its abdomen with its legs and flick hairs onto a person's skin.

Recognizing Tarantula Bites and Embedded Hairs

Tarantula bites and embedded hairs have the following characteristics:

- The bite causes pain—aching or stinging.
- The hairs cause itching and inflammation that can last several weeks.

Care for Tarantula Bites and Embedded Hairs

To care for a victim of a tarantula bite:

1. If possible, catch the spider to confirm its identity. Even if the body has been crushed, save it for identification (although most spider bite victims never see the spider). The species helps determine the treatment, so the dead spider (if it can be found) should be taken with the victim to the hospital.

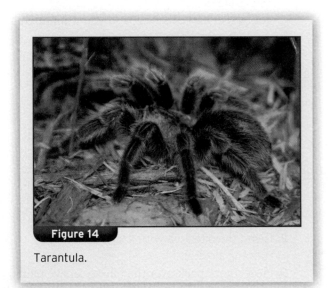

Figure 14

Tarantula.

2. Clean the bite area with soap and water or rubbing alcohol.
3. Place an ice pack over the bite to relieve pain and delay the effects of the venom.
4. Give aspirin (adults only), ibuprofen, or acetaminophen.
5. Seek medical care immediately.

To care for a victim of embedded tarantula hairs:

1. Remove the hairs from the skin with sticky tape (repeating as necessary).
2. Wash the area with soap and water.
3. Apply hydrocortisone cream.
4. Give the victim pain medication (aspirin—for adults only—or ibuprofen or acetaminophen)
5. Give the victim an antihistamine.

Common Aggressive House Spider (Hobo Spider)

Another biter is the common aggressive house spider, or hobo spider. It arrived in the Pacific Northwest in 1936 and slowly made its way across Washington State and into surrounding states. In those areas, the hobo spider is the most common large spider.

Recognizing Common Aggressive House Spider Bites

The signs and symptoms of the common aggressive house spider bite are similar to those of the brown recluse spider.

- Redness, blisters, and later, gangrene (dead tissue)
- Headache, visual problems, weakness

Care for Common Aggressive House Spider Bites

If someone has been bitten by a common aggressive house spider, you can help by doing the following:

1. If possible, catch the spider to confirm its identity. Even if the body has been crushed, save it for identification (although most spider bite victims never see the spider). The species helps determine the treatment, so the dead spider (if it can be found) should be taken with the victim to the hospital.
2. Clean the bite area with soap and water or rubbing alcohol.
3. Place an ice pack over the bite to relieve pain and delay the effects of the venom.
4. Give aspirin (adults only), ibuprofen, or acetaminophen.
5. Seek medical care immediately.

Spider Bites and Scorpion Stings

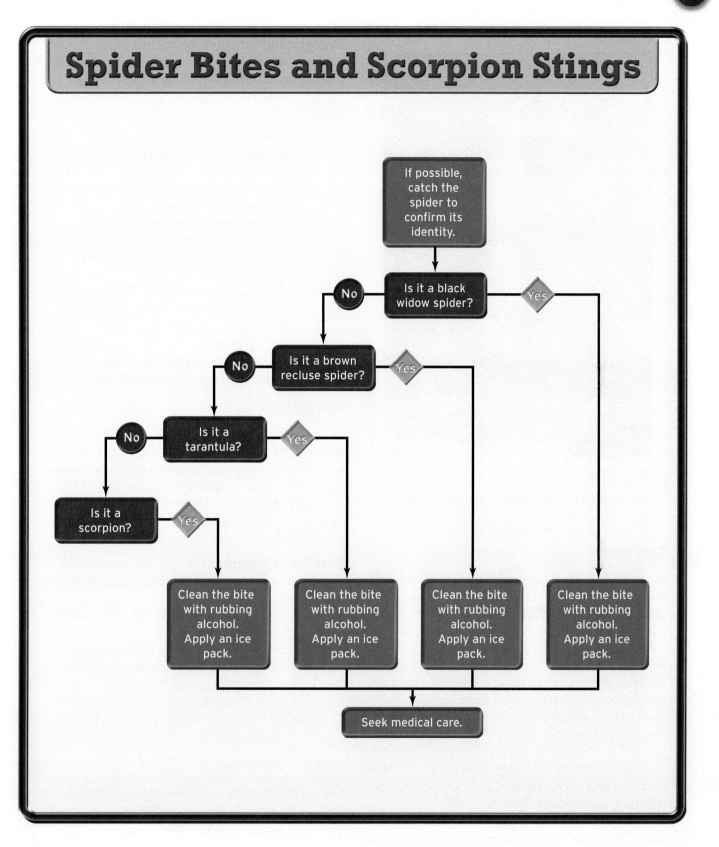

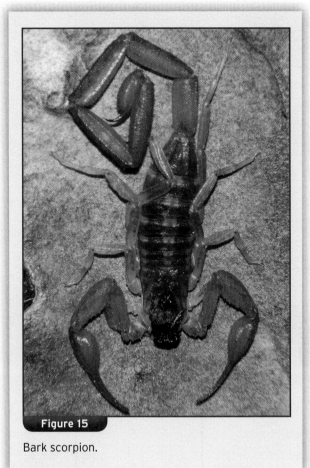

Figure 15

Bark scorpion.

Scorpions

Scorpions look like miniature lobsters, with lobsterlike pincers and a long, up-curved taillike appendage with a poisonous stinger **Figure 15**. Several species of scorpions inhabit the southwestern United States, but only the bark scorpion poses a threat to humans. Severe cases, which usually appear only in children, could include paralysis, spasms, or breathing difficulties. Death due to scorpion stings in the United States is rare.

The bark scorpion is found primarily in Arizona. Rare stings have been reported in other parts of the United States, after the scorpions traveled from Arizona as stowaways in luggage or in car trunks. The bark scorpion is pale tan and is ¾″ to 1¼″ long, not including the so-called tail.

Stings to adult victims usually are not life threatening. Stings to small children, however, are often dangerous. When a child is stung, every effort should be made to get the victim to medical care as quickly as possible. Pay close attention to make sure the victim's airway is open and that he or she is breathing.

Recognizing Scorpion Stings

The most frequent symptom of a scorpion sting, especially to an adult victim, is local, immediate pain and burning around the sting site. Later, numbness or tingling occurs.

Care for Scorpion Stings

Care for a scorpion sting victim by doing the following:
1. Monitor breathing.
2. Gently clean the sting site with soap and water or rubbing alcohol.
3. Apply an ice pack over the sting site to reduce pain and venom absorption.
4. Give aspirin (adults only), ibuprofen, or acetaminophen.
5. Seek medical care. Recently, bark scorpion antivenom production has been discontinued. Its use was controversial. The US Food and Drug Administration has given approval for clinical trials to evaluate a Mexican antivenom for use in the United States.

Mosquitoes

Mosquitoes bite millions of people. Mosquitoes are not only a nuisance, but they also carry many diseases. In developing countries, mosquitoes transmit malaria, yellow fever, and dengue fever; in the United States, they carry encephalitis. There is no evidence that mosquitoes transmit HIV, the virus that causes acquired immunodeficiency syndrome (AIDS).

Care for Mosquito Bites

You can care for someone who has mosquito bites in the following manner:
1. Wash the bitten area with soap and water.
2. Apply an ice pack.
3. Apply calamine lotion or hydrocortisone ointment to decrease redness and itching.
4. For a victim with a number of bites or a delayed allergic reaction, an antihistamine every 6 hours or a physician-prescribed cortisone might be useful.

Ticks

Some ticks produce a substance that helps cement them to the host. As they feed, some ticks increase in size 20 to 50 times **Figure 16**.

Care for Embedded Ticks

Remove ticks as soon as possible. If a tick is carrying a disease, the longer it stays embedded, the greater the chance of the disease being transmitted. Because

The Knot Method of Tick Removal

An embedded tick should be removed as soon as possible. The longer an infected tick stays embedded, the more likely it is to transmit a disease. An alternative to using tweezers and special commercial tick removal devices, especially when they are not available, is the knot method.

Use cotton thread or dental floss and tie an overhand knot (similar to a shoelace knot without the bows). The open overhand knot is placed over the tick as close as possible to the skin surface and then gently closed to form a loop around the tick. Lift the tick's body over its head in a somersault-type fashion to remove the tick. This method removes the entire tick and is simple and effective.

Source: Celensa A. 2002. The knot method of tick removal. Wilderness Environ Med 13(2):181.

its bite is painless, a tick can remain embedded for days before the victim realizes it. Most tick bites are harmless, although ticks can carry Lyme disease, Rocky Mountain spotted fever, and other serious diseases   Figure 17 .

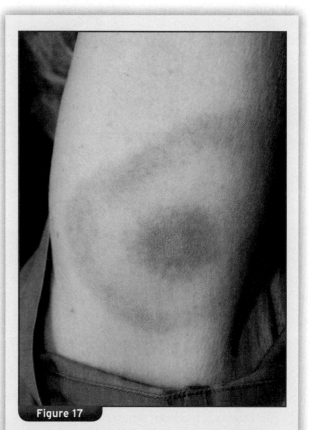

Figure 17

A bull's-eye rash is a distinctive finding in Lyme disease, but is not always present in victims.

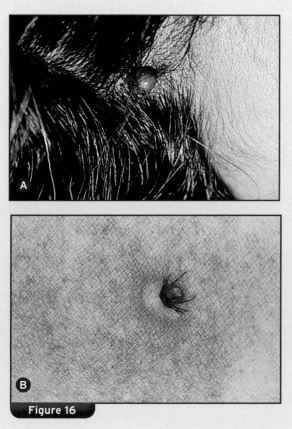

Figure 16

A. Tick embedded and engorged. **B.** Tick embedded.

CAUTION

DO NOT use the following popular methods of tick removal, which are ineffective:

- Applying petroleum jelly
- Applying fingernail polish
- Applying rubbing alcohol
- Touching a hot match to the tick
- Applying a petroleum product, such as gasoline

DO NOT grab a tick at the rear of its body. The internal organs could rupture, and the contents could be squeezed out, causing infection.

DO NOT twist or jerk the tick, which could result in incomplete removal.

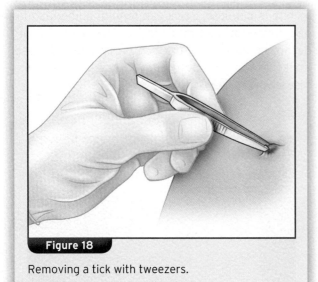

Figure 18

Removing a tick with tweezers.

To pull off a tick:
1. Use tweezers or a specialized tick removal tool.
2. Grasp the tick as close to the skin as possible, and lift it with enough force to tent the skin surface. Hold it in this position until the tick lets go (about 1 minute). Pull the tick away from the skin. Do not pull hard enough to break the tick apart because this will leave parts of the tick behind, which may cause infection **Figure 18** .

After the tick has been removed:
1. Wash the area with soap and water. Apply rubbing alcohol to further disinfect the area.
2. Apply an ice pack to reduce pain.
3. Apply calamine lotion to relieve itching. Keep the area clean.
4. For 1 month, continue to watch the bite site for a rash. If a rash appears, seek medical care. Watch for other signs such as fever, muscle aches, sensitivity to bright light, and paralysis that begins with leg weakness.

▶ Marine Animal Injuries

Most marine animals bite or sting in defense, rather than attack. Marine venoms are similar to many venoms found in reptiles and arthropods and can cause anaphylaxis or other types of reactions.

Sharks

Sharks are the most feared of all marine animals, but the chance of being attacked by a shark along the North American coastline is less than 1 in 5,000,000. Although exact figures are unavailable, it is estimated that, worldwide, more than 50 attacks and fewer than a dozen deaths occur each year. The number of unprovoked shark attacks has grown at a steady rate over the past century.

Most attacks occur within 100 feet of shore, and most victims are attacked by a single shark without warning. In the majority of attacks, the victim does not see the shark before the attack **Figure 19** . The leg is the most frequently bitten part. Sharks are clearly more attracted to people on the surface than to underwater scuba divers. The greatest attraction for sharks seems to be chemicals found in fish blood—sharks can detect them in quantities as small as one part per million parts of water. Shark bite wounds, among the most devastating of all animal bites, are similar to injuries caused by boat propellers and chainsaws. Immediate control of bleeding and treatment for shock are essential.

Recognizing a Shark Bite or Puncture

Most victims are attacked by single sharks, violently and without warning. In most attacks the victim does not see the shark before the attack. Signs include:
- Severe bleeding
- Large, open wounds, most often on the legs
- Abrasions caused by contact with sharkskin

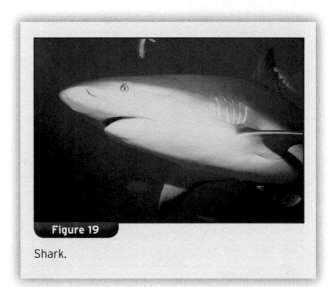

Figure 19

Shark.

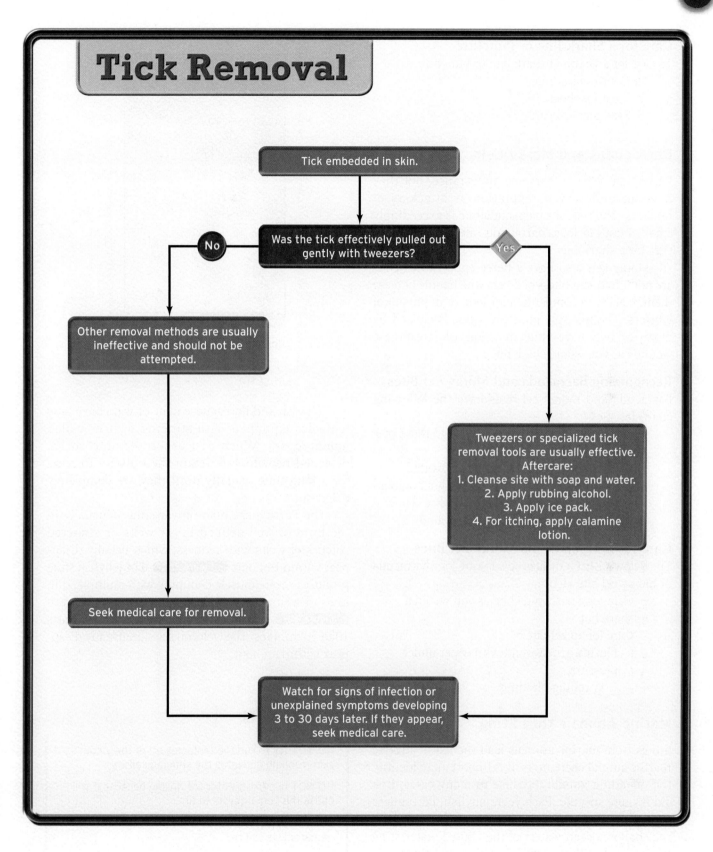

Tick Removal

Tick embedded in skin.

Was the tick effectively pulled out gently with tweezers?

No

Yes

Other removal methods are usually ineffective and should not be attempted.

Tweezers or specialized tick removal tools are usually effective.
Aftercare:
1. Cleanse site with soap and water.
2. Apply rubbing alcohol.
3. Apply ice pack.
4. For itching, apply calamine lotion.

Seek medical care for removal.

Watch for signs of infection or unexplained symptoms developing 3 to 30 days later. If they appear, seek medical care.

Care for a Shark Bite or Puncture

To care for a victim of shark bite or puncture:

1. Control bleeding.
2. Treat for shock.
3. Seek medical care.

Barracudas and Moray Eels

Barracudas have a fearsome appearance, but they have an undeserved reputation as attackers of humans. The risk of a barracuda bite is exceedingly small. First aid for a barracuda bite is identical to that for a shark bite.

Moray eels also have a fierce appearance. They are not infrequent biters of divers who handle or tease them, usually in competition for food or in pursuit of lobsters. The multiple puncture wounds created by moray eel bites have a high infection risk. Treat these wounds as you would shark bites.

Recognizing Barracuda and Moray Eel Bites

Barracuda and moray eel bites have the following characteristics:

- Barracuda lacerations are similar to those of a shark.
- Eel bites involve severe puncture wounds with their narrow jaws. Eels will hold onto a victim, rather than strike and release. They leave multiple, small puncture wounds.

Care for Barracuda and Moray Eel Bites

The following list indicates how to care for a barracuda or moray eel bite victim.

- Care for a barracuda bite as you would a shark bite.
- Care for an eel bite by:
  - Flushing the wound with water under pressure.
  - Controlling bleeding.

Marine Animals that Sting

Stings from marine animals lead the list of adverse marine animal encounters. It is important to identify the offending animal, because in many cases, first aid is quite specific. Each year, jellyfish, Portuguese man-of-wars, corals, and anemones that lie along the shallow ocean waters of the United States sting more than 1 million people. Reactions to being stung vary from mild dermatitis to severe reactions. Most victims recover without medical attention.

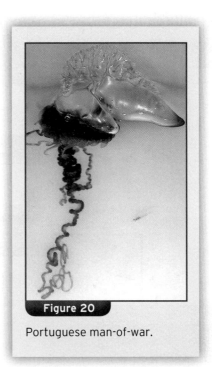

Figure 20

Portuguese man-of-war.

Jellyfish and Portuguese man-of-wars have long tentacles equipped with stinging devices called **nematocysts**. When cast ashore or onto rocks, detached nematocysts retain their ability to sting for a long time, usually until they are completely dried out.

The Portuguese man-of-war sting is usually in the form of well-defined linear welts or scattered patches of welts with redness, which usually disappear within 24 hours **Figure 20**. The jellyfish sting produces severe muscle cramping with multiple, thin lines of welts crossing the skin in a zigzag pattern **Figure 21**. Pain usually is a burning type that lasts 10 to 30 minutes. The welts on the skin usually disappear within an hour.

CAUTION

DO NOT try to rub the tentacles off of the victim's skin—rubbing activates the stinging cells.

DO NOT use fresh water for rinsing because it will cause the nematocysts to fire.

DO NOT apply cold packs—they also will cause the nematocysts to fire.

DO NOT touch the tentacles with your bare hands.

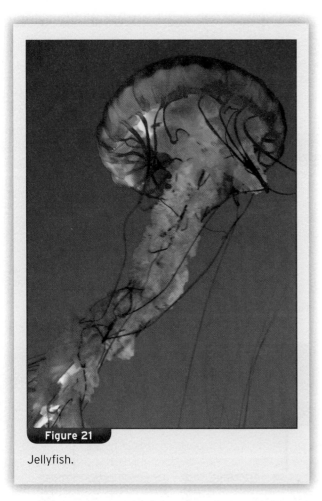

Figure 21

Jellyfish.

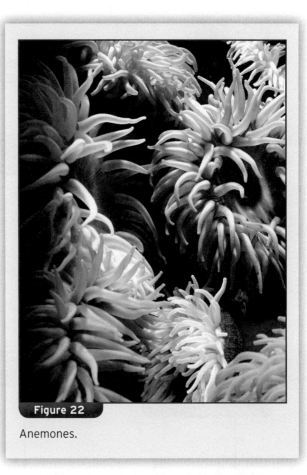

Figure 22

Anemones.

Anemones are beautiful but potentially dangerous **Figure 22** . Many anemone stings result from the improper handling of aquarium animals.

Recognizing Marine Stings

Marine stings cause the following symptoms:

- Stinging
- Severe itching, burning
- Prickling, tingling
- Blisters
- Severe allergic reaction
- Difficulty breathing
- Muscle cramping
- Nausea, vomiting

Care for Marine Stings

Follow these steps to care for a victim of a marine sting:

1. Apply vinegar to the sting area for at least 30 seconds; it deactivates the nematocysts. If vinegar is not available, use a baking soda paste.
2. Use hot water (110° F [43° C]) immersion for at least 20 minutes to reduce pain. If hot water is not available, use hot dry packs.
3. Apply a coating of hydrocortisone (1%) several times a day.

Stingrays

Stingrays, commonly found in tropical and subtropical waters, are peaceful, reclusive bottom feeders that generally lie buried in the sand or mud **Figure 23** . Most wounds inflicted by stingrays are produced on the ankle or foot when the victim steps on a ray. The ray reacts by thrusting its barbed tail upward and forward into the victim's leg or foot. At least 1,500 stingray injuries occur each year in coastal US waters. The stingray's venomous tail barb easily penetrates human skin. The sting usually is more like a laceration because the large tail barb can do significant damage. The venom causes intense burning pain at the site.

Marine Animal Injuries

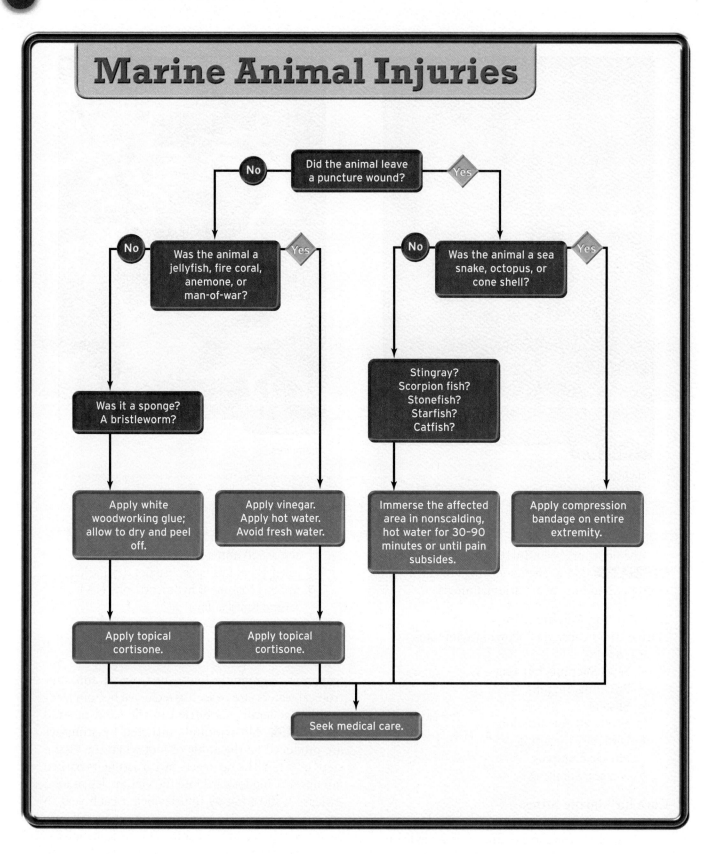

Did the animal leave a puncture wound?

No → Was the animal a jellyfish, fire coral, anemone, or man-of-war?

- **No** → Was it a sponge? A bristleworm? → Apply white woodworking glue; allow to dry and peel off. → Apply topical cortisone.
- **Yes** → Apply vinegar. Apply hot water. Avoid fresh water. → Apply topical cortisone.

Yes → Was the animal a sea snake, octopus, or cone shell?

- **No** → Stingray? Scorpion fish? Stonefish? Starfish? Catfish? → Immerse the affected area in nonscalding, hot water for 30–90 minutes or until pain subsides.
- **Yes** → Apply compression bandage on entire extremity.

Seek medical care.

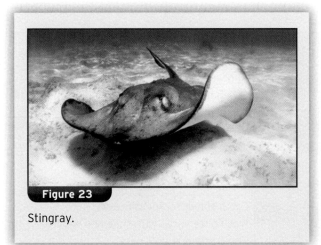

Figure 23

Stingray.

Care for Stingray Punctures

You can care for stingray puncture victims by doing the following:

1. Relieve pain by immersing the injured body part in hot water (110° F [43° C]) for 30 to 90 minutes. Make sure the water is not hot enough to cause a burn.
2. Wash the wound with soap and water.
3. Irrigate the area with water under pressure to wash out as much of the toxin and foreign material as possible.
4. Treat the wound like any puncture wound.

Recognizing Stingray Punctures

A stingray puncture results in the following:

- Sudden, intense pain
- An open wound
- Swelling

▶ Emergency Care Wrap-up

Condition	What to Look For	What to Do
Bites and stings	Animal and human bites Torn tissue Bleeding	Wash wound with soap and water. Flush wound thoroughly with water under pressure. Control bleeding. Seek medical care.
	Venomous snake bites Severe, burning pain Small puncture wounds Swelling Nausea, vomiting, sweating, weakness Discoloration and blood-filled blisters developing hours after the bite	Get away from the snake. Limit victim's movement and keep bitten extremity below heart level. Call 9-1-1. Gently wash area with soap and water. Apply mild pressure by wrapping the entire affected arm or leg with an elastic bandage.

Condition	What to Look For	What to Do
	Insect stings Pain Itching Swelling Severe allergic reaction, including breathing problems	Remove any stinger. Wash with soap and water. Apply an ice or cold pack. Give pain medication and an antihistamine and apply hydrocortisone cream. Observe for at least 30 minutes for signs of severe allergic reaction. Call 9-1-1 if a severe allergic reaction occurs. If victim has an epinephrine auto-injector, help victim use it.
	Spider bites Black widow May feel sharp pain Two small fang marks Severe abdominal pain Headache, chills, fever, sweating, dizziness, nausea Brown recluse and hobo Blister developing several days later Ulcer in skin Headache, fever, weakness, nausea	Catch spider for identification. Wash bitten area with soap and water. Apply an ice or cold pack. Seek medical care.
	Scorpion stings Pain and burning at sting site Later, numbness or tingling	Wash sting site with soap and water. Apply an ice or cold pack. Seek medical care.
	Tick bites Tick still attached Rash (especially one shaped like a bull's-eye) Fever, joint aches, weakness	Remove tick. Wash bitten area with soap and water. Apply rubbing alcohol. Apply an ice or cold pack. Watch bitten area for 1 month for rash. Seek medical care if rash or other signs such as fever or muscle joint aches appear.
Marine animal injuries	Bites, rips, or punctures from marine animals (for example, sharks, barracudas, moray eels)	Control bleeding. Treat for shock. Call 9-1-1.
	Stings from marine animals (for example, jellyfish, Portuguese man-of-war)	Apply vinegar (minimum of 30 seconds). Immerse in hot water for 20 minutes to reduce pain.
	Punctures from marine animal spines (for example, stingray)	Immerse injured part in hot water for 30 to 90 minutes. Wash with soap and water. Flush with water under pressure. Care for wound.

prep kit

▶ Ready for Review

- Almost half of all Americans will suffer a bite from either an animal or human.
- Throughout the world, about 50,000 people die each year of snake bites.
- The stinging insects belonging to the order of Hymenoptera include honeybees, bumblebees, yellow jackets, hornets, wasps, and fire ants.
- Most spiders are venomous, which is how they paralyze and kill their prey. However, most spiders lack an effective delivery system—long fangs and strong jaws—to bite a human.
- Most marine animals bite or sting in defense, rather than attack.

▶ Vital Vocabulary

antivenom An antiserum containing antibodies against reptile or insect venom.

nematocysts Stinging cells found on certain marine animals.

rabies An acute viral infection of the central nervous system transmitted by the bite of an infected animal.

▶ Assessment in Action

You are enjoying an overnight campout with your family in the springtime. As you get ready for bed, you notice a small lump on your belly and are startled to find an embedded tick.

Directions: Circle Yes if you agree with the statement; circle No if you disagree.

Yes   No   **1.** You should leave the tick alone because it will cause no harm to humans.

Yes   No   **2.** Covering the tick with petroleum jelly is very effective for removing the embedded tick.

Yes   No   **3.** You should touch a hot, blown-out match to the tick.

Yes   No   **4.** Grabbing the tick as close to the skin as possible with tweezers and pulling upward is usually effective.

Yes   No   **5.** After removing the tick, clean the wound and use an icepack to reduce pain.

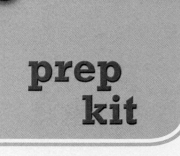

prep kit

▶ Check Your Knowledge

Directions: Circle Yes if you agree with the statement; circle No if you disagree.

Yes No **1.** Severe abdominal pain is a sign of a black widow spider bite.

Yes No **2.** Apply an ice or cold pack over a snake bite.

Yes No **3.** Use the cut and suck method for a snake bite.

Yes No **4.** Remove a bee's stinger by using tweezers to pull it out.

Yes No **5.** Apply an ice or cold pack over an insect sting or a suspected spider bite.

Yes No **6.** A baking soda paste can help reduce the itching and swelling from an insect sting.

Yes No **7.** A victim's prescribed auto-injector might have to be used if the victim has a life-threatening reaction to an insect sting.

Yes No **8.** Care for stings from marine animals (for example, jellyfish) by pouring hydrogen peroxide on the affected area.

Yes No **9.** Covering an embedded tick with petroleum jelly causes the tick to back out because of the lack of oxygen.

Yes No **10.** Ticks can transmit disease.

Cold-Related Emergencies

17

Cold-Related Emergencies

Heat flows from an area with a higher temperature to an area with a lower temperature. When a person is surrounded by air or water cooler than body temperature, the body loses heat. If heat escapes faster than the body produces heat, the body temperature falls. Normal body temperature is 98.6°F, and if the body temperature falls much below that, cold injuries can result.

▶ Freezing Cold Injuries

Freezing cold injuries can occur whenever the air temperature is below freezing (32°F). Freezing limited to the skin surface is **frostnip**. Freezing that extends deeper through the skin and into the flesh is **frostbite**.

Frostbite is prevalent during military campaigns and is a known hazard for outdoor workers, the homeless, mountain climbers, and explorers. As more people pursue cross-country skiing, snowmobiling, and other outdoor winter sports, the number of frostbite cases probably will increase. However, it is still thought to be rare in nonmilitary situations.

Frostnip

Frostnip is caused when water on the skin surface freezes. Frostnip should be taken seriously because it could be the first sign of impending frostbite.

Recognizing Frostnip

It is difficult to tell the difference between frostnip and frostbite. Signs of frostnip include:

- Skin appears red and sometimes swollen.
- Painful, but usually no further damage after rewarming.
- Repeated frostnip in the same spot can dry the skin, causing it to crack and become sensitive.

Care for a Frostnip Victim

To care for a frostnip victim:

1. Gently warm the affected area by placing it against a warm body part (for example, put bare hands under the armpits or on the stomach) or by blowing warm air on the area. After rewarming, the affected area can be red and tingling.
2. Do not rub the affected area.

Frostbite

Frostbite happens only in below-freezing temperatures.

Frostbite affects mainly the feet, hands, ears, and nose **Figure 1**. These areas do not contain large heat-producing muscles and are some distance from the body's heat-generation sources. The most severe consequences of frostbite occur when tissue dies (gangrene), and the affected part might have to be amputated. The longer the tissue stays frozen, the worse the injury. Check for hypothermia in any frostbitten victim.

Recognizing Frostbite

The severity and extent of frostbite are difficult to judge until hours after thawing. Frostbite can be classified as superficial or deep before thawing.

The signs and symptoms of superficial frostbite are as follows:

- The skin is white, waxy, or grayish yellow.
- The affected part feels very cold and numb. There might be tingling, stinging, or an aching sensation.
- The skin surface feels stiff or crusty and the underlying tissue soft when depressed gently and firmly.

The following signs and symptoms indicate deep frostbite:

- The affected part feels cold, hard, and solid and cannot be depressed—it feels like a piece of wood or frozen meat.

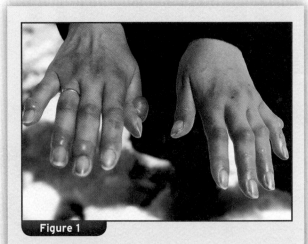

Figure 1

Frostbitten fingers 6 hours after rewarming in 108°F water.

- Blisters might appear after rewarming.
- The affected part is cold, with pale, waxy skin.
- A painfully cold part suddenly stops hurting.

After a part has thawed, frostbite can be categorized by degrees, similar to the classification of burns. First-degree frostbite is superficial, and second-, third-, and fourth-degree frostbite are deeper.

- First-degree frostbite: The affected part is warm, swollen, and tender.
- Second-degree frostbite: Blisters form minutes to hours after thawing and enlarge over several days **Figure 2** and **Figure 3**.
- Third-degree frostbite: Blisters are small and contain reddish blue or purplish fluid. The

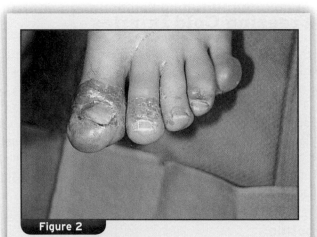

Figure 2

Second-degree frostbite.

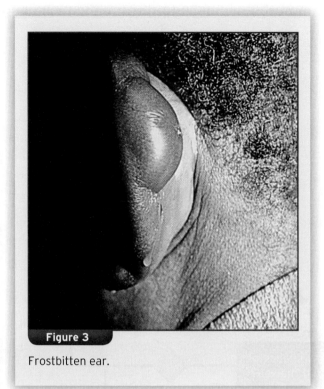

Figure 3

Frostbitten ear.

surrounding skin can be red or blue and might not blanch when pressure is applied.

- Fourth-degree frostbite: No blisters or swelling occur. The part remains numb, cold, and white to dark purple.

Care for a Frostbite Victim

All frostbite injuries require the same first aid treatment. Seek medical care immediately. Rewarming of frostbite should seldom be attempted outside a medical facility.

1. Get the victim out of the cold and to a warm place.
2. Remove any wet clothing or constricting items, such as rings, that could impair blood circulation.
3. Seek immediate medical care.
4. If the affected part is partially thawed, and you have warm water, use the following wet, rapid rewarming method. If there is risk of refreezing, do not rewarm. Place the frostbitten part in warm (100°F to 104°F) water. If you do not have a thermometer, pour some of the water over the inside of your arm or put your elbow into it to test that it is warm, not hot. Maintain water temperature by adding warm water as needed. Rewarming usually takes 20 to 40 minutes or until the tissues are soft. To help control the severe pain during rewarming, give the victim aspirin (adults only) or ibuprofen. For ear or facial injuries, it is best but may be difficult to apply warm, moist cloths, changing them frequently.
5. After thawing:
   - If the feet are affected, treat the victim as a stretcher case—the feet will be impossible to use after they are rewarmed.
   - Protect the affected area from contact with clothing and bedding.

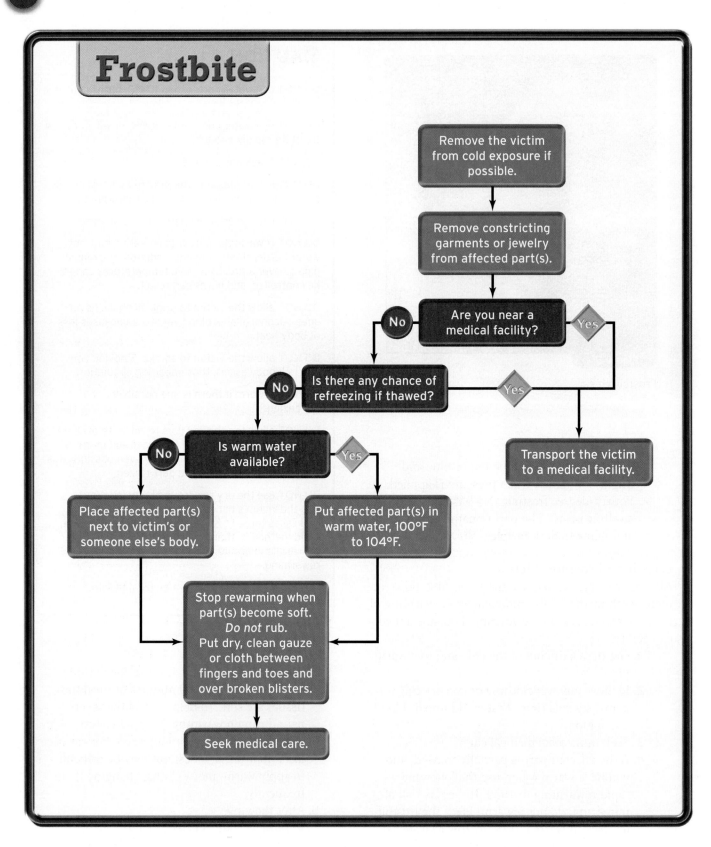

Frostbite

Remove the victim from cold exposure if possible.

↓

Remove constricting garments or jewelry from affected part(s).

↓

Are you near a medical facility?
— No
— Yes

No — **Is there any chance of refreezing if thawed?** — Yes

→ Transport the victim to a medical facility.

No — **Is warm water available?** — Yes

Place affected part(s) next to victim's or someone else's body.

Put affected part(s) in warm water, 100°F to 104°F.

Stop rewarming when part(s) become soft. *Do not* rub. Put dry, clean gauze or cloth between fingers and toes and over broken blisters.

↓

Seek medical care.

- Place dry, sterile gauze between the toes and the fingers to absorb moisture and keep them from sticking together.
- Slightly elevate the affected part to reduce pain and swelling.
- Apply aloe vera gel, if advised by a physician, to promote skin healing.
- Provide aspirin (adults only), ibuprofen, or acetaminophen to limit pain and inflammation.

▶ Hypothermia

Body temperature falls when the body cannot produce heat as fast as it is lost. **Hypothermia** is a life-threatening condition in which the body's core temperature falls below 95°F. Generally, the core temperature will not fall until after many hours of continuous exposure to cold air, if the person is healthy, physically active, and reasonably dressed. However, because wet skin and wind accelerate body heat loss and the body produces less heat during inactive periods, the core body temperature can fall even when the air temperature is above freezing if conditions are windy, clothing is wet, or the person is inactive.

Hypothermia can occur year round. Most people think of hypothermia as related only to cold outdoor exposure. It can happen indoors, in the southern states, and even on a summer day. It does not require subfreezing temperatures.

Recognizing Hypothermia

Consider hypothermia in all victims who have been exposed to cold and who have an altered mental status. Suspect hypothermia in any person who has a temperature of less than 95°F. (Keep in mind that some thermometers do not measure below 95°F.) Shivering is a good clue, but it could be suppressed when energy stores (glycogen) are depleted. Suspect hypothermia in people with frostbite and those injured in a cold environment.

Some people die of hypothermia because they or those around them do not recognize the symptoms, which are difficult to recognize in the early stages. Here are some signs to watch for:

- Change in mental status. This is one of the first symptoms of developing hypothermia. Examples are disorientation, apathy, and changes in personality, such as unusual aggressiveness.

- Shivering. Shivering is the first, and most important, body defense against a falling body temperature. Shivering starts when the body temperature drops 1°F and can produce more heat than many rewarming methods. As the core temperature continues to fall, shivering decreases and usually stops at about 86°F. Shivering also stops as body temperature rises. If shivering stops as responsiveness decreases, assume that the core temperature is falling. If, on the other hand, shivering stops while the victim is becoming more coordinated and feeling better, assume that the core temperature is rising.
- Cool abdomen. Place the back of your hand between the clothing and the victim's abdomen to assess the victim's temperature. When the victim's abdominal skin under clothing is cooler than your hand, consider the victim hypothermic until proven otherwise.
- Low core body temperature. The best indicator of hypothermia is a thermometer reading of the core body temperature. The ability to reliably measure core temperature depends on the availability of an appropriate thermometer and access to the victim's rectum. Normal thermometers do not register below 94°F and so do not indicate whether the hypothermia is mild or severe. Because first aid for mild hypothermia is different from that for severe hypothermia, it is helpful to have a rectal thermometer that registers below 90°F. Oral and axillary (armpit) temperatures are influenced by too many external factors to make them reliable.

Measuring rectal temperatures in wilderness or remote locations is seldom done, mainly because low-reading rectal thermometers usually are not readily available. Also, taking a rectal temperature can be difficult, inconvenient, and embarrassing to the victim and rescuer. If done outdoors, such a procedure can further expose the already cold victim.

Types of Hypothermia

The difference between mild and severe hypothermia is based on the core body temperature, but taking a rectal temperature often is not possible. The second most significant difference is that with severe hypothermia, the victim becomes so cold that shivering stops, which means the victim's body cannot rewarm itself internally and requires external heat for recovery. In fact, 50% to 80% of all victims of severe hypothermia die.

Recognizing Mild Hypothermia

Signs of mild hypothermia include the following:

- Vigorous, uncontrollable shivering
- Victim has the "umbles"
  - Grumbles—decreased mental skills
  - Mumbles—slurred speech
  - Fumbles—difficulty using fingers or hands
  - Stumbles—staggers while walking
- Has cool or cold skin on the abdomen, chest, or back
- Victims have a core body temperature above 90°F

Care for a Mild Hypothermia Victim

Do the following to care for victims of mild hypothermia:

1. Stop further heat loss:
   - Get the victim out of the cold.
   - Handle the victim gently.
   - Prevent heat loss by replacing wet clothing with dry clothing and placing insulation (blankets, towels, pillows, wadded-up newspapers) beneath and over the victim. Cover the victim's head (50% to 80% of the body's heat loss is through the head).
   - Cover the victim with a vapor barrier (such as a tarp, sheet of plastic, or trash bags). If you are unable to remove wet clothing, place a vapor barrier between clothing and insulation. For a dry victim, the vapor barrier can be placed outside of the insulation.
   - Keep the victim in a horizontal (flat) position. Do not raise the legs.
   - Do not let the victim walk or exercise. Do not massage the victim's body. Either activity could drive cold blood from the extremities to the torso and produce what is known as temperature after drop.
2. Call 9-1-1 for immediate medical transportation. Remember that hypothermia is more common in urban settings than in victims found in the wilderness.
3. Allow the victim to shiver—do not stop the shivering by adding heat to the victim. Shivering that generates heat will rewarm mildly hypothermic victims.
4. Give warm, sugary drinks, which can provide energy (calories) for the shivering

to continue. They may also provide a psychological boost. These drinks will not provide enough warmth to rewarm the victim.

Recognizing Severe Hypothermia

The following signs indicate severe hypothermia:

- No shivering.
- Skin feels ice cold and appears blue.
- Muscles can be stiff and rigid, similar to rigor mortis.
- Altered mental status—not alert.
- Breathing and pulse slow.
- Victim might appear to be dead.
- Victim has a core body temperature below 90°F.

Care for a Severe Hypothermia Victim

Care for someone with severe hypothermia by doing the following:

1. Stop further heat loss:
   - Get the victim out of the cold.
   - Handle the victim gently. Rough handling can cause cardiac arrest.
   - Prevent heat loss by replacing wet clothing with dry clothing and placing insulation (blankets, towels, pillows, wadded-up newspapers) beneath and over the victim. Cover the victim's head (50% to 80% of the body's heat loss is through the head).
   - Cover the victim with a vapor barrier (such as a tarp, plastic sheets, or trash bags). If you are unable to remove wet clothing, place a vapor barrier between clothing and insulation. For a dry victim, the vapor barrier can be placed outside of the insulation.
   - Keep the victim in a horizontal (flat) position. Do not raise the legs.
   - Do not let the victim walk or exercise. Do not massage the victim's body. Either activity could drive cold blood from the extremities to the torso and produce what is known as temperature after drop.
2. Call 9-1-1 for immediate medical transportation. Remember that hypothermia is more common in urban settings than in victims found in the wilderness.
3. When the victim is in a remote location and far from medical care, warm the victim by any available external heat source (such as body-to-body contact).

FYI

Wind Chill Chart

Effective 11/01/01

Calm	40	35	30	25	20	15	10	5	0	-5	-10	-15	-20	-25	-30	-35	-40	-45
5	36	31	25	19	13	7	1	-5	-11	-16	-22	-28	-34	-40	-46	-52	-57	-63
10	34	27	21	15	9	3	-4	-10	-16	-22	-28	-35	-41	-47	-53	-59	-66	-72
15	32	25	19	13	6	0	-7	-13	-19	-26	-32	-39	-45	-51	-58	-64	-71	-77
20	30	24	17	11	4	-2	-9	-15	-22	-29	-35	-42	-48	-55	-61	-68	-74	-81
25	29	23	16	9	3	-4	-11	-17	-24	-31	-37	-44	-51	-58	-64	-71	-78	-84
30	28	22	15	8	1	-5	-12	-19	-26	-33	-39	-46	-53	-60	-67	-73	-80	-87
35	28	21	14	7	0	-7	-14	-21	-27	-34	-41	-48	-55	-62	-69	-76	-82	-89
40	27	20	13	6	-1	-8	-15	-22	-29	-36	-43	-50	-57	-64	-71	-78	-84	-91
45	26	19	12	5	-2	-9	-16	-23	-30	-37	-44	-51	-58	-65	-72	-79	-86	-93
50	26	19	12	4	-3	-10	-17	-24	-31	-38	-45	-52	-60	-67	-74	-81	-88	-95
55	25	18	11	4	-3	-11	-18	-25	-32	-39	-46	-54	-61	-68	-75	-82	-89	-97
60	25	17	10	3	-4	-11	-19	-26	-33	-40	-48	-55	-62	-69	-76	-84	-91	-98

Wind (mph) — vertical axis label. Columns are air temperature.

Frostbite Times: 30 minutes, 10 minutes, 5 minutes

$$\text{Wind Chill (°F)} = 35.74 + 0.6215T - 35.75(V^{0.16}) + 0.4275T(V^{0.16})$$
Where, T=Air Temperature (°F) V=Wind Speed (mph)

How Cold Is It?

In addition to cold, two other factors account for body heat loss: moisture and wind. Moisture—whether from rain, snow, or perspiration—speeds the conduction of heat away from the body.

Wind causes sizable amounts of body heat loss. If the thermometer reads 20°F and the wind speed is 20 mph, the exposure is comparable to 4°F. This is called the windchill factor. Use the following rough measures of wind speed: if you feel the wind on your face, wind speed is at least 10 mph; if small branches move or if dust or snow is raised, it is 20 mph; if large branches are moving, it is 30 mph; and if a whole tree bends, it is about 40 mph.

To determine the windchill factor:

1. Estimate the wind speed by checking for the aforementioned signs.
2. Look at an outdoor thermometer reading (in degrees Fahrenheit).
3. Match the estimated wind speed with the actual thermometer reading in the following table.

Source: Courtesy of the National Weather Service/NOAA.

Hypothermia

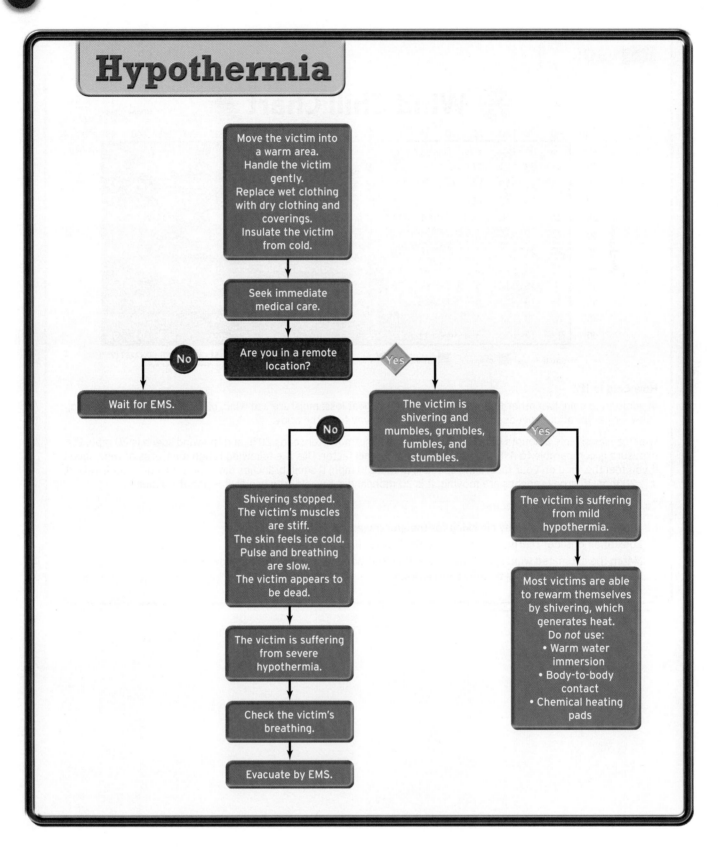

Move the victim into a warm area.
Handle the victim gently.
Replace wet clothing with dry clothing and coverings.
Insulate the victim from cold.

↓

Seek immediate medical care.

↓

Are you in a remote location?

No → Wait for EMS.

Yes → The victim is shivering and mumbles, grumbles, fumbles, and stumbles.

No → Shivering stopped.
The victim's muscles are stiff.
The skin feels ice cold.
Pulse and breathing are slow.
The victim appears to be dead.

↓

The victim is suffering from severe hypothermia.

↓

Check the victim's breathing.

↓

Evacuate by EMS.

Yes → The victim is suffering from mild hypothermia.

↓

Most victims are able to rewarm themselves by shivering, which generates heat.
Do *not* use:
• Warm water immersion
• Body-to-body contact
• Chemical heating pads

CAUTION

DO NOT allow the victim to exert himself or herself (no walking, no climbing).

DO NOT try to rewarm a hypothermic victim outside a medical facility. External measures to rewarm should not be used, especially on the extremities, because surface rewarming leads to vasodilation (wider blood vessels), which can lead to a drop in blood pressure and temperature after drop.

DO NOT try to rewarm a hypothermic victim outside a medical facility because rewarming the skin will stop shivering, which is the most effective way to rewarm.

DO NOT put an unconscious victim in a bathtub.

DO NOT give the victim alcohol. Alcohol interferes with shivering and accelerates heat loss by dilating the blood vessels in the skin. The victim might feel warmer temporarily, but there is a greater risk of hypothermia.

DO NOT give the victim a caffeine drink. Caffeine has a diuretic effect, and the victim probably is already dehydrated.

DO NOT rub or massage the victim's arms or legs. Rubbing the skin suppresses shivering, dilates the blood vessels in the skin (resulting in more heat loss), and produces temperature after drop.

DO NOT raise the victim's legs, which allows cold blood from the legs to flow into the body core and adversely affect the heart. Keep the victim in a flat position.

Q&A

What is the coldest body temperature?
The lowest recorded body temperature with a full recovery was 56.6°F (13.7°C). This was the temperature of D. Anna Bagenholm, age 29, who was trapped under ice for 80 minutes in May 2000, while skiing with friends near Narvik, Norway.

▶ Emergency Care Wrap-up

Condition	What to Look For	What to Do
Frostbite	White, waxy-looking skin Skin feels cold and numb (pain at first, followed by numbness) Blisters, which may appear after rewarming	Move victim to a warm place. Remove tight clothing or jewelry from injured part(s). Place dry dressings between toes and/or fingers. Seek medical care.
Hypothermia	**Mild** Uncontrollable shivering Confusion, sluggishness Cold skin even under clothing **Severe** No shivering Muscles stiff and rigid Skin ice cold Appears to be dead	**All victims:** Move victim to a warm place. Prevent heat loss by • Replacing wet clothing with dry clothing • Covering victim's head **Mild** Give warm, sugary beverages. Do not add anything warm to the skin—let the shivering rewarm the body. **Severe** Do not rewarm unless in a very remote location. Call 9-1-1.

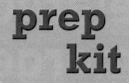

prep kit

▶ Ready for Review

- When a person is surrounded by air or water cooler than body temperature, the body loses heat.
- Humans protect themselves from cold primarily by avoiding or reducing cold exposure through the use of clothing and shelter.
- Nonfreezing cold injuries can occur when conditions are cold and wet and the hands and feet cannot be kept warm and dry.
- Freezing cold injuries can occur whenever the air temperature is below freezing.
- Hypothermia is a life-threatening condition in which the body's core temperature falls below 95°F.

▶ Vital Vocabulary

<u>frostbite</u> The damage to tissues as a result of prolonged exposure to extreme cold.

<u>frostnip</u> The superficial local tissue destruction caused by freezing; it is limited in scope and does not destroy the full thickness of skin.

<u>hypothermia</u> Decreased body temperature.

▶ Assessment in Action

You are on a winter hike with five friends high in the mountains. The snowshoeing has been great but it is very cold. At the trailhead, the temperature was 15°F (−9°C) and it has not warmed up much during your hike. One of your friends wore only tennis shoes but has not been complaining. When you return to the trailhead and begin to warm up in your car, your friend begins to complain of tingling and aching in his toes.

Directions: Circle Yes if you agree with the statement; circle No if you disagree.

Yes No **1.** It is difficult to determine if your friend has frostnip or frostbite.

Yes No **2.** Frostbite requires freezing temperatures (below 32°F [0°C]).

Yes No **3.** The skin and underlying tissue affected by superficial frostbite feel hard and solid.

Yes No **4.** As long as there is no danger of refreezing, you could begin warming his toes in warm water.

Yes No **5.** If you do not have warm water, you could rub his toes to increase circulation.

▶ Check Your Knowledge

Directions: Circle Yes if you agree with the statement; circle No if you disagree.

Yes No **1.** Shivering is a signal that clothing and shelter are inadequate to protect the body from the cold.

Yes No **2.** Up to 100% of the body's total heat production can be lost by radiation through a person's unprotected head.

Yes No **3.** Physically unfit people are more susceptible to cold injury.

Yes No **4.** Frostnip is caused when water on the skin surface freezes.

Yes No **5.** Shivering produces body heat.

Yes No **6.** Rub a frostbitten part to rewarm it.

Yes No **7.** Rewarm a hypothermic victim quickly in a hot shower or with chemical heat packs.

Yes No **8.** Replace any wet clothing with dry clothing for a hypothermic victim.

Yes No **9.** Seek medical care for a severe hypothermic victim.

Yes No **10.** Below-freezing temperatures are required for hypothermia to occur.

Heat-Related Emergencies

Heat-Related Emergencies

When the temperature goes up, a multitude of problems can—and do—arise. Given the right (or wrong) conditions, anyone can develop heat illness. Some victims are lucky enough to have only heat cramps, but less fortunate people could be laid low by heat exhaustion or devastated by heatstroke.

▶ Heat Illnesses

Heat illnesses include a range of disorders 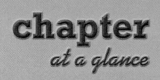 . Some of them are common, but only heatstroke is life threatening. Untreated heatstroke victims always die.

Heat Cramps

<u>Heat cramps</u> are painful muscle spasms that occur suddenly during or after vigorous exercise or activity. They usually involve the muscles in the back of the leg (calf and hamstring muscles) or the abdominal muscles. Some experts state they are caused by water and electrolyte losses during times of excessive sweating. Victims might be drinking fluids without adequate salt content. However, other experts disagree because the typical American diet is heavy with salt.

Table 1   Heat Illnesses

Condition	Symptoms	What to Do
Heat cramps	Painful muscle spasms Sweaty skin Normal body temperature	1. Sit or lie down in the shade. 2. Drink cool, lightly salted water or a sports drink. 3. Stretch affected muscles.
Heat exhaustion	Profuse sweating Flulike symptoms Clammy or pale skin Dizziness Nausea, vomiting Rapid pulse Thirst Normal or slightly above normal body temperature	1. Treat mild cases the same way as heat cramps (but do not stretch the muscles). 2. If persistent, gently apply wet towels and call 9-1-1.
Heatstroke	Unresponsiveness (if responsive, victim will be confused, stagger, be agitated) Hot skin, which can be dry or wet	1. Move person to a half-sitting position in the shade. 2. Call 9-1-1. 3. If humidity is below 75%, spray victim with water and vigorously fan. If humidity is above 75%, apply ice packs on neck, armpits, and groin.

World Record: Highest Body Temperature

The person with the highest body temperature who lived to tell about it is Willie Jones. On July 10, 1980, a day when the temperature reached 90°F (32.2°C) with 44% humidity, Mr. Jones was admitted to Grady Memorial Hospital, Atlanta, Georgia, with heatstroke. His temperature was 115.7°F (46.5°C). The record temperature was taken after he had been immersed for 25 minutes in cold water. The attending physician said that his body temperature may have exceeded 120°F when he first arrived at the hospital. After 24 days in the hospital, he was discharged. Body temperatures of 109°F can be fatal.

Source: *Guinness Book of World Records*. Bantam. 2008, page 112.

Recognizing Heat Cramps

Heat cramps have the following characteristics:
- Painful muscle spasms that happen suddenly
- Affect the muscles in the back of the leg or abdomen
- Occur during or after physical exertion

Care for Someone With Heat Cramps

To relieve heat cramps (it could take several hours), follow these steps:

1. Have the victim rest in a cool place.
2. Have the victim drink lightly salted, cool water (dissolve ¼ teaspoon salt in 1 quart of water) or a commercial sports drink. (A commercial sports drink is easier to absorb if diluted to half strength to reduce the sugar content.)
3. Stretch the cramped calf muscle. Place an ice bag (over a towel or cloth, to protect the skin) on the painful muscle. Also, try an acupressure method: pinch the upper lip just below the nose.

Heat Exhaustion

Heat exhaustion is characterized by heavy perspiration with a normal or slightly above-normal body temperature. Heavy sweating cause water and electrolyte losses. Some experts believe that a better term would be *severe dehydration*. Heat exhaustion affects workers and athletes who do not drink enough fluids while working or exercising in hot environments. The affected person often mistakenly believes he or she has the flu. Uncontrolled heat exhaustion can evolve into heatstroke.

Recognizing Heat Exhaustion

Heat exhaustion differs from heatstroke by having (1) no altered mental status and (2) skin that is not hot, but clammy. Heat exhaustion causes the following symptoms:

- Sweating
- Thirst
- Fatigue
- Flulike symptoms (headache and nausea)
- Shortness of breath
- Fast heart rate

Care for Heat Exhaustion Victims

Use the following guidelines to care for a victim of heat exhaustion:

1. Move the victim immediately out of the heat to a cool place.
2. Give cool liquids, adding electrolytes (lightly salted water or a commercial sports drink) if plain water does not improve the victim's condition in 20 minutes. Do not give salt tablets; they can irritate the stomach and cause nausea and vomiting.
3. Consider raising the victim's legs 6 to 12 inches (keep the knees slightly bent).
4. Remove excess clothing.
5. Sponge the victim with cool water and fan him or her; or, place ice bags on the sides of the chest, neck, and armpits.
6. If no improvement is seen within 30 minutes, seek medical care.

Heatstroke

Two types of heatstroke exist: classic and exertional Table 2 . Classic heatstroke, also known as the slow cooker, can take days to develop. It is often seen during summer heat waves and typically affects poor, elderly, chronically ill, alcoholic, and obese people. Because elderly people, who often have medical problems, are frequently afflicted, this type of heatstroke has a 50% death rate, even with medical care. It results from a combination of a hot environment and dehydration. Under normal conditions, temperature and humidity are the most important elements influencing

Table 2 Classic or Exertional Heatstroke?

Characteristics	Classic	Exertional
Age group usually affected	Elderly	Males 15-45 years
Claims many victims at the same time	During heat waves	During athletic competition
Health status of victims	Chronically ill	Healthy and physically fit
Activity at the time of incident	Sedentary	Strenuous exercise
Medication use	Common	Usually none
Sweating	Absent	Often present (50% of victims)

body comfort. The heat index compiled by the National Weather Service lists apparent temperatures (how hot it feels) at various combinations of temperature and humidity Table 3 .

Exertional heatstroke is also more common in the summer. It is frequently seen in athletes, laborers, and military personnel, all of whom often sweat profusely. This type of heatstroke is known as the fast cooker. It affects healthy, active people who are strenuously working or playing in a warm environment. Because its rapid onset does not allow enough time for severe dehydration to occur, 50% of exertional heatstroke victims usually are sweating. (Classic heatstroke victims are not sweating.)

There are several ways to tell the difference between heat exhaustion and heatstroke.

- If the victim's body feels extremely hot when touched, suspect heatstroke.
- Altered mental status (behavior) occurs with heatstroke, ranging from slight confusion and disorientation to coma. Between those extreme conditions, victims usually become irrational, agitated, or even aggressive, and they might have seizures.

Table 3 Heat Index

Temperature (°F)

Relative Humidity (%)	80	82	84	86	88	90	92	94	96	98	100	102	104	106	108	110
40	80	81	83	85	88	91	94	97	101	105	109	114	119	124	130	136
45	80	82	84	87	89	93	96	100	104	109	114	119	124	130	137	
50	81	83	85	88	91	95	99	103	108	113	118	124	131	137		
55	81	84	86	89	93	97	101	106	112	117	124	130	137			
60	82	84	88	91	95	100	105	110	116	123	129	137				
65	82	85	89	93	98	103	108	114	121	128	136					
70	83	86	90	95	100	105	112	119	126	134						
75	84	88	92	97	103	109	116	124	132							
80	84	89	94	100	106	113	121	129								
85	85	90	96	102	110	117	126	135								
90	86	91	98	105	113	122	131									
95	86	93	100	108	117	127										
100	87	95	103	112	121	132										

Likelihood of Heat Disorders with Prolonged Exposure or Strenuous Activity
■ Caution ■ Extreme Caution ■ Danger ■ Extreme Danger

- In severe heatstroke, a coma can occur in less than an hour. The longer a coma lasts, the lower the chance for survival.
- Rectal temperature can also distinguish heatstroke from heat exhaustion, although obtaining a rectal temperature is usually not practical. A responsive heatstroke victim might not cooperate, taking a rectal temperature can be embarrassing to the victim and the rescuer, and rectal thermometers are seldom available.

Recognizing Heatstroke

Signs of heatstroke include:

- Extremely hot skin when touched—usually dry, but can be wet from sweating related to strenuous work or exercise.
- Altered mental status ranging from slight confusion, agitation, and disorientation to unresponsiveness.

Care for Heatstroke Victims

Heatstroke is a medical emergency and must be treated rapidly! Every minute delayed increases the

CAUTION

DO NOT delay initiating cooling while waiting for an ambulance. The longer the delay, the greater the risk of tissue damage and prolonged hospitalization.

DO NOT continue cooling after the victim's mental status has improved. Unnecessary cooling could lead to hypothermia.

DO NOT use rubbing alcohol to cool the skin. It can be absorbed into the blood and cause alcohol poisoning. Also, the vapors are a potential fire hazard.

DO NOT give the victim aspirin or acetaminophen. The brain's control center is not elevated, as it is with fever caused by diseases, so these products are not effective for lowering body temperature.

likelihood of serious complications or death. Do the following:

1. Move the victim immediately to a cool place.
2. Remove clothing down to the victim's underwear.

3. Keep the victim's head and shoulders slightly elevated.

4. Call 9-1-1 immediately even if the victim seems to be recovering.

5. The only way to prevent damage is to cool the victim quickly and by any means possible. Cooling methods include the following:

 - Spraying the victim with water and then fanning **Figure 1**. This method is not as effective in high humidity (more than 75%) conditions.
 - Applying cool, wet sheets or cloths.

 - Placing ice bags against the large veins on the groin, armpits, and sides of the neck; this cools the body, regardless of humidity.
 - Placing the victim in an ice bath; this cools a victim quickly, but it requires a great deal of ice—at least 80 pounds—to be effective. The need for a big enough tub also limits this method.
 - Placing the victim in a cool water bath (less than 60°F) can be successful if the water is stirred to prevent a warm layer from forming around the body. This is the most effective method in high humidity (greater than 75%) conditions.

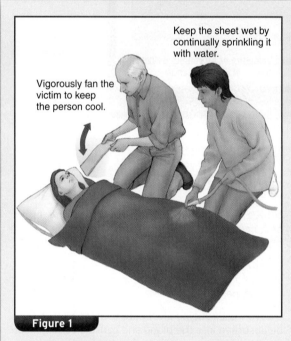

Keep the sheet wet by continually sprinkling it with water.

Vigorously fan the victim to keep the person cool.

Figure 1

Spraying with water and fanning are effective in low humidity conditions.

FYI

Other Heat Illnesses

Less serious heat illnesses include heat syncope, heat edema, and prickly heat.

- Heat syncope, in which a person becomes dizzy or faints after exposure to high temperatures, is a self-resolving condition. Victims should lie down in a cool place and, if not nauseated, drink water. Syncope may be associated with heat exhaustion.

- Heat edema, which is also a self-resolving condition, causes the ankles and feet to swell from heat exposure. It is more common in women who are not acclimatized to a hot climate. It is related to salt and water retention and tends to disappear after acclimatization. Wearing support stockings and elevating the legs could help reduce the swelling.

- Prickly heat, also known as a heat rash, is an itchy rash that develops because of unevaporated moisture on skin wet from sweating. Treat by drying and cooling the skin.

Heat-Related Emergencies

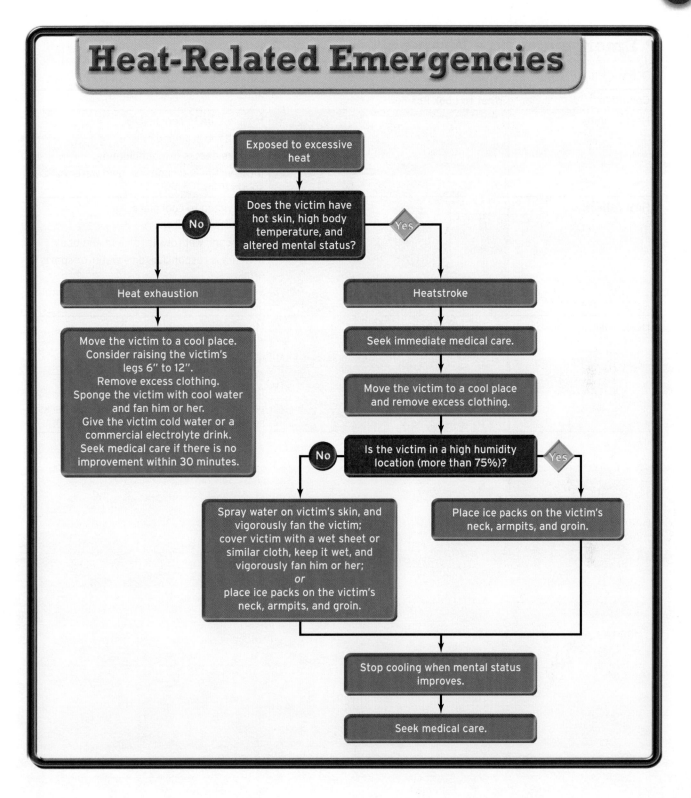

Exposed to excessive heat

Does the victim have hot skin, high body temperature, and altered mental status?

No

Yes

Heat exhaustion

Move the victim to a cool place.
Consider raising the victim's legs 6" to 12".
Remove excess clothing.
Sponge the victim with cool water and fan him or her.
Give the victim cold water or a commercial electrolyte drink.
Seek medical care if there is no improvement within 30 minutes.

Heatstroke

Seek immediate medical care.

Move the victim to a cool place and remove excess clothing.

Is the victim in a high humidity location (more than 75%)?

No

Yes

Spray water on victim's skin, and vigorously fan the victim;
cover victim with a wet sheet or similar cloth, keep it wet, and vigorously fan him or her;
or
place ice packs on the victim's neck, armpits, and groin.

Place ice packs on the victim's neck, armpits, and groin.

Stop cooling when mental status improves.

Seek medical care.

▶ Emergency Care Wrap-up

Condition	What to Look For	What to Do
Heat Cramps	Painful muscle spasm during or after physical activity Usually lower leg affected	Move victim to cool place. Stretch the cramped muscle. Remove excess or tight clothing. If the victim is responsive, give water or sports drink.
Heat Exhaustion	Heavy sweating Severe thirst Weakness Headache Nausea and vomiting	Move victim to cool place. Have victim lie down. Apply cool, wet towels to head and body. If victim is responsive, give water or sports drink. Seek medical care if no improvement within 30 minutes.
Heatstroke	Extremely hot skin Dry skin (may be wet at first) Confusion Seizures Unresponsiveness	Move victim to cool place. Call 9-1-1. If unresponsive, open airway, check breathing, and provide appropriate care. Rapidly cool victim by whatever means possible (cool, wet sheets; ice or cold packs against armpits, side of neck, and groin).

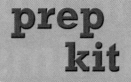

prep kit

▶ Ready for Review

- Given the right conditions, anyone can develop a heat illness.
- The human body is constantly dispersing the heat that it produces.
- Heat illnesses include a range of disorders from heat cramps to heatstroke. Heatstroke is life threatening.

▶ Vital Vocabulary

<u>heat cramps</u> A painful muscle cramp resulting from excessive loss of salt and water through sweating.

▶ Assessment in Action

You decide to watch your local high school football team practice before its first game in late August. The coach has the defense running sprints for the last 30 minutes without rest breaks. At the end of the sprints, all but one player walk over to the water station. That player falls to the ground and you are the first to respond. The victim is responsive and his skin is moist and clammy.

Directions: Circle Yes if you agree with the statement; circle No if you disagree.

Yes No **1.** The victim is most likely suffering from heatstroke.

Yes No **2.** The first thing you should do is to help the coach and athletic trainer move the victim out of the heat and to a cool place.

Yes No **3.** The victim should drink cool water or a sports drink.

Yes No **4.** Giving several salt tablets, if available, should always be considered.

Yes No **5.** Removing the player's jersey, shoulder pads, and helmet and sponging him with cool water is recommended.

Yes No **6.** The coach and/or athletic trainer should seek medical care if there is no improvement within 30 minutes.

▶ Check Your Knowledge

Directions: Circle Yes if you agree with the statement; circle No if you disagree.

Yes No **1.** For heat cramps in the legs, stretch the cramped muscle.

Yes No **2.** Commercial sports drinks can be given to victims of heat-related emergencies.

Yes No **3.** Move victims of heat-related illness to a cool place.

Yes No **4.** Victims of heatstroke need immediate medical care—it is a life-threatening condition.

Yes No **5.** Cool heatstroke victims rapidly, including the use of ice packs applied to the neck, armpits, and groin.

Yes No **6.** Fruit juices are digested quickly and rehydrate the body most rapidly.

Yes No **7.** You can drink too much water and cause water intoxication.

Yes No **8.** Humidity cannot significantly reduce evaporative cooling.

Yes No **9.** Certain medications predispose to heatstroke.

Yes No **10.** Heat exhaustion can feel like the flu.

Rescuing and Moving Victims

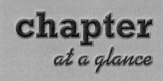

19

Victim Rescue

▶ Water Rescue

Reach-throw-row-go identifies the sequence for attempting a water rescue. The first and simplest rescue technique is to reach for the victim. Reaching requires a lightweight pole, ladder, long stick, or any object that can be extended to the victim. Once you have your "reacher," secure your footing and have a bystander grab your belt or pants for stability. Secure yourself before reaching for the victim.

You can throw anything that floats—an empty picnic jug, an empty fuel or paint can, a life jacket, a floating cushion, a piece of wood, or an inflated spare tire—whatever is available. If there is a rope handy, tie it to the object to be thrown so you can pull the victim in, or, if you miss, you can retrieve the object and throw it again. The average untrained rescuer has a throwing range of about 50 feet.

If the victim is out of throwing range and there is a rowboat, canoe, motor boat, or boogie board nearby, you can try to row to the victim. Maneuvering these craft requires skill learned through practice. Wear a personal flotation device for your own safety. To avoid capsizing, never pull the victim in over the side of a boat; instead, pull the victim in over the stern (rear end) or tow the victim to safety.

If reach, throw, and row are impossible and you are a capable swimmer trained in water lifesaving procedures, you can go to the drowning victim by swimming. Entering even calm water makes a swimming rescue difficult and hazardous. All too often a would-be rescuer becomes a victim as well.

Care for Drowning

1. Survey the scene (see the chapter entitled Action at an Emergency), then carry out a water rescue **Figure 1**.
2. If the victim was diving (or it is unknown whether he or she was diving), suspect a possible spine injury. Keep the victim in-line floating on the water surface until properly trained rescuers arrive with a backboard.
3. Check breathing and treat accordingly. Any nonbreathing victim who has been submerged in cold water should be resuscitated unless submerged for more than 60 minutes.
4. If no spinal injury is suspected, after the victim has been resuscitated, place the victim on his or her side to allow fluids to drain from the airway.

Cold-Water Immersion

Immersion in cold water is a potential hazard for anyone who participates in activities in the oceans, lakes, and streams of all but the tropical regions of the world. The US Coast Guard defines cold water as water with a temperature of less than 70°F. However, water does not need to be that cold for a person to become hypothermic. A person can become hypothermic in water that is 77°F. Most North American lakes, rivers, and coasts are colder than that year-round. The risk of immersion hypothermia in North America is nearly universal most of the year. A person immersed in cold water loses heat about 25 times faster than someone exposed to cold air.

The US Coast Guard and other rescue organizations recommend that survivors get as much of their bodies out of the water as possible to minimize cooling rate and maximize survival time. A widespread misunderstanding of the concept of wind chill often causes people to conclude that survivors have higher heat losses if they are exposed to wind, especially if they are wet, than if they are immersed in water. During recreational activities at beaches, lakes, and swimming pools, most people have experienced feeling colder after leaving the water than they do while swimming. That reinforces the misunderstanding, which has sometimes led accident victims to abandon a safe position atop a capsized vessel and reenter the water, usually with tragic results.

Cold-water immersion is associated with two potential medical emergencies: drowning and hypothermia. Numerous case histories and statistical evidence document the prominence of cold-water immersion as a cause of drowning and hypothermia.

A *heat escape lessening position* (HELP) has been devised, in which the victim draws the knees up close to the chest, presses the arms to the sides, and remains as quiet as possible **Figure 2**. For two or more people, huddling quietly and closely together (huddle position) will decrease heat loss from the groin and the front of the body. Both of these positions require personal flotation devices (life jackets).

▶ Ice Rescue

If a person has fallen through the ice near the shore, extend a pole or throw a line with a floatable object attached to it. When the person has hold of the object, pull him or her toward the shore or the edge of the ice. If the person has fallen through the ice away from the shore and you cannot reach him or her with a pole or a throwing line, lie flat and push a ladder, plank, or similar object ahead of you **Figure 3**. You can also tie a rope to a spare tire and the other end to an anchor point on the shore, lie flat, and push the tire ahead of you. Pull the person ashore or to the edge of the ice.

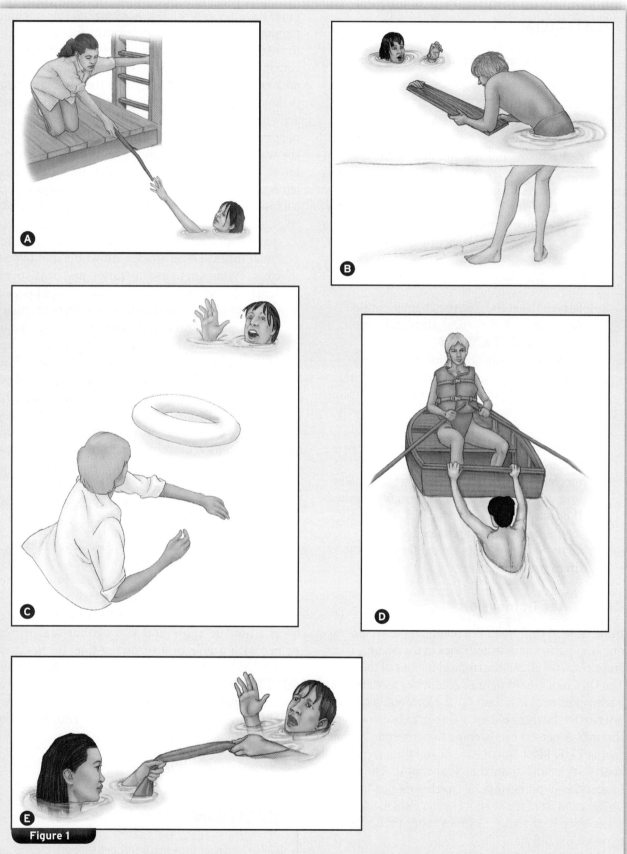

Water rescue. **A.** Reach the victim from shore. **B.** If you cannot reach the victim from shore, wade closer. **C.** If a floating object is available, throw it to the victim. **D.** Use a boat if one is available. **E.** If you must swim to the victim, use a towel or board for the victim to grab and hold onto. Do not let the victim grab you.

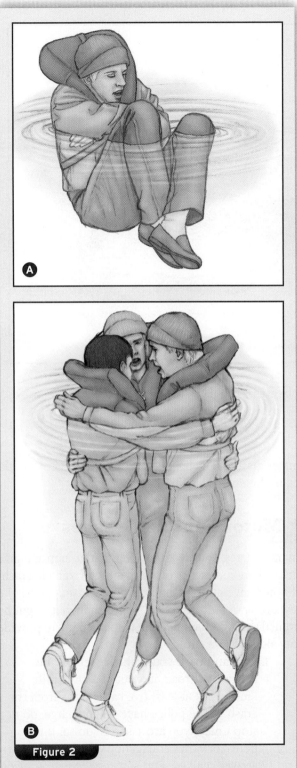

Figure 2

HELP or huddle. **A.** A person wearing a flotation device can minimize heat loss and increase chances of survival by assuming the heat escape lessening position (HELP) in which the knees are pulled up to the chest and the arms crossed. **B.** Groups of three or more can conserve heat by wrapping their arms around one another and pulling into a tight circle or huddle.

▶ Electrical Emergency Rescue

Electrical injuries can be devastating. Just a mild shock can cause serious internal injuries. A current of 1,000 V or more is considered high voltage, but even the 110 V of household current can be deadly.

When a person receives an electrical shock, electricity enters the body at the point of contact and travels along the path of least resistance (nerves and blood vessels). The current travels rapidly, generating heat and causing destruction.

Most indoor electrocutions are caused by faulty electrical equipment or the careless use of electrical appliances. Before you touch the victim, turn off the electricity at the circuit breaker, fuse box, or outside switch box or unplug the appliance if the plug is undamaged.

If the electrocution involves high-voltage power lines, the power must be turned off before anyone approaches the victim. If you approach a victim and feel a tingling sensation in your legs and lower body, stop. You are on energized ground, and an electric current is entering one foot, passing through your lower body, and leaving through the other foot. You should raise one foot off the ground, turn around, and hop to a safe place. Wait for trained personnel with the proper equipment to cut the wires or disconnect them. If a power line falls over a car, tell the driver and passengers to stay in the car. A victim should try to jump out of the car only if an explosion or fire threatens and then without making contact with the car or the wire.

CAUTION

DO NOT touch an appliance or the victim until the current is off.

DO NOT try to move downed wires.

DO NOT use any object, even dry wood (broomstick, tools, chair, stool) to separate the victim from the electrical source.

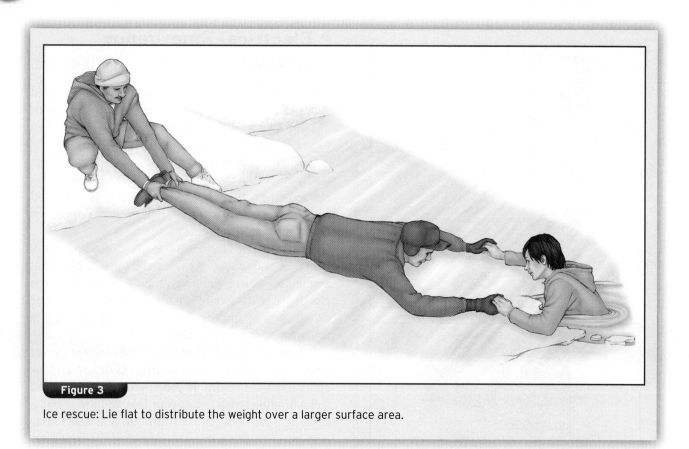

Figure 3

Ice rescue: Lie flat to distribute the weight over a larger surface area.

▶ Hazardous Materials Incidents

Almost any highway crash scene involves the potential danger of hazardous chemicals. Clues that indicate the presence of hazardous materials include the following:

- Look for warning signs on the vehicle (for example, "explosive," "flammable," "corrosive"). If you are unable to read the placard or labels, do not move closer and risk exposure. If you are able to read the placard with the naked eye, you may be too close and should consider moving farther away. **Figure 4** shows a chart illustrating the hazardous materials warning placards, and **Figure 5** shows a chart illustrating the warning labels.
- Watch for a leak or spill from a tank, container, truck, or railroad car with or without hazardous material placards or labels.
- A strong, noxious odor can denote a hazardous material.
- A cloud or strange-looking smoke from the escaping substance "says" stay away.

Stay well away and upwind from the area. Only people who are specially trained in handling hazardous materials and who have the proper equipment should be in the area.

▶ Motor Vehicle Crashes

In most states, you are legally obligated to stop and give help when you are involved in a motor vehicle crash. If you arrive at a crash shortly after it happens, the law does not require you to stop, although it might be argued that you have a moral responsibility to provide any aid that you can.

1. Stop and park your vehicle well off the highway or road and out of active traffic lanes. Park at least five car lengths from the crash. If the police have taken charge, do not stop unless you are asked to do so. If the police or other emergency vehicles have not arrived, call or send someone to call 9-1-1 or the local emergency number as soon as possible. Ways to call include the following:
   - Finding a pay phone or roadside emergency phone
   - Using a cellular phone or CB (citizen's band) radio
   - Using a phone at a nearby house or business

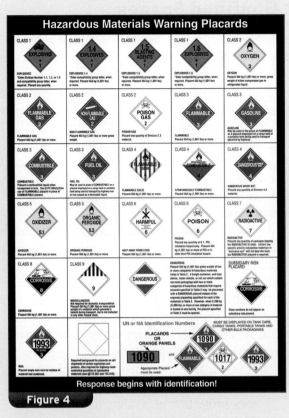

Hazardous materials warning placards.

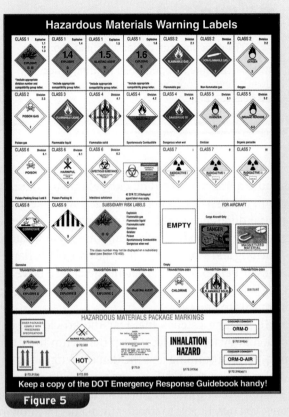

Hazardous materials warning labels.

2. Turn on your vehicle's emergency hazard flashers. Raise the hood of your vehicle to draw more attention to the scene.

3. Make sure everyone on the scene is safe.
   - Ask the driver to turn off the ignition or turn it off yourself.
   - Ask bystanders to stand well off the roadway.
   - Place flares or reflectors 250 to 500 feet behind the crash scene to warn oncoming drivers of the crash. Do not ignite flares around leaking gasoline or diesel fuel.

4. If the driver or passenger is unresponsive or might have spinal injuries, use your hands to stabilize the person's head and neck.

5. Check and keep monitoring the victim's breathing. Treat any life-threatening injuries.

6. Whenever possible, wait for EMS personnel to extricate the victims from vehicles because they have training and the proper equipment. In most cases, keep the victims' conditions stabilized inside the vehicle.

7. Allow the EMS ambulance to take victims to the hospital.

CAUTION

DO NOT rush to get the victims out of a car that has been in a crash. Contrary to opinion, most vehicle crashes do not involve fire, and most vehicles stay in an upright position.

DO NOT move or allow victims to move unless there is an immediate danger such as fire or oncoming traffic.

DO NOT transport victims in your car or any other bystander's vehicle.

▶ Fires

Should you encounter a fire, you should:

1. Get all the people out of the vehicles and area quickly.

2. Call the emergency telephone number (usually 9-1-1).

Then—and *only* then—if the fire is small and if your own escape route is clear, should you fight the fire yourself with a fire extinguisher. You may be able to

> **CAUTION**
>
> DO NOT let victims run if their clothing is on fire.
>
> DO NOT become trapped while fighting a fire. Always keep a door behind you so you can exit if the fire gets too big.

put out the fire or at least hold damage to a minimum. Because a fire can spread quickly, efforts to contain it within the first 5 minutes of a blaze can make a substantial difference in the eventual outcome.

To use a fire extinguisher, aim directly at whatever is burning and sweep across it at the base of the flames. Extinguishers expel their contents quickly; it takes just 8 to 25 seconds for most home models containing dry chemicals to empty.

If clothing catches fire, tear the article off, in a motion away from the face. Keep the victim from running, because running fans the flames. Wrap a rug or a woolen blanket around the victim's neck to keep the fire from the face or throw a blanket on the victim. In some cases, you may be able to smother the flames by throwing the victim to the floor and rolling him or her in a rug.

▶ Threatening Dogs

When you enter any emergency scene, look for signs of a dog and proceed with caution if the animal is not threatening. Ask the owner to control a threatening dog. If you cannot be delayed, consider using a fire extinguisher, water hose, or pepper spray. For a vicious dog, call the police for assistance.

▶ Farm Animals

Emergencies involving farm animals can be dangerous to rescuers. Horses kick and bite. Cattle kick, bite, gore, or squeeze people against a pen or barn. Pigs can deliver severe bites.

- Approach a situation involving animals with caution.
- Do not frighten an animal. Speak quietly to reassure it.
- If food is available, use it to lure the animal away from the victim.

▶ Confined Spaces

A *confined space* is any area not intended for human occupancy that may have or develop a dangerous atmosphere. They have limited openings for entrance and exit. There are three types of confined spaces: below ground, ground level, and above ground. Below-ground confined spaces include manholes, below-ground utility vaults and storage tanks, old mines, cisterns, and wells. Ground-level confined spaces include industrial tanks and farm storage silos. Above-ground confined spaces include water towers and legged storage tanks.

An accident in a confined space demands immediate action. If someone enters a confined space and signals for help or becomes unresponsive, follow these steps:

1. Call 9-1-1 for immediate assistance.
2. Do not rush in to help.
3. When help arrives, try to rescue the victim without entering the space.
4. If rescue from the outside cannot be done, only trained and properly equipped (respiratory protection plus safety harnesses or lifelines) rescuers should enter the space and remove the victim.
5. Once the victim is removed, provide care. Additional training is required if first aiders may be on-call in helping rescue confined space victims.

Triage: What to Do With Multiple Victims

You may encounter emergency situations in which there are two or more victims. This often occurs in multiple vehicle accidents or disasters. After making a quick scene survey, decide who must be cared for and transported first. This process of prioritizing or classifying injured victims is called **triage**. Triage comes from the French word trier, to sort. The goal is to do the greatest good for the greatest number of victims. Triage may require unpleasant decisions to withhold care from victims who are unlikely to survive so that lifesaving care can be given to those more likely to survive.

▶ Finding Life-Threatened Victims

A variety of systems are used to identify care and transportation priorities. To find the people needing immediate care for life-threatening conditions, first tell all victims who can get up and walk to move to a specific area. Victims who can get up and walk rarely have life-threatening injuries. These victims (walking wounded) are classified as needing delayed care (see the following definitions). Do not force a victim to move if he or she reports pain.

Find the life-threatened victims by performing only a primary check on all remaining victims. Assess motionless victims first. You must move rapidly (spend less than 60 seconds with each victim) from one victim to the next until all have been assessed. Classify victims according to the following care and transportation priorities:

1. Immediate care: Victim needs immediate care and transport to medical care as soon as possible.
   - Breathing difficulties
   - Severe bleeding
   - Severe burns
   - Signs of shock
   - Open chest or abdominal injuries
2. Delayed care: Care and transport can be delayed up to 1 hour.
   - Burns without airway problems
   - Major or multiple bone or joint injuries
   - Back injuries with or without suspected spinal cord damage
3. Walking wounded: Care and transportation can be delayed up to 3 hours.
   - Minor fractures
   - Minor wounds
4. Dead: Victim is obviously dead or unlikely to survive because of the type and extent of the injuries. This includes most cases of cardiac arrest due to injury.

Do not become involved in treating the victims at this point, but ask knowledgeable bystanders to provide care for immediate life-threatening problems (eg, bleeding).

Reassess victims regularly for changes in their condition. Only after victims with immediate life-threatening conditions receive care should people with less serious conditions be given care.

You may have to care for multiple victims without adequate help until more highly trained emergency personnel arrive. You will usually be relieved when more highly trained emergency personnel arrive on the scene. You may then be asked to provide first aid, to help move victims, or to help with ambulance or helicopter transportation.

Moving Victims

A victim should not be moved until he or she is ready for transportation to a hospital, if required. All necessary first aid should be provided before moving a victim. A victim should be moved only if there is an immediate danger, such as the following:

- There is a fire or danger of a fire.
- Explosives or other hazardous materials are involved.
- It is impossible to protect the scene from hazards.
- It is impossible to gain access to other victims in the situation who need lifesaving care (such as in a vehicle crash).

A cardiac arrest victim is usually moved unless he or she is already on the ground or floor because CPR must be performed on a firm, level surface.

FYI

Principles of Lifting

- Know your capabilities. Do not try to handle a load that is too heavy or awkward; seek help.
- Use a safe grip. Use as much of your palms as possible.
- Keep your back straight. Tighten the muscles of your buttocks and abdomen.
- Bend your knees to use the strong muscles of the thighs and buttocks.
- Keep your arms close to your body and your elbows flexed.
- Position your feet shoulder width apart for balance, one in front of the other.
- When lifting, keep and lift the victim close to your body.
- While lifting, do not twist your back; pivot with your feet.
- Lift and carry slowly, smoothly, and in unison with the other lifters.
- Before you move a victim, explain to him or her what you are doing.

CAUTION

DO NOT move a victim unless absolutely necessary, such as if the victim is in immediate danger or must be moved to shelter while waiting for EMS personnel to arrive.

DO NOT make the injury worse by moving the victim.

DO NOT move a victim who could have a spinal injury unless absolutely necessary due to other threats to life such as fire.

DO NOT move a victim without stabilizing the injured part.

DO NOT move a victim unless you know where you are going.

DO NOT leave an unconscious victim alone except for taking a short time to call 9-1-1.

DO NOT move a victim when you can send someone for help. Wait with the victim.

DO NOT try to move a victim by yourself if other people are available to help.

▶ Emergency Moves

The major danger in moving a victim quickly is the possibility of aggravating a spinal injury. In an emergency, every effort should be made to pull the victim in the direction of the long axis of the body to provide as much protection to the spinal cord as possible. If the victims are on the floor or ground, you can drag them away from the scene by using the various techniques shown in Figure 6 to Figure 19.

▶ Nonemergency Moves

All injured parts should be stabilized before and during moving. If rapid transportation is not needed, it is helpful to practice on another person about the same size as the injured victim.

Stretcher or Litter

The safest way to carry an injured victim is on some type of stretcher or litter, which can be improvised. Before using it, test an improvised stretcher by lifting a rescuer about the same size as the victim.

- Blanket-and-pole improvised stretcher. If the blanket is properly wrapped, the victim's

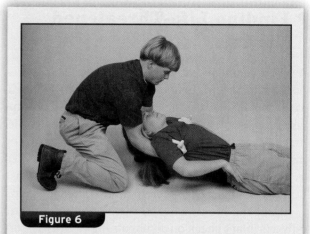

Figure 6

Shoulder drag. Use for short distances over a rough surface; stabilize the victim's head with your forearms.

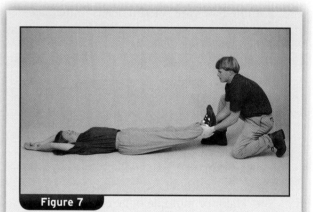

Figure 7

Ankle drag. This is the fastest method for a short distance on a smooth surface.

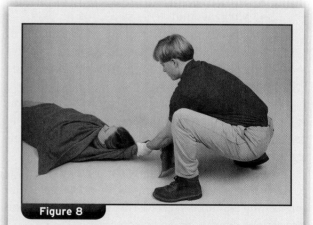

Figure 8

Blanket pull. Roll the victim onto a blanket, and pull from behind the victim's head.

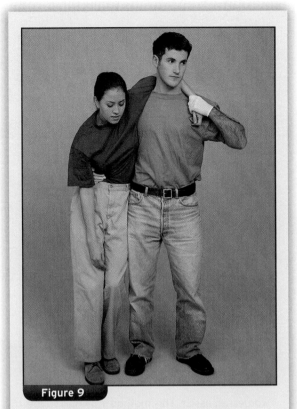

Figure 9

Human crutch (one person helps victim to walk). If one leg is injured, help the victim to walk on the good leg while you support the injured side.

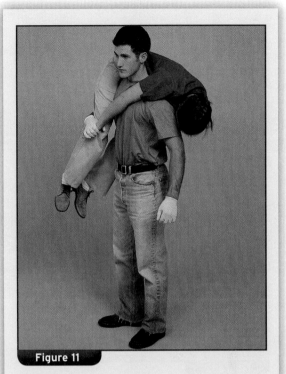

Figure 11

Fire fighter's carry. If the victim's injuries permit, you can travel longer distances if you carry the victim over your shoulder.

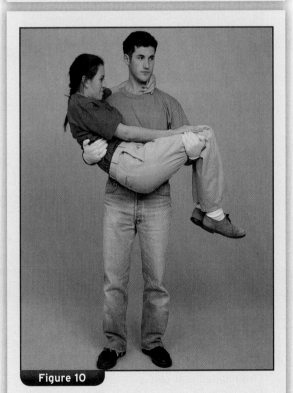

Figure 10

Cradle carry. Use this method for children and lightweight adults who cannot walk.

weight will keep it from unwinding **Figure 20**.

- Blanket with no poles. The blanket is rolled inward toward the victim and grasped for carrying by four or more rescuers.
- Board-improvised stretcher. These are sturdier than a blanket-and-pole stretcher but heavier and less comfortable. Tie the victim on to prevent him or her from rolling off **Figure 21**.
- Commercial stretchers and litters. These usually are not available except through EMS.

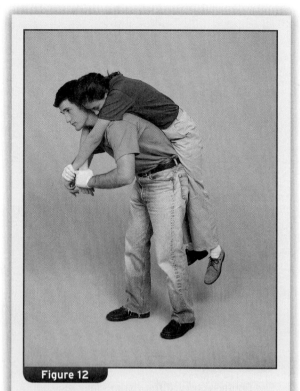

Figure 12

Pack-strap carry. When injuries make the fire fighter's carry unsafe, this method is better for longer distances.

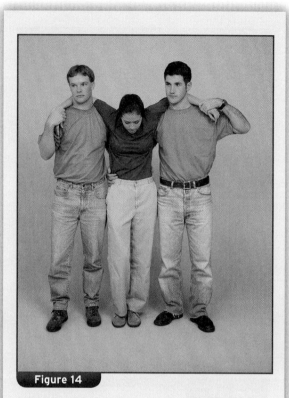

Figure 14

Two-person assist. This method is similar to the human crutch.

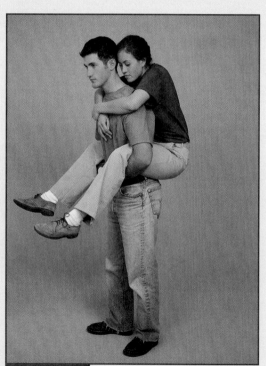

Figure 13

Piggyback carry. Use this method when the victim cannot walk but can use the arms to hang onto the rescuer.

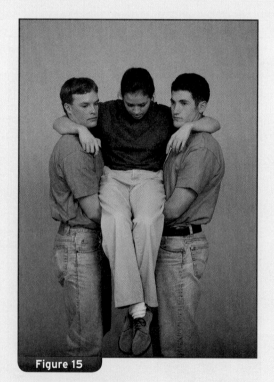

Figure 15

Two-handed seat carry.

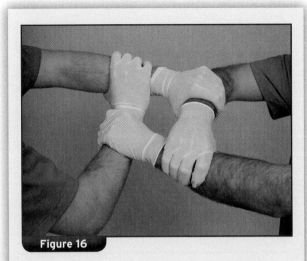

Figure 16

Four-handed seat carry. This is the easiest two-person carry when no equipment is available and the victim cannot walk but can use the arms to hang onto the two rescuers.

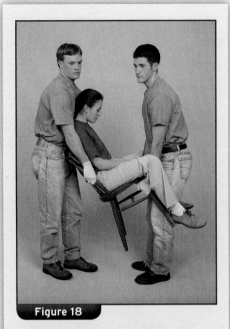

Figure 18

Chair carry. This method is useful for a narrow passage or up or down stairs. Use a sturdy chair that can take the victim's weight.

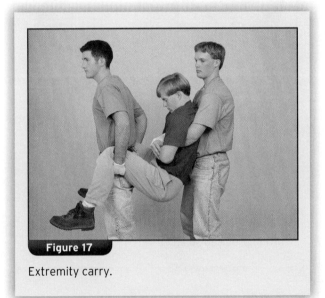

Figure 17

Extremity carry.

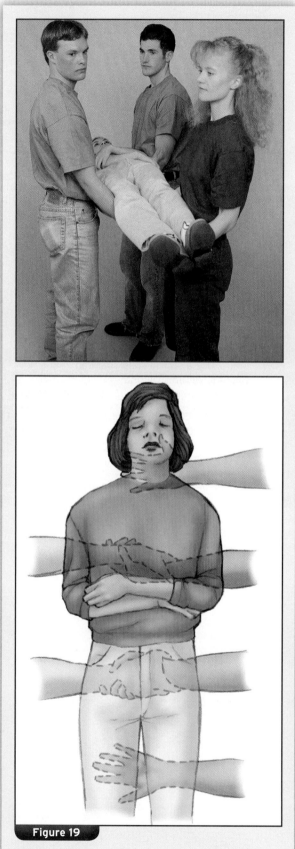

Figure 19

Hammock carry. Three to six people stand on alternate sides of the injured person and link hands beneath the victim.

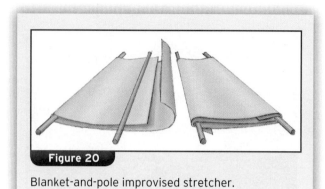

Figure 20

Blanket-and-pole improvised stretcher.

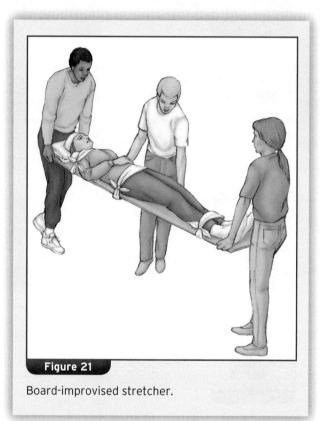

Figure 21

Board-improvised stretcher.

▶ Ready for Review

- Reach-throw-row-go identifies the sequence for attempting a water rescue.
- If a person has fallen through the ice near the shore, extend a pole or throw a line with a floatable object attached to it.
- Electrical injuries can be devastating.
- Almost any highway crash scene involves the potential danger of hazardous chemicals.
- In most states, you are legally obligated to stop and give help when you are involved in a motor vehicle crash.
- Should you encounter a fire, you should:
  - Get all people out fast.
  - Call 9-1-1.
- When you enter any emergency scene, look for signs of an animal and proceed with caution if the animal is not threatening.
- Emergencies involving farm animals can be dangerous to rescuers.
- A confined space is any area not intended for human occupancy that may have or develop a dangerous atmosphere.
- The goal of triage is to do the greatest good for the greatest number of victims.
- A variety of systems are used to identify care and transportation priorities.
- A victim should not be moved until he or she is ready for transportation to a hospital, if required.
- The major danger in moving a victim quickly is the possibility of aggravating a spinal injury.
- All injured parts should be stabilized before and during moving.

▶ Vital Vocabulary

<u>triage</u> A system used for sorting victims to determine the order in which they will receive medical attention.

prep kit

▶ Assessment in Action

You are fishing at the nearby lake. Several swimmers and others in canoes are also enjoying the lake. One swimmer decides to swim to the other side but begins to struggle about 30 feet off shore.

Directions: Circle Yes if you agree with the statement; circle No if you disagree.

Yes   No   1. This type of drowning situation is called distressed nonswimmer.

Yes   No   2. You are a very strong swimmer so you should immediately jump in the lake to rescue the victim.

Yes   No   3. You could try throwing a floating object to the victim.

Yes   No   4. The best option in this situation would be to use a canoe to rescue the victim.

▶ Check Your Knowledge

Directions: Circle Yes if you agree with the statement; circle No if you disagree.

Yes   No   1. You should attempt to move downed power lines away from a victim by using a broom or other wooden object.

Yes   No   2. Strong, unusual odors or clouds of vapor are possible indications of the presence of hazardous materials.

Yes   No   3. To keep from becoming trapped while attempting to extinguish a fire, you should always keep a door behind you for rapid exit.

Yes   No   4. In a situation involving several victims, those with breathing difficulties need immediate attention.

Yes   No   5. A major concern in moving a victim quickly is the possibility of aggravating a spinal injury.

Yes   No   6. "Row-throw-reach-go" represents the safe order for executing a water rescue.

Yes   No   7. In most states, you are legally obligated to stop and give help when you are involved in a motor vehicle crash.

Yes   No   8. The first thing to do in case of a fire is to use a fire extinguisher and try to put out the fire.

Yes   No   9. When using a fire extinguisher, aim it at the base of the flames.

Yes   No   10. When several people are injured, those crying or screaming should receive your attention first.

▶ Medication Information

As a first aider, you might be in a situation that requires you to give a victim certain medications (or to assist a victim in taking his or her own medication). A knowledgeable first aider should be familiar with the following medications:

Over-the-counter pain relievers:
- Acetaminophen
- Aspirin
- Ibuprofen
- Naproxen

Physician-prescribed medications:
- Metered-dose inhaler
- Nitroglycerin
- Epinephrine

Over-the-counter medications carried in a first aid kit or available from the victim:
- Oral glucose

▶ Pros and Cons of Popular Pain Relievers

Acetaminophen

Brand name: Tylenol
Advantages: Relieves pain and fever, does not irritate stomach
Disadvantages: Heavy or prolonged use can damage liver

Aspirin

Brand names: Bufferin, Anacin, Bayer
Advantages: Relieves pain, fever, inflammation; useful for heart attacks and their prevention
Disadvantages: Interferes with blood clotting; might trigger stomach bleeding; can cause Reye's syndrome in children with viral infections

Ibuprofen

Brand names: Advil, Nuprin, Motrin
Advantages: Relieves pain, fever, and inflammation
Disadvantages: Interferes with clotting; can cause stomach bleeding, ulcers, irritation; heavy or prolonged use can damage liver and kidneys

Naproxen

Brand name: Aleve
Advantages: Relieves pain, fever, and inflammation; one dose lasts 8 to 12 hours
Disadvantages: Can cause stomach bleeding, ulcers, irritation; prolonged use can harm kidneys

▶ Nitroglycerin

Give a victim nitroglycerin (trade name Nitrostat) if the following conditions exist:
- The victim is an adult.
- The victim has chest pain.
- The victim has physician-prescribed sublingual tablets or spray.

Do not give a victim nitroglycerin if any of the following conditions applies:
- The victim has a head injury.
- The victim is an infant or a child.
- The victim has already taken three doses.

Medication forms: tablet (about one tenth the size of an aspirin), sublingual spray, and patch.
Dosage: One dose.

Procedure

1. Once you have decided to administer nitroglycerin, follow these steps:
2. Check the expiration date of nitroglycerin.

3. Ask the victim about the last dose taken. Ask the victim to lift his or her tongue. Place the tablet or spray dose under the tongue or have the victim do so. Do not touch the tablet—wear gloves because your skin can absorb nitroglycerin and your blood pressure may be affected.
4. Have the victim keep his or her mouth closed (if doing so will not interfere with easy breathing) with the tablet under the tongue (without swallowing) until the tablet dissolves and is absorbed.

Actions

Nitroglycerin takes the following actions:
- Relaxes (dilates) blood vessels
- Reduces the workload of the heart

Side Effects

Side effects of nitroglycerin include the following:
- Lower blood pressure (victim should sit or lie down)
- Headache
- Heart rate changes

▶ Epinephrine Auto-Injector

Give a victim epinephrine (trade name Adrenaline, Epi-pen) if both of the following conditions exist:
- The victim exhibits signs of a severe allergic reaction (includes breathing distress or shock).
- The victim has physician-prescribed medication.

Medication form: liquid from automatic needle-and-syringe injection system.

Dosage

- Adult: One adult auto-injector (0.3 mg)
  Figure A-1
- Child/infant: One infant/child auto-injector (0.15 mg)

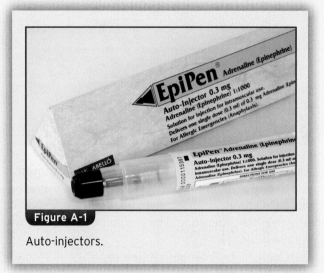

Figure A-1

Auto-injectors.

Procedure

Use these steps when administering epinephrine:
1. Obtain the victim's physician-prescribed auto-injector.
2. Remove the safety cap.
3. Place the tip of the auto-injector against the victim's thigh.
4. Push the injector firmly against the thigh to inject medication.
5. Hold the injector in place for 10 seconds.
6. Call 9-1-1.

Actions

Epinephrine takes the following actions:
- Dilates the bronchioles (small tubes in lungs)
- Constricts blood vessels

Side Effects

Epinephrine has the following side effects:
- Increased heart rate
- Dizziness
- Headache
- Chest pain
- Nausea
- Vomiting
- Anxiety

▶ Metered-Dose Inhaler

Give a victim a metered-dose inhaler (trade names Albuterol, Proventil, Ventolin) if the victim is experiencing asthma, difficulty breathing with wheezing.

Dosage

- Adult/child: 1 to 2 inhalations

Procedure

Use these steps when administering a metered-dose inhaler:

1. Obtain the victim's physician-prescribed inhaler.
2. Coach the victim to take one to two inhalations while pressing the inhaler. The victim must inhale all medication in one breath.
3. Coach the victim to hold breath for 5 seconds after inhalation.
4. Wait 5 minutes before repeating dose.

Actions

A metered-dose inhaler takes the following actions:

- Stimulates the nervous system
- Causes bronchodilation

Side Effects

A metered-dose inhaler has the following side effects:

- Hypertension
- Increased heart rate
- Anxiety
- Restlessness

▶ Oral Glucose

Give a victim oral glucose if all of the following conditions exist:

- The victim has low blood glucose (hypoglycemia, insulin reaction).
- The victim is able to swallow.
- The victim is alert and able to follow instructions.

Dosage

Adult: 1 tube of gel or three tablets

Procedure

Use these steps when administering oral glucose:

1. Coach the victim to squeeze oral glucose between a cheek and the gum, then let it dissolve.
2. If the victim experiences a decline in responsiveness or there is no improvement in the low glucose after 15 minutes, call 9-1-1. If the patient remains alert, repeat the dose while awaiting EMS arrival.

Actions

When oral glucose is absorbed by the body, it provides glucose for cell use.

Side Effects

Oral glucose has the following side effects:

- Nausea
- Vomiting

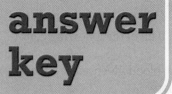

answer key

Assessment in Action

Chapter 1
1. No; 2. Yes; 3. No; 4. No

Chapter 2
1. Yes; 2. No; 3. Yes; 4. Yes

Chapter 3
1. No; 2. Yes; 3. No; 4. Yes; 5. Yes

Chapter 4
1. Yes; 2. No; 3. No; 4. Yes; 5. No; 6. Yes

Chapter 5
1. Yes; 2. Yes; 3. No; 4. Yes; 5. No

Chapter 6
1. Yes; 2. Yes; 3. No; 4. No

Chapter 7
1. Yes; 2. Yes; 3. No; 4. Yes

Chapter 8
1. No; 2. No; 3. Yes; 4. No

Chapter 9
1. No; 2. No; 3. Yes; 4. Yes; 5. Yes

Chapter 10
1. No; 2. Yes; 3. Yes; 4. No

Chapter 11
1. Yes; 2. Yes; 3. Yes; 4. No; 5. Yes

Chapter 12
1. Yes; 2. Yes; 3. Yes; 4. No; 5. Yes

Chapter 13
1. Yes; 2. Yes; 3. No; 4. No

Chapter 14
1. No; 2. Yes; 3. No; 4. Yes

Chapter 15
1. No; 2. No; 3. Yes; 4. Yes

Chapter 16
1. No; 2. No; 3. No; 4. Yes; 5. Yes

Chapter 17
1. Yes; 2. Yes; 3. No; 4. Yes; 5. No

Chapter 18
1. No; 2. Yes; 3. Yes; 4. No; 5. Yes; 6. Yes

Chapter 19
1. No; 2. No; 3. Yes; 4. Yes

Check Your Knowledge

Chapter 1
1. No; 2. Yes; 3. No; 4. No; 5. Yes; 6. No; 7. Yes; 8. Yes; 9. Yes; 10. No

Chapter 2
1. Yes; 2. No; 3. Yes; 4. Yes; 5. Yes; 6. Yes; 7. Yes; 8. No

Chapter 3
1. Yes; 2. Yes; 3. No; 4. Yes; 5. No; 6. No; 7. Yes; 8. No; 9. Yes; 10. Yes

Chapter 4
1. Yes; 2. Yes; 3. Yes; 4. Yes; 5. No; 6. Yes; 7. Yes; 8. Yes; 9. No; 10. Yes

Chapter 5
1. Yes; 2. Yes; 3. No; 4. No; 5. No; 6. Yes; 7. No; 8. Yes; 9. Yes; 10. No

Chapter 6
1. No; 2. Yes; 3. No; 4. No; 5. Yes; 6. Yes; 7. Yes; 8. Yes; 9. Yes; 10. No

Chapter 7

1. No; 2. No; 3. Yes; 4. Yes; 5. Yes; 6. No; 7. Yes; 8. Yes; 9. Yes; 10. No

Chapter 8

1. Yes; 2. No; 3. Yes; 4. Yes; 5. Yes; 6. No; 7. Yes; 8. No; 9. No; 10. Yes

Chapter 9

1. No; 2. No; 3. Yes; 4. No; 5. Yes; 6. Yes; 7. Yes; 8. No; 9. Yes; 10. No

Chapter 10

1. No; 2. No; 3. No; 4. Yes; 5. No; 6. Yes; 7. No; 8. Yes; 9. Yes; 10. No

Chapter 11

1. Yes; 2. Yes; 3. No; 4. No; 5. Yes; 6. Yes; 7. No; 8. Yes; 9. No; 10. Yes

Chapter 12

1. Yes; 2. Yes; 3. Yes; 4. Yes; 5. No; 6. No; 7. No; 8. Yes; 9. No; 10. Yes

Chapter 13

1. Yes; 2. No; 3. Yes; 4. No; 5. No; 6. Yes; 7. Yes; 8. No; 9. No; 10. Yes

Chapter 14

1. Yes; 2. Yes; 3. Yes; 4. Yes; 5. Yes; 6. No; 7. Yes; 8. No; 9. Yes; 10. Yes

Chapter 15

1. Yes; 2. No; 3. No; 4. No; 5. No; 6. No; 7. Yes; 8. Yes; 9. Yes; 10. Yes

Chapter 16

1. Yes; 2. No; 3. No; 4. Yes; 5. Yes; 6. Yes; 7. Yes; 8. No; 9. No; 10. Yes

Chapter 17

1. Yes; 2. No; 3. Yes; 4. Yes; 5. Yes; 6. No; 7. No; 8. Yes; 9. Yes; 10. No

Chapter 18

1. Yes; 2. Yes; 3. Yes; 4. Yes; 5. Yes; 6. No; 7. Yes; 8. No; 9. Yes; 10. Yes

Chapter 19

1. No; 2. Yes; 3. Yes; 4. Yes; 5. Yes; 6. No; 7. Yes; 8. No; 9. Yes; 10. No

index

drowning victim, care for, 241
positioning the victim, 21, 23
recognizing, 120–121, 122–124, 127
secondary check, 24
victims, moving, 248
victims, not moving, 122
vital vocabulary, 128
Splints
applying, 155–156
defined, 154, 157
types of, 154
Sprains
care for, 145, 147
defined, 145, 148, 150, 157
recognizing, 145, 147
Spray poisons, 183
Standard precautions, 12, 15
Status epilepticus, 173, 181
Stingray injuries, 215, 216, 217, 218
Stings. *See* bites and stings
STOP (Sugar, seizures, stroke, shock, Temperature, Oxygen, Poisoning, pressure on brain) reasons for change in responsiveness, 159, 160
Strains
care for, 145, 147
defined, 150, 157
recognizing, 145, 147
Stroke
acquired brain injury, 108
care for, 166, 179
described, 163, 165, 181
recognizing, 165–166, 167, 179
responsiveness, change in, 160
types of, 165
Sucking chest wound, 132, 133, 137, 138
Superficial (first-degree) burns, 90, 93–94, 96, 102, 103
Sutures, 78, 85
Swathe, 156, 157
Swelling, checking for, 24, 25, 32
Symptoms
defined, 24, 32
SAMPLE history, 30
Syncope, 170, 181. *See also* fainting

T

Tarantula bites, 208, 209
Teeth. *See* dental injuries
Tenderness, checking for, 24, 25, 32
Tendinitis, 150, 157
Tetanus
animal bites, 195, 198
inoculation, 78
Thermal burns. *See also* burns
defined, 89, 103
electrical, 97
Third-degree (full-thickness) burns, 90, 91, 93, 95, 102, 103
Tick bites, 210–212, 213, 218

Tongue
airway obstruction, 40
bitten, 117, 127
Triage
described, 31, 32, 246, 253
victim classification, 247
Tripod position, 23, 168
True electrical injuries, 97, 99, 101
Tumors, brain, 108
Two-handed seat carry, 250
Two-person assist, 250

V

Venous bleeding, 67, 68, 73
Ventricular fibrillation (V-fib), 49, 50
Ventricular tachycardia (V-tach), 49, 50
Vision problems, after head injuries, 108
Vomiting
head injury, 108
poisoning victims, 185

W

Walking wounded, as triage category, 31, 247
Wasp stings, 203, 204, 205
Water
AED use, 53
chemical burns, 97, 98
cold, for burns, 93, 94
Water moccasin (cottonmouth) snakes, 199, 200
Water rescue
cold-water immersion, 241, 243
drowning, 241, 242
reach-throw-row-go, 240–241, 242
Wheezing, 21
Wind chill chart, 227
Wounds
amputations, 74, 76, 79–81, 86, 87
blisters, 81–83
chapter review, 87
cleaning, 76–77
closed, 84
dressings and bandages, 77–78, 85, 87
high-risk, 77, 78
impaled (embedded) objects, 83–84, 86
infection, 78–79
medical care, requiring, 84–85
open, 74–79, 86, 87
scalp, 104–105, 126
vital vocabulary, 87
wound care, myths about, 79

Y

Yellow jacket stings, 203, 204, 205

photo credits